Breastfeeding and Culture

Funded by the Government of Canada
Financé par la gouvernement du Canada | Canada

Demeter Press
140 Holland Street West
P. O. Box 13022
Bradford, ON L3Z 2Y5
Tel: (905) 775-9089
Email: info@demeterpress.org
Website: www.demeterpress.org

Demeter Press logo based on the sculpture "Demeter" by Maria-Luise Bodirsky, www.keramik-atelier.bodirsky.de

Printed and Bound in Canada

Front cover photo: Tamara Nicole Skilbred, Tammy Nicole Photography, Munich, Germany,

Library and Archives Canada Cataloguing in Publication

Breastfeeding & culture : discourses and representations / edited by Ann Marie Short, Abigail L. Palko, and Dionne Irving.

Includes bibliographical references.
ISBN 978-1-77258-155-3 (softcover)

1. Breastfeeding—Social aspects. I. Short, Ann Marie, 1979–, editor II. Palko, Abigail L., editor III. Irving, Dionne, 1979–, editor IV. Title: Breastfeeding and culture.

RJ216.B68 2018 649'.33 C2018-900641-2

Breastfeeding and Culture
Discourses and Representation

EDITED BY
Ann Marie A. Short, Abigail L. Palko,
and Dionne Irving

DEMETER
DEMETER PRESS

Table of Contents

Acknowledgements

The idea for this collection started with a gender and women's studies brownbag discussion during my first year at Saint Mary's College about what was then a work in progress on Emma Donoghue's novel *Room*. Fortunately, I am a member of an amazingly supportive GWS faculty, and their feedback was instrumental in developing my kernel of an idea into a conference paper about the depiction of breastfeeding in the novel and critics' and readers' reactions to it. I can safely say that that paper would never have evolved into a book had it not been for my colleague's enthusiasm about my work and their encouragement to expand it into a larger project. Many thanks to Stacy Davis, Laura Elder, Laura Haigwood, Phyllis Kaminski, Bettina Spencer, Jamie Wagman, and Laura Williamson Ambrose.

I also owe a huge thank you to Saint Mary's College's Center for Academic Innovation for a summer grant that allowed me to spend an extended period of time on the project, and to my student Alyssa Santos, whose complementary independent research project on birthing choices inspired me to think in more complex ways about feminist advocacy, health care choices, and cultural constructions of "natural" when it comes to pregnancy, childbirth, and breastfeeding.

My co-editors, Abigail L. Palko and Dionne Irving, have lent so much of their time, energy, and love to this collection, and I cannot imagine the project without them. When Abby and I first discussed the possibility of collaborating over brunch at NWSA in 2015, I immediately sensed her passion for the topic and knew that I would love working with such an intelligent, fierce, and compassionate academic-mama-activist. We were thrilled when, a few months later, Dionne agreed to join our efforts. Each of us brings our own experiences as researchers, writers, and breastfeeding mothers to the project, and I could not have asked for a better team, or for better friends.

Additionally, everyone at Demeter has been such a pleasure to work with, and their support and patience have been invaluable since the very first time I contacted the press to find out if there was any interest in publishing a collection on this topic. Thank you so very much, Dr. Andrea O'Reilly, for believing in this project and providing it a home. Moreover, thank you to the peer reviewers for their generous insights and suggestions, and to everyone else behind the scenes at the press, without whom this book would not have been published. I would also like to note my gratitude for the work of Tamara Nicole Skilbred, of Tammy Nicole Photography of Munich, Germany, whose beautiful photo graces the cover of *Breastfeeding and Culture: Discourses and Representation.*

Finally, a humble and heartfelt thank you to our contributors. The collection boasts an array of insightful, intelligent, and passionate analyses covering a broad range of fascinating topics. I am honoured that these scholars trusted me with their projects, and I truly enjoyed the privilege of working with each of them.

Ann Marie A. Short
Saint Mary's College, Notre Dame, IN
January 2018

For our children, with so much love and gratitude—
Coraline Moon, Ellison Headley, Nora Grace,
and Willow Jade Lee

Introduction

Contextualizing *Breastfeeding and Culture: Discourses and Representation*

ANN MARIE A. SHORT

> "The *real* heroics of the breast-is-best revolution happen not in government buildings or laboratories, but rather in online chat rooms, playgroups, and prenatal classes, in the pages of parenting magazines, and in the headlines of daily news feeds."
> (Barston 14, emphasis in original)

This collection attends to diffuse discourses and cultural representations of infant feeding, and to interrogate—using feminist methodologies—essentializing ideologies suggesting that women's bodies are the natural choice for infant feeding. These interdisciplinary and methodologically diverse analyses—which include history, law, art history, literary studies, sociology, critical race studies, media studies, communication studies, and history—are meant to represent a broader conversation about how society understands infant feeding and maternal autonomy. In particular, our goal as editors is to facilitate deeper and more complex discussions about how "natural" as a construct informs breastfeeding discourse and representation at a moment when there is much interest in and concern about how babies are fed.

Since 1995, when Patricia Stuart Macadam and Katherine A. Dettwyler published *Breastfeeding: Biocultural Perspectives,* the body of scholarship on breastfeeding and culture has steadily grown, including, most recently, books by Joan B. Wolf, Bernice L. Hausmann, and Katherine Foss.[1] In addition, such books as *Lactivism* (Jung) and *Bottled Up* (Barston), and Hanna Rosin's

Atlantic article "The Case against Breastfeeding," alongside the rise of digital connectedness and social media, have all invited more public engagement with debates around infant feeding and motherhood. This collection is less interested in positioning itself on a particular side of the "is breast best?" debate, however. Instead, through the variety of analytical approaches taken by the authors herein, we hope to show just how wide-ranging and complex these conversations are.

The authors in this collection are interested in engaging with the construction of "natural," as it continues to be employed in breastfeeding discourse and representation. Questions about what is "natural" about breastfeeding get articulated implicitly and explicitly in a wide range of cultural spaces, and the ubiquity of these discussions reveals the countless ways women's bodies continue to be subjected to moralizing public scrutiny. As a scientific term, "natural" is unstable, and its meaning is often misleading. It was named one of the top seven "misused science words" by *Scientific American* in 2013, and in 2016, an article published by the American Association of Pediatrics specifically warns about the dangers of invoking the idea of "natural" in promoting breastfeeding among new mothers. The authors advise that "this messaging plays into a powerful perspective that 'natural' approaches to health are better" and that "promoting breastfeeding as 'natural' may be ethically problematic, and, even more troublingly, it may bolster this belief that 'natural' approaches are presumptively healthier" (Martucci and Barnhill). Although these authors are most concerned that using the term "natural" in breastfeeding promotion will dilute the faith people put in medical interventions (pharmaceuticals, vaccinations) considered unnatural, their article quite validly points to the linguistic appeal—and power—of the term. Feminists know all too well how problematic "natural" can be when employed to connote normative gendered or sexual behaviour, particularly when that behaviour is connected to biological sex or reproduction. Breastfeeding and, indeed, the institution of motherhood are all too often attached to the oppressive dictum of biology-as-destiny, and the essays in this collection explore the varied ways in which this tension makes itself felt in the way breastfeeding is represented and discussed in contemporary culture.

ENGAGING WITH CURRENT DISCUSSIONS ABOUT LACTATION AND BREASTFEEDING: WHAT'S AT STAKE?

In May 2012, when *Time* magazine featured a mother breastfeeding her three-year-old son on its cover, I had just secured my first tenure-track job and was still nursing my two-year-old daughter between teaching at various institutions and preparing for a cross-country move. Given my personal and professional interest in mothering discourse, I pored over the commentary that proliferated online in the weeks and months that followed. As the mother of a nursing toddler, I cringed defensively at the disgust, rage, and accusations of sexual abuse directed at Jamie Lynne Grumet, the twenty-six-year-old mother on the *Time* cover. As a feminist, I understood—with as much intellectual objectivity as I could muster—that at the heart of these reactions were deeply held cultural anxieties about the female body and the underlying tension between maternal and sexualized interpretations of its function. Still, I chafed at the provocative question posed in all caps, the final two words emphasized in red, in the middle of the page: "ARE YOU MOM ENOUGH?" Why, I wondered, did the editor have to go *there?*

The answer probably has more to do with the bottom line than ideology, but the question was clearly meant to hit a nerve, and it most definitely did. And although the article accompanying the photo was about attachment parenting, the ensuing debates were by and large focused on issues related to breastfeeding: is breast best? how old is too old to nurse? is it okay to nurse in public? covered or uncovered? Various iterations of these questions swirled around the comments sections of news sites, throughout the parenting blogosphere, and on social media, and the emotional intensity of these conversations suggested that they were long overdue.

The controversy surrounding the *Time* cover is instructive because of how clearly it reflects the terms of debates over breastfeeding in the U.S. The visual impact of the cover (the boy was placed on a stool to appear older than his three years; the mother is youthful, stylish, and attractive), with its suggestion of sexuality, speaks to cultural anxiety over the meaning of women's breasts. As Marilyn Yalom notes in *A History of the Breast*, "the breast has been coded with both 'good' and 'bad' connotations since the beginning of time"; thus, "good" breasts nourish, whereas "bad" breasts sexually entice" (4). I would argue that the photograph featured on the *Time* cover renders that distinction unclear, which helps to explain the outpouring of negative responses to it.[2] Additionally, in the context of Kathy Dettwyler's research about sexuality and breastfeeding, in which she argues that the misinterpretation of breasts as sexual objects has (negatively) shaped breastfeeding discourse in the U.S., the *Time* cover reinforces the prevailing belief in the separation of sexuality and motherhood.

Moreover, in the provocative question it poses, the cover engages with the decidedly unfeminist debate over what makes a so-called good mother. The question "Are you mom enough?"—though ostensibly addressing the demands of attachment parenting—is easily applicable to the countless other ways in which mothering has become competitive and divisive. It is more important than ever for motherhood scholars and activists to remember that the terms of these debates have emerged out of patriarchal structures and have been shaped by patriarchal values. In that spirit, contributors throughout this collection cite Linda Blum, Bernice Hausman, Joan Wolf, as well as other scholars—all of whom have worked to dismantle damaging discourses tying maternal value to specific mothering practices such as breastfeeding and attachment parenting.

The past decade has brought these conversations into the public arena in unprecedented ways thanks to digital connectivity and social media. In some ways, online manifestations of this discourse have intensified its divisiveness. Take, for instance, the way that the "Fed is best" campaign—which began in response to messaging from the World Health Organization (WHO) and the March of Dimes promoting breastfeeding as the "best" way to feed babies—turned into a hashtag war. In other ways, the digital age has encouraged solidarity and has allowed mothers to find support from online communities and message boards, seemingly innumerable Facebook groups, and ever-popular mommy blogs. These virtual communities exist for countless parenting niches, which, among many other things, reflect a wide variety of infant-feeding situations. Breastfeeding activists (or "lactivists," as they have come to be called) also use online spaces to organize "nurse-ins," which have become an increasingly popular way to shame establishments, such as restaurants, that ask breastfeeding mothers to leave or cover up. Unsurprisingly, several chapters in this collection speak to the role that the Internet and social media play in facilitating contemporary parenting culture. Although online spaces have the potential to become echo chambers for the like-minded and are still overwhelmingly cis and/or heteronormative, the Internet show no signs of receding as force that both disseminates and shapes breastfeeding discourse.

For myriad reasons, breastfeeding and breastfeeding advocacy are fraught and contentious not just in the U.S. but also around the world. Although most of the recent scholarship on breastfeeding discourse focuses on North America, the U.K., and Ireland, this collection also features two chapters about breastfeeding in India. The editors agreed that India is one of the most logical places to examine how U.K. and North-American-centered mothering practices have been globally exported. Moreover, we were fascinated by the continuity of concerns related to how breastfeeding is talked about, advocated, and represented. These chapters engage with questions about what is natural about breastfeeding and concerns over the problematic conflation of the natural and biological in specific cultural and economic contexts, such as India's growing assisted reproductive technologies industry.

Breastfeeding raises many important concerns surrounding gendered embodiment, reproductive rights and autonomy, essentializing discourses, and public policies that undermine parents—especially mothers. Although many experts have written about breastfeeding since the publication of that notorious *Time* cover, further need for feminist-academic-activist work in addressing the complexity of contemporary breastfeeding discourse remains. This collection responds to that need, and the essays within it engage with the varied and complicated ways in which cultural attitudes about mothering and female sexuality inform the way people understand, embrace, reject, and talk about breastfeeding, as well as with the promises and limitations of feminist breastfeeding advocacy.

BREASTFEEDING AND CULTURE: THE CHALLENGES AND LIMITATIONS OF DISCOURSE, REPRESENTATION, AND ADVOCACY

The collection is divided into four sections, which represent the breadth and complexity of breastfeeding discourse in contemporary culture. Section One, "Historicizing Cultural Representations of Lactation and Breastfeeding," includes essays examining cultural constructions of breastfeeding and lactation in the West from the medieval period to the present. In Chapter One, "'Big Mother': Breastfeeding Rhetoric and the Panopticon in Popular Culture, 1700 to Present," Elizabeth Johnston compares popular culture to a modern-day panopticon that shames mothers who do not breastfeed and undermines the promises of maternal choice and agency. Johnston traces contemporary attitudes about nursing back to the latter half of the eighteenth century, which brought about a new conception of the body politic that necessitated surveillance of and power over women's reproductive functions, the professionalization of medicine, and the idealization of motherhood as women's "natural" privilege. In Chapter Two, "'Milk for Gall': Elizabethan Power Strategies in *Macbeth*," Eileen Sperry historicizes Lady Macbeth's refusal to accept the maternalization of her body in Shakespeare's popular tragedy. Sperry argues that Lady Macbeth "divorces political power from reproduction" by refusing to breastfeed, an act that she associates with political weakness. Moreover, understood in the context of Elizabethan reproductive politics, Lady Macbeth's rejection of corporeal motherhood suggests a "new model of female agency not dependent on biological reproduction." In Chapter Three, "Same-Sex Lactations in European Art and Literature (ca. 1300-1800): Allegory, Melancholy, Loss," Jutta Sperling considers artistic and literary depictions of women breastfeeding their own mothers, which became popular in medieval and early modern Europe. Using Judith Butler's account of gendered melancholia, Sperling argues that these same-sex lactation scenes provide commentary on mother-daughter love and the ways in which it has historically been circumscribed by patriarchal and heteronormative imperatives. In the last chapter of this section, Elaine McDevitt's chapter, "Latch: The Object of the

Breast Pump," explores the development of the breast pump in the context of material culture, and uses its design and social history to consider contemporary discourse surrounding infant feeding. McDevitt argues that the breast pump is a deeply significant object that has provided "a new experience of motherhood"—one that is far more complicated than a question of "bottle or breast."

Section Two of this collection focuses on representations of breastfeeding and lactation in recent popular culture, including literature, film, and television. In Chapter Five, "'That's Not a Beer Bong; It's a Breast Pump!': Representations of Breastfeeding in Prime-Time Fictional Television," Katherine Foss examines fifty-four depictions of breastfeeding on television between 1974 and 2012. She argues that in representations of so-called normal breastfeeding—a "certain group of women" nursing newborns, in a private space—nursing is presented as "natural, beautiful and easy"; however, representations of breastfeeding that fall outside these norms are depicted as "absurd, unnecessary, socially unacceptable, or deviant." As with the other chapters in this section, Foss's research suggests that when narrow boundaries delineate what is natural or unnatural, normal or abnormal behaviours in breastfeeding, cultural perceptions of lactation and nursing become similarly limited and limiting. In Chapter Six, Abigail L. Palko's "(Breast)Milking the Situation: Interracial Wet-Nursing in Sherley Anne Williams's *Dessa Rose*" explores breastfeeding as embodied "othermothering" in Williams's 1986 historical neoslave narrative. Palko argues that the novel, unique in its depiction of a white woman serving as a wet nurse for a black infant, emphasizes the ubiquity of race and class in cultural constructions of motherhood. In an "idealistic reconfiguring of history," Palko suggests, *Dessa Rose* offers interracial maternal bonding as a site of resistance against patriarchy and racialized oppression. In Chapter Seven, Tatiana Prorokova's "Gender, Psychology, and Breastfeeding as 'Perverse': From *A Clockwork Orange* to *Game of Thrones*" continues to explore the implications of the natural-unnatural binary as it pertains to breastfeeding discourse. She argues that when breastfeeding occurs outside of the mother-infant dyad it is understood as perverse and, therefore, represented as either comical or horrific. Finally, my own chapter, "'In This Whole Story, That's the Shocking Detail?':

Extended Breastfeeding in Emma Donoghue's *Room,*" focuses on a 2010 novel in which a five-year-old boy narrates his experiences being raised in captivity by his mother. In particular, my analysis examines the novel's depiction of extended breastfeeding and the reading public's response to it, and I ultimately argue that the novel forces readers to contend with questions related to what is natural, especially in parent-child relationships.

The essays in Section Three examine how breastfeeding discourse is both personal and political, which suggests the pressing need for intersectional feminist intervention in conversations surrounding infant feeding choices. Dionne Irving's powerful personal essay, "My Black Breast Friend," explores the essentializing narratives that reduced her black breasts to sex objects, and the manner in which her struggle to nurse her son allowed her to reclaim what her breasts mean to her. The essay emphasizes the importance of mother-to-mother support, but argues that for Black women, navigating the spaces that offer such support is complicated by race, class, and history. In Chapter Ten, "Breastfeeding in the Military: A Communicology Analysis," Patty Sotirin examines breastfeeding done by military mothers through using the frames of everyday interactions, identity performance, military culture, and representational politics. Paying particular attention to visual culture, Sotirin argues that a feminist communicology analysis reveals complex "dynamics of marginalization and resistance" for breastfeeding mothers in the U.S. armed forces. Dana Lloyd's essay on "Legal Representations of Breastfeeding" focuses on the case of Angela Ames, a mother who lost her job at Nationwide Insurance Company in 2012 because she was breastfeeding and needed to take time from her work day to pump milk. Lloyd argues that the Ames case is not just a legal document; it also serves to show just how "socially constructed and culturally situated" motherhood and breastfeeding really are and to emphasize the profound implications on social policy. Chapter Twelve, "The Politics of Mothers' Milk in Modern India," by Sucharita Sarkar, connects Ayurvedic texts to official government documents supporting breastfeeding to examine how they idealize motherhood and construct the "good mother" as "responsible citizens"—effectively excluding women who cannot or will not breastfeed from these categories. Sarkar traces the effects of this discourse in posts on popular "mommy blogs," and shows the potential of virtual spaces to provide more inclusive mother-to-mother support.

Finally, essays in Section Four of the collection address some of the challenges emerging in feminist breastfeeding discourse. In Chapter Thirteen, "'We Chose the Hardest Road': Examining Self-Representations of the Exclusive Pumper," Lee Ann Glowzenski examines online self-representations of "exclusive pumpers," or "EPers"—women who "as a result of circumstance, perform the labour of breastfeeding via pumping and bottle-feeding." Since most women who pump and bottle-feed also directly breastfeed, Glowzenski points out that the experiences of EPers are under-represented in academic research about breastfeeding and in popular culture, and she argues that their self-representation in online communities works to "reframe discussions about their work and reimagine previously negative representations of their bodies." In Chapter Fourteen, "Surrogacy and Breastfeeding—A Puzzle to Solve: A Case Study on the Surrogacy Industry in India," Anindita Sengupta examines what it means for breastfeeding to be "a site where constructions of 'bad' and 'good' motherhood are created" for surrogate mothers in India, where assisted reproductive technology has become increasingly common. She argues that although most new mothers are encouraged to breastfeed, surrogate mothers are often prohibited from doing so; the "denial of breastfeeding is part of the process of controlling and disciplining" these "reproductive workers" who are not meant to establish a maternal bond with the babies they birth. In the final chapter of the collection, "Framing Breastfeeding as 'Natural' and the Implications for Mothers' Identities," Laura Fitzwater Gonzales presents findings gathered from interviews with new mothers and their partners about their understanding of the word "natural," their reasons for choosing to breastfeed their children, and their breastfeeding experiences. Because breastfeeding has become an important marker of a mother's self-definition, Gonzales argues, mothers who understand breastfeeding to be natural suffer negative effects on their identities when breastfeeding is difficult or impossible. She concludes that in feminist breastfeeding advocacy, it is imperative to frame breastfeeding as a learned rather than instinctual experience. Although in addressing these challenges the essays in this section engage in various ways with the limitations of breastfeeding advocacy, they serve to remind us how fluid these discourses are. Moreover, like all of the chapters in this collection suggest, they demonstrate that as a discipline, motherhood studies must keep up with the evolving landscape of twenty-first-century parenting and remain inclusive in its approach to the challenges that will undoubtedly emerge.

ENDNOTES

[1]Hausmann's most recent book is a collection of essays co-edited with Paige Hall Smith and Miriam Labbock. Although some of its commitments intersect with this collection, the collection's contributors are more specifically interested in exploring the numerous and multifaceted factors that influence a mother's decision whether or not to breastfeed.

[2]In an interview with Feifei Sun, the photographer Martin Schoeller describes his choice to have the boy stand on the chair: "to underline the point that this was an uncommon situation."

WORKS CITED

Blum, Linda. *At the Breast: Ideologies of Breastfeeding and Motherhood in the Contemporary United States*. Beacon Press, 1999.

Dettwyler, Katherine A. "Beauty and the Breast." *Breastfeeding: Biocultural Perspectives*, edited by Patricia Stuart Macadam and Katherine A. Dettwyler, Aldine de Gruyer, 1995, pp. 167-215.

Foss, Katherine A. *Breastfeeding and Media: Exploring Conflicting Discourses That Threaten Public Health*. Palgrave Macmillan, 2017.

Ghose, Tia. "'Just a Theory': 7 Misused Science Words." *Scientific American*, 2 April 2013, www.scientificamerican.com/article/just-a-theory-7-misused-science-words/. Accessed 10 Dec. 2017.

Hausman, Bernice L. *Mother's Milk: Breastfeeding Controversies in American Culture*, Routledge, 2003.

Jung, Courtney. *Lactivism*, Basic Books, 2015. New York.

Macadam, Patricia Stuart and Katherine A. Dettwyler, editors.

Breastfeeding: Biocultural Perspectives, Aldine de Gruyer, 1995.

Martucci, Jessica and Anne Barnhill. "Unintended Consequences of Invoking the 'Natural' in Breastfeeding Promotion." *Pediatrics: Official Journal of the American Academy of Pediatrics*, vol. 137, no. 4, March 2016, pp. 1-3, http://pediatrics.aappublications.org/content/early/2016/03/02/peds.2015-4154. Accessed 10 Dec. 2017.

Smith, Paige Hall, Bernice L. Hausman, and Miriam Labbock, editors. *Beyond Health, Beyond Choice: Breastfeeding Constraints and Realities*. Rutgers UP, 2012.

Sun, Feifei. "Behind the Cover: Are You Mom Enough?" *TIME*, 10 May 2012, www.time.com/3450144/behind-the-cover-are-you-mom-enough. Accessed May 2015.

TIME Magazine, TIME, Inc., 21 May 2012. Cover.

Wolf, Joan B. *Is Breast Best? Taking on the Breastfeeding Experts and the New High Stakes in Motherhood*. New York University Press, 2010.

Yalom, Marilyn. *A History of the Breast*, Alfred A. Knopf, 1997.

I.
Historicizing Cultural Representations of Lactation and Breastfeeding

1.
Big Mother

Breastfeeding Rhetoric and the Panopticon in Popular Culture, 1700 to Present

ELIZABETH JOHNSTON

> "Breastfeeding is a natural negotiation between mother and baby and you interfere with it at your peril."
> —Mary Renfrow, Director of the Mother and Infant Research Unit at the University of York, 2006 (qtd. in Thomas)

I am four months into my first pregnancy and grossed out by the idea of breastfeeding. There is something animal in it, I tell my mother-in-law who agrees. Cows are for milking, I say.

As my due date approaches, I change my mind. I'll give it a try. All the literature says, "Breast is best." I don't want to give my child something inferior. And I am curious.

Ava delivers herself into the world at 10:00 a.m., two days before Christmas. I am delirious with joy and morphine. "Let her try to breastfeed," the nurse says handing her bundled body to me. I am amazed that she instinctively turns to my nipple. I have nothing to offer but colostrum, but Ava is too tiny and weak to suck hard anyway. I discover that I love breastfeeding.

Rather, I love the idea of breastfeeding. Ava is having trouble "latching on." Instinct is not enough. Nurses come in, pinch my nipple between their sandpapery fingers, and thrust it into her mouth. She sucks until they leave. Then, as if she knows they're gone, she spits me out, shakes her head.

I take her home where she still can't latch on. She is losing weight. We return to the lactation consultant. "She's fine," the nurse says. "You have plenty of milk." She eyes my swollen breasts accusingly. Abashed, I swaddle Ava back into her blanket and return to our apartment where I wrestle her wiggling body against my nipple. Breastmilk squirts into her eye, runs down her cheek, and spurts across the room. She whimpers impatiently. Why is this so hard to do? Animals can do it. Dogs. Pigs. Why can't I?

Ava is three weeks old. I can kind of get her to nurse, but when she does she projectile vomits. We change her spit-up-soaked onesie six times a day. I smell like sour milk. My hair is coated with it. She spits up on my student papers. On my briefcase. On the couch. I worry her belly hurts because I have too much milk; it comes out too fast, too hard. Or I've eaten something wrong, so I cut out dairy. I cut out Mexican food and Indian food. On the days I'm teaching, my husband stays home with Ava; on those days, he feeds her from a bottle. He says she doesn't spit up for him.

Three a.m. Class in four hours, and Ava and I are two hours into a marathon nursing session. She won't stop crying, but she refuses my nipple. "Why are you doing this?" my husband asks from the door. He motions for me to move from the rocking chair, takes her, and gives her the bottle he has warmed. She guzzles it. He burps her and lays her in the crib where she instantly falls asleep. My breasts weep filmy, useless milk.

I want to be like the woman in the Mary Cassatt painting on my OBGYN's wall—her diaphanous robe swelling around her, her generous breasts discretely offered to the baby in her arms, his mouth around her nipple, his plump little hands on her skin. How gratefully he gazes up at her.

But my daughter doesn't want my breast; I am afraid she doesn't want me.

BREASTFEEDING IDEOLOGY IN MEDICAL AND ADVICE LITERATURE: A BRIEF HISTORY

Breastfeeding, popular culture informs us, cements the sacred relationship between child, mother, and breast. Yet sitting behind my office door with an electronic machine sucking milk from my nipples through plastic tubing, I felt more cyborg than Madonna. So why was I, a feminist scholar of eighteenth-century literature with eyes laser-trained on cultural indoctrination, so committed to the maternal ideal and so devastated by my inability to attain it? Why did I find it nearly impossible to separate my objective analysis of breastfeeding rhetoric from the pressure I felt to nurse my daughters and the ensuing guilt I experienced when I could not? Certainly, I recognized my feelings of inadequacy as evidence of my acculturation by heteronormative, class-based gender mythologies. Yet every time I discretely pulled a bottle from my diaper bag or skulkingly placed a can of formula on the grocery store conveyer belt, I winced beneath what felt like a panopticon of censuring eyes.

In my use of the term "panopticon," I am invoking cultural critic and social historian Michel Foucault. The panopticon was, literally, an architectural design by eighteenth-century philosopher Jeremy Bentham of a circular prison within which everyone inside could be observed at any given time without realizing it. The idea was this: the inmates, because they did not know when they were being observed, would internalize the belief that they were always under observation; therefore, they would behave on their own. For Foucault, however, the panopticon becomes a symbol of how regulatory ideology functions. The structure works "to induce in the inmate a state of conscious and permanent visibility that assures the automatic functioning of power ... in short, that the inmates should be caught up in a power situation of which they are themselves the bearers" (*Discipline* 205). Having studied Foucault and how we interpellate and then perform our ideologically sanctioned subjectivities, I knew full well that no one was forcing me to breastfeed. Yet I still found myself an "inmate" of a regulatory fiction created in and consistently reproduced since the eighteenth century. A fiction, in fact, that I had long studied.

While still an undergraduate in the field of English studies, I happened on Anna Laetitia Barbauld's poem "The Rights of Women," a biting response to Mary Wollstonecraft's *Vindication of the Rights of Women*, both written in 1792. In her poem, Barbauld lampoons Wollstonecraft's view that women, as a means to independence from male subjection, should breastfeed their own children rather than farming them out to wet nurses, as was the practice of many women in the middle and upper classes. Wollstonecraft had complained that women rejected the role of motherhood and allowed themselves to be treated like "rattles" by their childish husbands—a role that often led to them being abandoned when their husbands grew bored. Barbauld opens her poem parodying Wollstonecraft:

> Yes, injured Woman! rise, assert thy right!
> Woman! too long degraded, scorned, opprest;
> O born to rule in partial Law's despite,
> Resume they native empire o'er the breast! (lines 1-4)

Her poem concludes by suggesting that women who experience mutual love will not feel the need to assert their independence. Because I was interested in representations of female rivalry, I was drawn to this exchange between these two women writers. That interest, in turn, led to a fascination with how breastfeeding was represented in eighteenth-century discourse.

Although women have always breastfed, it was only with the onset of the European enlightenment that, in public discourse, breastfeeding became inextricably linked to women's virtue and became explicitly tied to their compulsory role as citizen in the local, state, and federal communities. How and why did this happen? Much of the answer to this question lies in understanding how the breast functions historically as a site of symbolic meaning. Marilyn Yalom, author of *A History of the Breast,* explains that during the European Renaissance literature and art had increasingly eroticized the breast—an impulse that led to a decrease in maternal breastfeeding among the upper class and to an increase in the reliance on wet nurses from the working class. Wet nursing freed up wealthy women's attention and bodies so they might better satisfy their husbands' desires; furthermore, not breastfeeding meant their breasts could more closely meet standards of beauty celebrated by Renaissance culture. Consequently, the burgeoning middle-class population, in a desire to separate itself from the working class, emulated the behaviour of the upper class. Thus, as Yalom notes, by 1700, more than half of all women living in England were using wet nurses.[1]

However, the European attitude toward wet nursing changed during the latter half of the eighteenth century. Suddenly, breastfeeding advocacy took on "the aspect of a cult" (Yalom 114) and choosing to use a wet nurse invited nearly universal scorn. Why the change? At least part of this transition can be explained by understanding how the conception of the body politic arose and how individual choice and autonomy were reimagined as bound up in and essential to the functioning of the new republic. In his landmark text *The History of Sexuality: An Introduction,* Foucault argues that "one of the great innovations in the techniques of power in the eighteenth century was the emergence of 'population' as wealth, population as manpower or labor capacity, population balanced between its own growth and the resources it commanded" (25). As such, government and its ideological apparatus became deeply invested in collecting data studying and regulating what had hitherto been the private functions of its populations; among these newly scrutinized functions were the marriage practices and fertility issues so vital to the production and reproduction of populations.

In particular, women's bodies—as the site of reproduction—were imagined as in need of constant surveillance. Foucault argues that in order to regulate women's bodies, female sexuality was first pathologized, which then justified its need to be supervised by medical and governmental entities; these entities, in turn, imagined that the only way to "cure" the female body of its pathology was to situate it within the desexualized sphere of home and family.[2] Where before maternity had been overseen by midwives and understood as a ritual associated with female community, the professionalization of medicine meant that a growing body of medical literature—written by men—increasingly imagined women's bodies not as the province of women but under the jurisdiction of the patriarchal state.[3] William Cadogan's enormously influential *Essay on Nursing* (1748) exemplifies this discourse of male appropriation. In a letter to the governors of his foundling hospital, he congratulates the men who are running it, and explains that under their educated governance, infants will be better fed:

> It is with great Pleasure I see at last the Preservation of Children become the Care of Men of Sense: It is certainly a matter that well deserves their Attention, and, I doubt not, the publick [sic] will soon find the good use of it. The *Foundling Hospital* may be of more Use to the World, than was perhaps at first imagin'd by the Promoters of it;

> it will be a Means not only of preventing the Murder of many, but of saving more, by introducing a more reasonable and more natural Method of Nursing. In my Opinion, this Business has been too long fatally left to the Management of Women, who cannot be supposed to have proper Knowledge to fit them for such a Task, notwithstanding they look upon it to be their own Province. What I mean, is a Philosophic Knowledge of Nature, to be acquired only by learned Observation and Experience, and which therefore the Unlearned must be incapable of. (3)

In the hierarchy Cadogan establishes, male doctors are positioned as knowing more than female nurses about reproduction and childrearing. Infant feeding, left to the "management of women" results in the "murder" of infants; this is not because women are malicious, Cadogan says, but because they are "unlearned."

But Cadogan is not simply concerned with the inadequate care of nurses for orphans; he extends his view into the domestic space of families to advocate for male governance of infant feeding there as well: "I would earnestly recommend it to every Father to have his Child nursed under his own Eye to make use of his own Reason and Sense in superintending and directing the Management of it; nor suffer it to be made on of the Mysteries of the *Bona Dea*, from which the Men are to be excluded" (24). Cadogan's implicit bias extends beyond his belief that education makes men better parents; instead, men are, by virtue of being men, better aware of and more suited to govern what is right. At the same time, Cadogan warns that women cannot be left to their own devices, since "most Mothers, of any Condition, either cannot, or will not undertake the troublesome Task of suckling their own Children ... [But] were it rightly managed, there would be much Pleasure in it, to every Woman that can prevail upon herself to give up a little of the Beauty of her Breast to feed her Offspring" (24). Thus, Cadogan's discourse establishes men as possessing reason, and women, frivolous and uninformed, as in need of their governance.

Cadogan just as importantly makes explicit that breastfeeding is not a private issue but a public one. He notes that the breastfed child of a mother "in the lower Class of Mankind" is "healthy and strong, and very soon able to shift for itself" ; in contrast, "the puny Insect, the Heir and Hope of a rich family lies languishing" because his mother has fed her child rich but nutrient-weak substitutes (7). Here, very clearly, Cadogan uses a class-competitive argument to advocate for breastfeeding as a means to increase population among the wealthy, since "a multitude of inhabitants is the greatest strength and best support of a commonwealth" (6). Breastfeeding, then, is a "publick" good.

In Émile (1762), Jean Jacque Rousseau, too, links the breastfeeding body to the body politic. Rousseau sees the deterioration of the public sphere as directly related to the deterioration of family life.

> Do you wish to bring everyone back to his first duties? Begin with mothers.... Everything follows from this first depravity [wet nursing]. The whole moral order degenerates, but let mothers deign to nurse their own children, then morals will reform themselves, nature's sentiment will be awakened in every heart, the state will be repeopled. This first point, this point alone, will bring everything back together. (46)

For writers like Rousseau, breastfeeding was inextricably bound up in the family's commitment to a political and moral revolution. Both Rousseau and Cadogan's discourse exemplify what Foucault means by "bio-power": "For the first time in history, no doubt, biological existence was reflected in political existence ... Power would no longer be dealing simply with legal subjects over whom the ultimate dominion was death, but with living beings...[I]t was the taking charge of life, more than the threat of death, that gave power its access even to the body" (*History* 143). The maternal body, because it reproduces future citizens, demands state control.

However, as Foucault has made clear, that control comes about most effectively when the subject internalizes her own governance. It's important to note that Rousseau describes breastfeeding as the mother's choice (albeit, an overdetermined one). Encouraging women to experience breastfeeding not as a law imposed on them but as a choice they make of their own free will is essential to ideological success. In the eighteenth century, a growing body of conduct-book literature idealized the mother figure as at the heart of the modern, middle-class family that, in turn, anchored the newly enlightened public sphere.[4] Accordingly, breastfeeding was reimagined as an opportunity for middle-class women to define themselves against those both beneath and above them. In fact, this so-called opportunity was frequently aligned with female agency—an early feminist cause in line with the Enlightenment's revolutionary and emancipatory ideals.

As I have already noted, Wollstonecraft writes about breastfeeding in her early feminist work *Vindication of the Rights of Woman* (1792). There, she criticizes the woman who relied on wet nurses: "Her parental affection, indeed, scarcely deserves the name, and have when it does not lead her to suckle her children" (227). But Wollstonecraft sees breastfeeding as a means to power—an act by which they may assert their worth outside the patriarchal sexual economy that oppressed and devalued them. Women, she argues, needed to reimagine their bodies not as entertaining "rattles" but as the locus of a domestic virtue that could reform the family and, by extension, civil society. She points to women who care only to "preserve their beauty, and wear the flowery crown of the day" because they think "that gives them a kind of right to reign for a short time over the sex"; however, these women "neglect to stamp impressions on their husbands' hearts" (214). In contrast, she offers her readers the idealized vision of "a woman nursing her children, and discharging the duties of her station with, perhaps, merely a servant maid to take off her hands the servile part of the household business" (215). She continues, "I have seen her prepare herself and children, with only the luxury of cleanliness, to receive her husband, who returning weary home in the evening found smiling babes and a clean hearth" (215). This middle-class version of maternity would come to dominate nineteenth-century discourse in England and America, and is perhaps best exemplified by Coventry Patmore's narrative poem *The Angel in the House* (1854-62). Of course, as a number of scholars have argued that this idealizing of domesticity also functioned to coax women away from the moderate equality they had enjoyed with husbands prior to the rise of the nuclear family.[5] Still, powerless everywhere else, women were encouraged to imagine mothering, and in particular, breastfeeding, as a locus of agency and self-determination.[6]

Determined, I enter my second pregnancy swollen with the promise that this time I can do this. This time I will do this. But my new daughter has other plans. In the postdelivery room, Christina screams, her tiny face pink with rage, or pain, or hunger. I don't know. But she won't take my milk. The nurses come in, one by one, take my breast, and squash my nipple into her mouth. Christina shakes her head: "Uh, uh, uh, uh." The nurses shrug. They don't know what to do. One gives me a plastic medicine cup and tells me to hand express my milk into it. I tug and pull at my breast while the nurse watches like a prison guard.

A week later. Another visit to the consultant. This time she sends us home with a supplemental nursing system. My husband and I are instructed to tape small plastic tubing along my engorged breast to my nipple; at the other end of the tube is a syringe full of breastmilk I've earlier expressed. I hold Christina's mouth to my nipple while he threads the opposite end of the tube into her mouth. He is in charge of the syringe, I of her mouth. When she attempts to suck, I tell him "Go," and he plunges the syringe so that she gets a mouthful of milk. When she quits, I say "stop" and he ceases the flow. The idea is that she will learn to suck for her reward. Go. Stop. Go. Stop. Go. Stop. Go. Stop.

Night two. 2:00 a.m. "Enough," he says, tossing the syringe down in disgust. He heads to the kitchen and returns with a bottle.

It is no use. Like Ava, Christina can't breastfeed. And this time, her stomach issues are worse. So for three more months, I pump. I don't want to dry up. My nipples swell and split. The milk in the plastic bags is tinged pink with blood. The doctor tells me that it's safe for her to drink my blood. My nipples scab over. I treat them with lanolin, douse them with hydrogen peroxide. Pumping hurts so much I have to practise breathing exercises before I hook myself up. I am trying to think good thoughts. I don't want to stress out the baby, don't want stress hormones contaminating my milk. I position the plastic funnels over my nipples and count backward from ten, willing my body to relax. Good thoughts. Good thoughts. Good thoughts. I brace for the first agonizing pull of the suction and switch the machine on. Everything goes white as I dig my fingernails into my thighs and bite my lip.

Of course, there are worse kinds of agony. One night while pumping, I am watching HBO's Rome, *and one of the female characters reaches for a crying baby. Expertly, she pushes aside her robes and a soft, full breast spills out. She pulls the baby to her, cooing, "There, there, my little piglet." My heart throbs watching the actor pretend to nurse a baby. I unplug the breast pump and unsuction the plastic cups from my nipples; my breasts sag, deflated.*

We celebrate the holidays. We invite friends and their families over for a cookie swap. Two of my girlfriends also have babies. On the couch, one lifts her shirt to her eighteen-month-old's wandering fingers, deftly pulling him beneath it to nurse. I feel the strain of my milk dropping. My useless breasts push against my nursing bra. They are an amputee's ghost limbs—so full but so very empty.

BREASTFEEDING IN MODERN ADVERTISING

In *A History of the Breast*, Marilyn Yalom posits that "it is not too far-fetched to argue that Modern Western democracies invented the politicized breast and have been cutting their teeth on it ever since" (105). In her fascinating, deeply-researched, and compelling book, she offers a wide-ranging history that examines representations of the breast across history, culture, and mediums. I refer readers to it for a broader discussion of the ways in which breastfeeding discourse evolved over the nineteenth and twentieth century in the Western imagination. For the purposes of this essay, however, I want to focus attention on a variety of themes in contemporary Western breastfeeding discourse inherited from eighteenth-century rhetoric. One of these themes is the notion that a woman's failure to breastfeed puts her children's health and intellectual futures at risk. Yet this kind of risk-centred discourse is not only misleading and unethical, but rooted in sexist assumptions about traditional divisions of labour.[7]

The most militant of breastfeeding rhetoric argues for exclusive breastfeeding for at least the first year of a child's life and makes clear that failure to do so imperils children. Lactivist Stephanie Ondrack argues that we should not even call "breastmilk" breastmilk, but only "milk" to separate it both from its site of origin and eliminate any suggestion that formula is milk. She goes on to say that mothers who give their children formula are "denying" them their "normal projected potential" (51), and claims that we need to eliminate from culture any and all references to bottle-feeding, since "baby-shower paraphernalia—wrapping paper, gift bags, decorated streamers, cards, e-cards—is lousy with images of baby bottles" (51). She points to toy bottles filled with bubble gum in the candy aisle, bottle-shaped Christmas tree ornaments, and baby dolls that come prepackaged with bottles and pacifiers, and she includes as evidence of a culture that "maligns" breastfeeding a newspaper article showing a little boy bottle-feeding a doll. This is "breast envy," she says; we should neither encourage nor allow boys and men to force their way into "the exclusive feeding relationship of mother and child" (56). Despite the fact that more than half of the workforce is now made up by women, Ondrack urges mothers to "sink fully into the attachment of parenting day and night" and complains about mothers who selfishly enjoy the convenience of bottles (56). She includes in her article a caricature of a defiant woman raising a baby bottle in the air while holding in her other arm a computer. Ironically, her parodying of women who choose not to breastfeed as militant ideologues recalls Barbauld's own eighteen-century parodying of women who do breastfeed.

Ondrack's article might be considered extreme; indeed, most breastfeeding advocates emphasize breastfeeding as "choice." An example of this is when Mayor Bloomberg debuted Latch-On NYC in 2012. The program asked hospitals to pledge to lock up formula, remove any references to formula from the hospital, and urge new mothers to breastfeed instead. In response to the program, women across the state, even self-proclaimed breastfeeding activists, vociferously protested. Op-ed columnist Amy Tuteur noted similarities between the program and laws requiring ultrasounds before abortions, saying, "When it comes to breastfeeding, Mr. Mayor, here's a good rule of thumb: Her baby, her body, her breasts, her choice." One blogger even called Bloomberg "a modern day Rousseau" because of the parallels between *Emile's* stance on breastfeeding and the program's regulations (Braverman).

Of course, in modern society, breastfeeding campaigns must depict breastfeeding as an act of empowerment and control. Yet as with the eighteenth century maternal ideal, the modern mother's "choice" translates as no choice. She is either choosing or abandoning social approbation, either protecting or neglecting her child's health and future. One example of the rhetoric of pseudo-authority lies in the 2008 "Be a Star" campaign commissioned by the Central Lancashire Primary Care Trust (PCT), in partnership with Little Angels breastfeeding peer support organization and The Hub social marketing agency. In these ads, regular women are dressed like models and depicted breastfeeding. Copy across the front of the ads reads, "She's not a celebrity; she's a star"; "She's not a model; she's a star"; and "She's not an actress; she's a star." In the semiotic context of our Reality TV-obsessed world, these ads imagine the breastfeeding mother as an idol, front and centre in the public eye. Breastfeeding is an act in which ordinary women can call attention and applause to themselves. Yet their empowerment lies in being approved of by their imagined audience; they do what is expected of them because they imagine themselves on stage and screen—a modern panopticon.

These ads also include quotations of affirmation from the people in the breastfeeding women's lives, many of them men. As with Cadogan's supervising father, one partner is quoted as saying: "Look at my girlfriend. She's gorgeous. Just when I thought I couldn't love her anymore, our son arrived and I fell even deeper." He adds, "By choosing to breastfeed she's protecting him against ear infections whilst burning up to 500 calories a day." It's clear that the breastfeeding mother's power is measured by her partner's desire for her, which, in turn, depends on her ability to keep her child healthy and her body thin.

Breastfeeding ads also rely on a longstanding tradition that objectifies women's bodies and reduces those bodies to parts. The Ad Council, under contract with the U.S. Department of Health and Human Services on Women's Health, sponsored the "Babies Were Born to Be Breastfed" national campaign from 2004 until 2006 ("Public"). Its ads visually substitute for women's breasts pairs of round objects: pocket watches, scoops of ice cream, dandelion heads, pediatric otoscopes. Beneath these images, the copy explains that by breastfeeding, women can head off such childhood illnesses as allergies, obesity, and ear infections. In a similar 2015 campaign titled "Your Child Is What You Eat," by the Brazilian Pediatric Society of Rio Grande organization, babies breastfeed from headless torsos, whose breasts have been replaced with round junk food: donuts, ice cream sundaes, and cheeseburgers. In both these campaigns, the woman is doubly displaced. If the breast is metonym for woman, the breast's use value becomes metonym for the breast. As an autonomous, thinking and feeling subject, the woman disappears altogether.

In other campaigns, the woman's role is similarly reduced to her use value as conduit of breastmilk. In a campaign commissioned by the New Zealand Ministry of Health, women breastfeed in public places. Copy across the image asks viewers to imagine the future of the babies as causally linked to their mothers' choice to breastfeed: "Future entrepreneur getting his order filled"; "Future internet whiz kid downloading"; "Future astronaut preparing for liftoff." Beneath each ad is more copy: "Wherever they're headed, a healthy start in life will help them get there." In these ads, the mother, though pictured in the ad, is in essence absent. What matters is her milk, that commodity which her infant, already possessing full subjectivity, needs. As in the eighteenth century, her role is to nurture and bring to full fruition productive, economically stable citizens.

How, given all the gains made by women during the first, second, and third waves of feminism, have we wound up regurgitating and recirculating the same tired, misogynistic ideals? Judith Warner, author of *Perfect Madness: Motherhood in the Age of Anxiety*, offers one explanation:

> Feminism filtered down and diluted by the mass media, came to be not about a redefinition of womanhood or a reorganization of family life and society, but about questions of performance and control ... For the emphasis on control of the body hid the fact that a larger politics that would have given women more permanent and far-reaching control of their lives—with real choices to carry them through

> all the phases of their lives, including motherhood—was nonexistent. (46)

Rather than considering why women choose not to breastfeed after they leave the hospital—for example a dearth of family-friendly policies for working women—women are urged to imagine "control" and "choice" at the site of their bodies. As in the eighteenth century, women are compensated for their losses with false autonomy and pseudo-power. But what of those women unable (or unwilling) to perform breastfeeding? How will they be compensated? How will they feel whole?

I nurse Christina with a nipple shield to protect my cracking nipples. Every few minutes she gets mad, punches at my breast with one of her balled fists, and the shield goes flying through the air. I crawl around on the carpet looking for it, rinse it, and stick it back on like a stripper's tassel. Christina swings her arm, and flings it again. Sometimes the cat finds the shield first, carries it around in her mouth like a mouse. I continue to use the shields after I stop nursing and start pumping. I buy extras because I keep losing them or leaving them—on my desk at work, slipped between the pillows of the couch at my in-laws, in the car wedged between the armrest and the passenger seat. A long trail of evidence of my guilt. My maternal inadequacy.

A week before Christina's first birthday, my free issue of Babytalk *arrives. I flip the pages past an advertisement for a "Women's Health and Breastfeeding Fair" sponsored by Babies-R-Us to an article titled "5 Ways to Nurse on the Go." At the top is a photo of a woman breastfeeding while unloading the dishwasher. The next day, the mail brings me a certificate of "Congratulations" for breastfeeding Christina. I feel the guilt lapping warmly at my cheeks; my breast pump is collecting dust in the closet and my nipples have fully healed. The certificate reads: "Your milk protects your child and your breastfeeding encourages other mothers to choose breastfeeding for their child. Thank you for promoting breastfeeding in our community." It is signed by my well-child nurse. She has misspelled my name (although she gets my daughter's name right). Across the top of the certificate are the words "World Breastfeeding Week 2006: Code Watch: 25 years of Protecting Breastfeeding." Later that afternoon my husband and I take Ava and Christina to Hamlin Beach Park for a picnic. The park charges a small fee for use; the woman who takes our money hands us two pamphlets: one about testing our house for lead, the other a breastfeeding pamphlet.*

It is Orwellian: Big Mother.

SUPERWOMAN

Recently a friend on Facebook posted a newspaper article about a "superwoman" who was photographed pumping while running a half-marathon. Beneath the photo, bloggers celebrated the runner's devotion to motherhood as evidence that women can do it all. Mothers who don't breastfeed, the commenters either explicitly said or implied, are simply not trying hard enough. A runner myself, however, I couldn't help but wonder what it means that this mother felt she couldn't take three hours off from breastfeeding.

Breastfeeding advocate Bernice Hausman, certainly a more reasonable voice in the debate, concludes in *Mother's Milk: Breastfeeding Controversies in American Culture* that "Breastfeeding advocacy must pay more attention to the structural impediments to breastfeeding—economic barriers, lack of support from medical personnel, and work/family patterns—that mothers face" (227). However, even given the removal of these impediments, we must do a better job of making clear that there are a lot of ways to raise healthy children; giving them breastmilk is only one of many choices parents might make. And parents—a word I use to degender these choices—should not be made to feel less adequate because they opt for some choices over others. Finally, we must also pay attention to evidences that for some women—perhaps for many—breastfeeding does not come naturally.

Foucault says of confession that it is an effect of power; we view confessing as "the infinite task of extracting from the depths of oneself, in between the words, a truth which the very form of the confession holds out like a shimmering mirage" (59). In this essay, I have "confessed" my failings as a mother unable to breastfeed my daughters. I have "confessed" my failings as a feminist academic unable to disentangle what I think I know about ideology and my position as a subject within that ideology. Yet I do not practise this confession to achieve absolution or to offer readers some final truth. Nor do the sections of this essay within which I historicize and deconstruct breastfeeding discourse provide a definitive "aha!" moment. Instead, my confessions interrupt my historicizing and my historicizing interrupts my confessions, disrupting any hierarchy that would suggest one form of storytelling (narrative, academic discourse) is truer than the other. No one text retains the truth about what it means to mother or mother well, although they may, on their own, each offer a version of truth.

My daughters are twelve and fourteen now. Neither their health nor our mother-daughter bond appears to have been affected by what seemed at the time the do-or-die practice of breastfeeding. My daughters still get colds. They still threaten to move in with their father when I tell them to clean their rooms. Sometimes they dazzle me with their brilliance; sometimes I'm certain they've been lobotomized. The kids are all right. I am all right. We are all right. Whatever that means.

ENDNOTES

[1]Also see Emily Stevens et al. for an additional discussion of the history of wet nursing.

[2]Foucault identifies "a threefold process whereby the feminine body was analyzed—qualified and disqualified—as being thoroughly saturated with sexuality; whereby it was integrated into the sphere of medical practices, by reason of a pathology intrinsic to it; whereby, finally, it was placed in organic communication with the social body ... the family space ... and the life of children" (*History* 104).

[3]For a discussion of this ideological shift see Ruth Perry and Susan Greenfield. Although her focus is not exclusively on breastfeeding, Marilyn Francus also provides an excellent overview of ways in which transgressive mothers were imagined during the eighteenth century.

[4]See Nancy Armstrong's canonical text *Desire and Domestic Fiction* for a discussion of how conduct-book literature uses the figure of

the woman to circulate and establish middle-class ideals.

[5]Elizabeth Kowaleski-Wallace specifically addresses Wollstonecraft's problematic alliance with the male medical industry (103). See also works by Armstrong; Perry; Greenfield.

[6]For an earlier example of this emerging rhetoric, Rachel Muers points to a seventeenth-century conduct book called *The Compleat Mother: An Earnest Perswasive to All Mothers (Especially Those of Rank and Quality) to Nurse Their Own Children*. Muers summarizes the text's argument: "The avoidance of risk to the child and the family—as a maternal responsibility--is rendered harmonious with the mother's self-fulfillment as a 'compleat mother,' of which the endurance of pain or inconvenience is an expected, or even a necessary, part" (11-12).

[7]Although there is not time in this essay to provide a critique of the literature, a good example is by Joan Wolf who conducted a study of the National Breastfeeding Awareness Campaign of 2005, an advertising campaign that focused on the risks associated with not breastfeeding. The highly controversial campaign was informed by the belief that breastfeeding is a public health policy. However, after reviewing the medical literature, Wolf concludes that the causal link between breastfeeding and infant health is not fully proved and "by most measures the [National Breastfeeding Awareness Campaign] did not meet the evidentiary standards for ethical public health practice set by multiple institutions" (610). Also see Jules Law's excellent analysis of the gender bias in lactivist rhetoric. Laws notes that

> a father's career may locate a family closer to various industrial or automotive toxins without being calculated a 'risk' ... City air is clearly more toxic than infant formula, but families rarely uproot their lives for incremental reductions in an infant's exposure to carbon monoxide, sulfur dioxide, or lead, and pediatricians are more likely to recommend a practice that will disrupt a woman's career than a relocation that may affect a man's commute. (415)

WORKS CITED

"5 ways to ... Nurse on the Go." *Babytalk*, Aug. 2006, p. 17.

Armstrong, Nancy. *Desire and Domestic Fiction.* Oxford University Press, 1987.

Barbauld, Anna. "The Rights of Woman." *The Poems of Anna Letitia Barbauld*, edited by William McCarthy and Elizabeth Kraft, University of Georgia Press, 1994, pp. 120-22.

Braverman. "Bloomberg's Breastfeeding Appeal is Strangely Reminiscent of Rousseau's Emile," *CNN iReport* 31 July 2012, www.ireport.cnn.com/docs/DOC-822865/. Accessed 10 May 2016.

Cadogan, William. *An Essay Upon Nursing and the Management of Children: From Their Birth to Three Years of Age.* 1748.

Foucault, Michel. *Discipline & Punish: The Birth of the Prison.* Vintage Books, 1995.

Foucault, Michel. *The History of Sexuality: An Introduction.* Vintage Books, 1990.

Francus, Marilyn. *Monstrous Motherhood: Eighteenth-Century Culture and the Ideology of Domesticity.* John Hopkins University Press, 2012

Greenfield, Susan. *Inventing Maternity: Politics, Science, and Literature* 1650-1865. University Press of Kentucky, 1999.

Hausman, Bernice. *Mother's Milk: Breastfeeding Controversies in American Culture.* Routledge, 2003.

Kowaleski-Wallace, Elizabeth. *Their Fathers Daughters: Hannah More, Maria Edgeworth, and Patriarchal Complicity.* Oxford University Press, 1991.

Law, Jules. "The Politics of Breastfeeding: Assessing Risk, Dividing Labor." *Signs* vol. 25, no. 2, 2000, pp. 407-450.

Muers, Rachel. "The Ethics of Breastfeeding: A Feminist Theological Exploration," *Journal of Feminist Studies,* vol. 26, no. 1, 2010, pp. 7-24.

Ondrack, Stephanie. "Taking Down the Almighty Bottle." *Mothering,* vol. 137, July/August 2006, pp. 48-56.

Patmore, Coventry. *The Angel in the House.* 2nd ed. John W. Parker and Son, 1858.

Perry, Ruth. "Colonizing the Breast: Sexuality and Maternity in Eighteenth-Century England," *Journal of the History of Sexuality,* vol. 2, no. 2, 1991, pp. 204-34.

"Public Service to Promote Breastfeeding Awareness Launched." *Ad Council: News Release*, 4 June 2004, HHS Press Office, www.archive.hhs.gov/news/press/2004pres/20040604.html/. Accessed 1 May 2016.

Rousseau, Jean Jacque. Émile*: Or, Concerning Education.* 1748. Translated by Eleanor Worthington. D.C. Heath & Co, 1889.

Stevens, Emily, et al. "A History of Infant Feeding," *The Journal of Perinatal Education,* vol. 18, no. 2, 2009, pp. 32-39.

Thomas, Pat. "Breast milk vs. 'formula' food," *The Ecologist* 1 Apr. 2006, www.theecologist.org/trial_investigations/268337/breastmilk_vs_formula_food.html/. Accessed 1 May 2016.

Tuteur, Amy. "Breastfeeding Wars: Why Locking Up Baby Formula Is a Bad Idea," *Time Online—Public Health* 3 Aug. 2012, www.hideas.time.com/2012/08/03/why-locking-up-formula-is-a-bad/?iid=op-article-mostpop1/. Accessed 17 June 2017.

Warner, Judith. *Perfect Madness: Motherhood in the Age of Anxiety*. Riverhead Press, 2005.

Wolf, Joan. "Is Breast Really Best? Risk and Total Motherhood in the National Breastfeeding Awareness Campaign," *Journal of Health Politics, Policy, and Law,* vol. 32, no. 4, 2007, pp. 595-36;

Wollstonecraft, Mary. *A Vindication of the Rights of Woman: With Strictures on Political and Moral Subjects.* 1792. New Edition with an Introduction by Mrs. Henry Fawcett. T.Fisher Unwin, 1891.

2.
"Milk for Gall"

Elizabethan Power Strategies in *Macbeth*

EILEEN SPERRY

Shakespeare's *Macbeth* is, at its core, a play concerned deeply with questions of fertility and reproduction. Images of childbirth, both successful and abortive, fill the text: Macbeth's mad rage, for instance, originates with the initial prophecies of the Weird Sisters, who declare that it is Banquo and not Macbeth who "shall get kings," dooming his line to a quick and sterile end (1.3.67). That end is subsequently brought about by Macduff, whose Caesarean origins—"from his mother's womb / untimely ripped"—signal the manifestation of raw reproductive potentiality, of vitality triumphing over mortality (5.7.45-46). The play's male characters are linked to the question of reproductive power writ large on the historical scale: whether or not their power will be continued by future generations or whether the political dynasty they have been associated with will endure. *Macbeth*'s female characters, however, engage this subject on the individual corporeal register, wielding power in the reproductive actions of their bodies.

Although the tragedy presents a number of different manifestations of femininity, from the androgynously bearded Weird Sisters to the expressly maternal nature of Lady Macduff, this chapter will focus on one central figure—Lady Macbeth—and the way she negotiates her own reproductive identity. In contrast to the perpetual lineage promised to Banquo, Lady Macbeth is associated throughout the play with a ruling strategy that divorces political power from biological reproduction, which is achieved, most notably, in her vocal rejection of breastfeeding.

Lady Macbeth repeatedly disassociates herself from the practice of nursing, declaring it a symbol of political weakness.

First staged only three years after Elizabeth I's death, Shakespeare's tragedy engages residual anxieties of the late Elizabethan period. During this time, the Virgin Queen's aging body and failure to produce or name an heir provoked debates about the appropriate forms of female political power. Although by most standards the Elizabethan era was a remarkably successful reign, marked by stability and significant cultural productivity, critics of the queen saw her refusal to marry and bear children as a failure to exercise her most potent form of feminine political agency—her reproductive potential. Elizabeth's actions reject this logic, however, and produce a model of leadership that divorces her political agency from her biological potentiality. This chapter examines the relationship between these political debates and Lady Macbeth's own model of leadership as articulated in *Macbeth*. This is not to suggest, of course, that Lady Macbeth is simply an allegorical stand-in for Elizabeth. It would have been politically disastrous for Shakespeare and for James I, the play's patron, to represent the late queen in such a villainous light; to do so would have risked alienating audience members and would have damaged James's claims to legitimacy. Taking seriously the influence of Elizabethan politics on the play, however, opens up new ways of understanding Lady Macbeth's character. After examining the representation of breastfeeding in *Macbeth* in the context of Elizabeth's legacy, this chapter concludes by suggesting alternative ways of interpreting Lady Macbeth in light of emerging models of political agency.

Recent work in Shakespeare studies has demonstrated that the figure of Lady Macbeth stands at the centre of important conversations about early modern gender, women's embodiment, and power. Janet Adelman's influential reading of Lady Macbeth, for example, places the character within an overarching system of male anxiety over maternal influence in Shakespeare's works. Stephanie Chamberlain has also argued that Lady Macbeth's rejection of nursing is reflective of "a generalized cultural anxiety about women's roles in the transmission of patrilineage" (73). Likewise, Christina León Alfar has posited that *Macbeth* "interrogates the tyranny of absolute monarchical practices ... divorce[d] from naturalized gender by placing Lady Macbeth at the center of the play's violence" (179). Moreover, Alfar argues that although Lady Macbeth "is often read as rupturing her designated gender function," she, in fact, "provides a parodic inversion of the ideal wife and allows Shakespeare to put pressure on masculinist ... structures of relations that depend on women's abject confirmation" (179-180). However, even as all these accounts demonstrate how Shakespeare, through Lady Macbeth, probes the construction of gender in systems of power and authority, none have done so with specific attention to the lingering legacy of Queen Elizabeth's rule. Indeed, most studies focused on Lady Macbeth's gender and its performance have done so in the broader (though still important) contexts of sixteenth and seventeenth century English medical and social discourses. Those studies stressing the importance of narrow historical context have focused almost exclusively on the Jacobean qualities of the play: the influence of James's *Daemonologie*, for instance, or the traces of Scottish politics. Although both of these lines of inquiry are indeed crucial for understanding the historical conversations into which *Macbeth* entered in 1606, the absence of any sustained consideration of Queen Elizabeth's signals a significant unexplored factor in the play's composition and reception.

Breastfeeding, as Lady Macbeth represents it, is associated with weakness, inaction, and political passivity. Having first received news of the Weird Sisters' prophecy, Lady Macbeth expresses her initial concern over Macbeth's lack of ambition through the language of nursing.

> Glamis thou art, and Cawdor, and shalt be
> what thou art promised; yet I do fear thy nature,
> it is too full o'th'milk of human kindness.
> to catch the nearest way. Thou wouldst be great,
> art not without ambition, but without
> the illness should attend it. (1.5.14-19)

Associating her husband with breastmilk, Lady Macbeth implies his potential reticence to usurp the king. He will not take "the nearest way" to power by murdering Duncan, but will instead be overruled by his reactive nature; he will await the realization of the Weird Sisters' prophecies rather than actively intervening in the political order to bring those realities into being. The particular kind of inactivity Macbeth is accused of here is dependent upon Lady Macbeth's reference to breastmilk—the "milk of human kindness." In addition to implying goodwill or affection, "kindness" in seventeenth-century usage would also have signified "kinship ... or special relationship" (*OED* def. 3). In early modern obstetrics, breastmilk was understood to be the medium in which the kinship between mother and child materialized. One sixteenth-century birth manual, *The Byrth of Mankynde, Otherwyse Named the Womans Booke,* stresses that the mother's milk would be more effective than that of a wet nurse because of the connection already existing between mother and child: "it shalbe best that the mother gives her child sucke her selfe, for the mothers milke is more convenient and agreeable to the Infant, then any other womans, and more doth it nourish it, for in the mothers belly it was wont to the same, and fedde with it, and therefore also it doth more deliciously covet the same, as that with the which it is best acquainted" (Roeslin 152-53).[1] The connection implied here is not one of active bonding but of passive association: breastfeeding is not represented as a behaviour by which connections can be formed, but as a response dictated by preexisting and involuntary exchange. By associating her husband with breastmilk, Lady Macbeth articulates a concern that Macbeth's response to his potential kingship will be affected by—and perhaps even prevented by—an unwillingness to intervene for himself.

By linking breastfeeding with this kind of political passivity, Lady Macbeth frames nursing as antithetical to the "illness" of action required by Macbeth to overthrow Duncan.[2] But the threat of being overcome by passivity is not limited to Macbeth alone—if he, a man, can be accused of being metaphorically milky and, therefore, feminized, Lady Macbeth's female body is even more vulnerable to such charges. Recognizing her physicality as the source of the traits she rejects, Lady Macbeth subsequently disavows female corporeality:

> Come, you spirits
> that tend on mortal thoughts, unsex me here,

> and fill me from the crown to the toe, top-full
> of direst cruelty. Make thick my blood,
> stop up th'access and passage to remorse,
> that no compunctious visitings of nature
> shake my fell purpose, nor keep peace between
> th'effect and it. Come to my woman's breasts
> and take my milk for gall, you murd'ring ministers.
> (1.5.39-47)

In this prayer, Lady Macbeth invites the separation of her sex from her speaking self. Adelman, in her reading of this moment, notes Lady Macbeth's plea to eradicate her reproductive potential. "In the play's contexts of unnatural births," she writes, "the thickening of the blood and the stopping up of access and passage to remorse ... sound like attempts to undo reproductive functioning and perhaps to stop the menstrual blood that is the sign of its potential"; it is "an attack on the reproductive passages of her own body, on what makes her specifically female" (134).[3] Although Lady Macbeth is not inviting masculinity—she is not asking to be made male, but rather to be unsexed entirely—she is striving to separate herself from what she portrays as the inherent docility of the female body, a physical composition that might cause her to stray from her "fell purpose" of advancement.

Even more so than the reproductive or menstruous aspects of her body, Lady Macbeth's breastmilk seems to represent the entirety of her female physicality. Linked to the passive connections of kinship rather than the active changes of her planned coup, this material is indicative of the political model she seeks to avoid. Lady Macbeth demands that the spirits exchange her "milk for gall" as the culmination of her transformation.[4] The specific bodily fluids named in this trade say much about the model of power Lady Macbeth works to claim. Whereas breastmilk has already been established in her rhetoric as indicative of political inaction, gall, or yellow bile, would have represented an opposing set of traits to an early modern audience. In Galenic medicine, yellow bile was the humor linked with choler, aggression, and rashness—a predisposition to violent or impulsive action, a sense still attached to "gall" in its current usage. Lady Macbeth is not the only Shakespearean character to bemoan an absence of gall; Hamlet, notably, describes himself as deficient in this particular humor. Considering his inability to revenge his father's death, Hamlet declares "I am pigeon-livered and lack gall" (2.2.554).[5] As a figure famously overwhelmed by his own passivity, Hamlet embodies everything that Lady Macbeth rejects in this moment: a lack of political initiative originating in bodily composition. But whereas Hamlet's insufficiency is simply a transient imbalance, Lady Macbeth's is a congenital state created by her sex. Inviting the exchange of milk for gall, she declares her desire to move beyond the type of agency dictated by her female body; rather than being controlled by a reactive or even inactive nature, she envisions a new model of political agency in which she may assume the ability to act out in order to seize the future she envisions.

The culmination of Lady Macbeth's denunciation of breastmilk and, with it, the kind of power afforded by the female body occurs as the king's murder transitions from plan to action. As she and her husband approach the chamber where Duncan lies asleep and vulnerable, Macbeth's momentary hesitation prompts Lady Macbeth to deliver an invective against inaction. She derides Macbeth's indecision, and, as a means of stressing the importance of action, she compares his commitment to murder to an imagined act of infanticide.

> I have given suck, and know
> how tender 'tis to love the babe that milks me;
> I would, while it was smiling in my face,
> have plucked my nipple from his boneless gums
> and dashed the brains out, had I so sworn
> as you have done to this. (1.7.49-59)

This moment, which has been at the centre of many past critical conversations, provides the most vivid and violent of Lady Macbeth's many characterizations of nursing.[6] Breastfeeding, and the bonds of kinship associated with it, are not rejected outright; Lady Macbeth claims ownership of the practice and describes her familiarity with the emotional connections developed in the physical exchange between mother and baby. It is, in fact, the inherent goodness and innocence of such an image that underscores the force of her conditional phrase in this moment. Even in the face of such a connection, this iconic image of motherhood, Lady Macbeth declares that the commitment to act should surpass any other obligation. By deprioritizing breastfeeding, Lady Macbeth rejects the condition of inactivity implied by her female corporeality. Without vilifying the act of nursing itself, Lady Macbeth asserts that her priority is not the passive associations of familial connection but the ability to claim power of her own accord.

Lady Macbeth's denunciation of breastfeeding has, historically, been read as a marker of her moral depravity. As *Macbeth* ultimately resolves by privileging reproductive power, these moments place her squarely outside the boundaries of the social order reestablished at the play's close. However, the model of ruling articulated in these scenes—a model prioritizing active intervention over the passive corporeality Lady Macbeth associates with breastfeeding—must be read not only in conjunction with the discourses of power within the play, but also within the context of ongoing political conversations of the early seventeenth century. The most obvious influence on *Macbeth* is that of the newly crowned King James, who had taken the throne and begun his role as patron of The King's Men, Shakespeare's theatre company, in 1603, three years prior to the play's first performance. The inclusion of such a significant occult element, as well as the play's overt concern with the etiology of the Stuart line in Banquo and Fleance, have long been recognized as elements of Shakespeare's tragedy intended to appeal to the new king. But equally important is the influence of James's predecessor, Elizabeth I. With her death at the age of sixty-nine still fresh in national memory, Elizabeth remained a prominent figure in English politics and a significant influence on *Macbeth*.

Elizabeth's political legacy was indelibly marked by her refusal to produce an heir, a decision seen as a failure to rule in a way befitting her gender. Ascending to the throne on the heels of her sister Mary's reign of violence, Elizabeth was met with a country already gripped by a pronounced suspicion of female rulers. Carol Levin notes that "ambivalence to the idea of a woman ruler" was oriented around "the conflict between her rule and her femininity." Levin writes, "If a queen were confidently to demonstrate the attributes of her power, she would not be acting in a womanly manner; yet womanly behavior would ill-fit a queen for the rigors of rule" (3). The most popular solution proposed to this perceived conflict of interest was reproduction. The widespread hope was that Elizabeth, twenty-five years old and unmarried at the time of her coronation, would quickly select a husband and have children. In doing so, she could ensure the stable future of the country without acting outside her prescribed social role. Especially with the relatively recent dynastic crisis of the War of the Roses and Henry VIII's multiple marriages in an attempt to generate a legitimate male heir, England was deeply concerned about the longevity of the Tudor line. Reproductivity and nurturing were the expected mode of female political power, the acceptable means by which a leader like Elizabeth might effectively rule and ensure the country's future.

Given these expectations, Elizabeth's lifelong refusal to marry was, unsurprisingly, met with great criticism.[7] Many speculated about her reproductive health, surmising that the only reason that a female leader might reject proposal after proposal, and thus refuse a child-centred approach to ruling, would be shame over an inability to conceive. As Anne Somerset notes in her biography of Elizabeth, the desire to know the queen's health was so great that "that inquisitive foreign ambassadors, who wished to find out whether or not the Queen was fertile, were sometimes driven to bribe royal laundrymaids or chamberwomen who could pass on details as to the frequency of Elizabeth's periods" as a way of verifying that a potential marriage would indeed prove productive (98). But even as rumours of barrenness circulated, contrary gossip also emerged accusing the queen of excessive sexuality and of an insatiable libido that exceeded the limits of any monogamous relationship. Reports of affairs with courtiers included allegations that not only was the Virgin Queen a false moniker for Elizabeth, but she had also secretly given birth many times and—in the most extreme stories—had ordered those illegitimate children murdered to conceal her secret (Levin 3-4).While these rumors seemed to contradict those implying the queen's infertility, both strands of gossip shared a common goal of reducing the queen's political power to her ability to bear children. Elizabeth's refusal to engage in the systems of marriage and reproduction was seen as an indication of non-normative sexuality and, therefore, as a threat to national stability.

Elizabeth's rejection of a reproductive approach to ruling extended as far as her refusal to officially declare a successor to the throne in the absence of a direct heir. Although, as biographer J.E. Neale notes, the queen's correspondence with James VI of Scotland during the later years of her reign revealed "in unmistakable if veiled phrases her intentions" that he would follow her on the throne, those plans were never made public (402-03). This decision may have in part been an attempt to ensure the safety of both the queen and of James. To have openly declared the Stuart monarch's place as heir apparent "would have been to invite all rivals and enemies to set about forestalling his succession, thus jeopardizing both his rights and [Elizabeth's] domestic peace" (Neale 403). The dangerous state of being next in line for the throne was one Elizabeth knew well; her experience during her sister's reign, when she was imprisoned in the Tower of London on suspicion of collaborating with a rebellion against the queen, "had left her with the unshakeable conviction that, involuntarily or otherwise, the sovereign's heir presumptive automatically became the fulcrum for treasonous intrigue, and she was determined not to provide plotters with a focus for their energies" (Somerset 103). But even beyond consideration for James's safety, Elizabeth's refusal to establish an official line of succession reinforced her attempts to consolidate power. The authority of the monarchy was not to be diffused by an act of reproduction—biological or metaphorical—but would rather remain concentrated in the person of the queen alone.

Discerning the rationale behind Elizabeth's choice not to marry or declare an heir is, of course, impossible. Although the queen made several statements over her lifetime regarding the virtue of chastity, Levin reminds us that "Elizabeth often was carefully crafting her statements for public consumption, and they reveal not so much what she felt about marriage but what she felt would be politic for her to *say* about marriage" (44, emphasis in the original). However, the effect of Elizabeth's choices is undeniable. In refusing marriage, and therefore reproduction, the queen effectively opened up a space between her biological and her political selves. As feminist phenomenologists from Simone de Beauvoir onward have noted, women's corporeality has been disproportionately emphasized as a way of justifying unequal systems of power. Elizabeth Grosz, in her account of female embodiment, argues that patriarchal structures have "found a convenient self-justification for women's secondary social positions by containing them within bodies that are represented, even constructed, as frail, imperfect, unruly, and unreliable" (13). Specifically, she continues, "women's powers of reproduction are the defining (cultural) characteristics of women, and, at the same time, these very functions render women vulnerable, in need of protection or special treatment" (13-14). Queen Elizabeth's natural body and her reproductive potential constantly threatened to overtake her political authority, even in the symbolic reproduction of naming an heir in the absence of a child of her own. In resisting the reproductive act, Elizabeth effectively created an alternative mode of feminine political power— one that deemphasized female corporeality and instead stressed a nongendered individual authority. No longer was the queen's sole power the power of reproduction, an act in which the future of the lineage was paramount. Now, England was faced with a queen whose rule was focused squarely on her own present authority.

The legacy of Elizabeth's innovative ruling strategy was mixed, especially in the early years of James's reign. During the final years of her life, "the grumblings about woman's rule were louder" than they had ever been, as the country's future was clouded in unease and uncertainty (Levin 9). Even with a smooth transition of power to James, residual resentment over Elizabeth's refusal to participate in a reproductive system of power remained; the Tudor line that had brought England out of war and into a period of prolonged prosperity had ended, and even a peaceful dynastic shift was in itself a kind of cultural trauma and a major transformation of national identity. But even with these lingering fears, the overall memory of the queen was largely positive. Many emphasized the peace of the queen's tenure and cited her chastity as a major contributing factor to the country's stability. And, as satisfaction with James began to wane, England's former queen began to be lifted up as figure of national pride. "Within two or three years of Elizabeth's death there began to be a nostalgia for 'good Queen Bess' and the glories of her reign," Levin notes (168-69). In this shift from resentment to elevation, Elizabeth's reproductive politics were slowly but consistently deemphasized. No longer was the absence of an heir or the lack of a husband mentioned. By the 1620s, a new cult of Elizabeth had emerged that celebrated the memory of a monarch whose corporeal identity had finally been set aside.

Macbeth first appears in the midst of this transition. It is embedded in a culture whose attitudes about the role of reproductivity in female power were deeply affected by the mixed and quickly shifting public image of the late Elizabeth. Lady Macbeth's representations of breastfeeding and their commentary on female identity and authority must, therefore, be considered in light of this specific political climate. Previous studies, such as those by Adelman and Chamberlain, have emphasized Lady Macbeth's performance of gender as a factor contributing to her reception as a villain. But rather than garnering reactions of only horror or disgust, Lady Macbeth, especially in light of any perceived similarity to Elizabeth, may well have been a much more ambivalent figure on the early Jacobean stage, a fact modern critics have overlooked. As twenty-first century readers of Shakespeare, we must be attentive to what Phillis Rackin describes as the internalized misogyny of Shakespearean criticism. Generalizations regarding the role of early modern women as "chaste, silent, and obedient," Rackin writes, "probably occur more frequently in recent scholarship than they did in the literature of Shakespeare's time; the connections between female speech and female sexual transgression are retraced and the anxieties evoked by the possibility of female power are discovered in play after play" (44). The result of this emphasis on entrenched misogyny has resulted in the creation of a distinctly masculine reading practice. Readers of Shakespeare are "taught to read from the subject position of a man, and a misogynist man at that" and to look for the ways in which the plays confirm already entrenched expectations of female subservience (Rackin 47). But if we regard *Macbeth* not from the perspective of a critic of Elizabeth but as a supporter—male or female—who sympathized with the late monarch's approach to ruling, Lady Macbeth takes on new possibilities. She explores the potential of a new model of female political agency not dependent upon biological reproduction or mediated through the use of her body. She separates reproductive potential from political authority, and denounces breastfeeding as an action indicative of a system responsible for reducing female leaders to transient figures in a larger dynastic line. Lady Macbeth, like Elizabeth, refuses to adopt a passive approach to ruling; instead, she elects to overcome the body threatening to obscure her. She, like Elizabeth, looks for an escape from reproductive politics.

But just as Lady Macbeth attempts to separate her political authority from her corporeality, she is immediately reinscribed within the system of bodily power. Only a few lines after Lady Macbeth delivers her analogy comparing infanticide and action, Macbeth responds by remarking upon her physicality. "Bring forth men-children only," he tells her, "for thy undaunted mettle should compose / nothing but males" (1.7.72-74). Macbeth's response first and foremost rejects Lady Macbeth's attempts to position herself outside of reproductivity. The female corporeality she has so diligently attempted to cast aside returns, and the whole of her character is summed up in her ability to bear children. But, notably, that fertility is not unqualified. As a direct result of Lady Macbeth's rejection of breastfeeding, Macbeth now regards her body as undeniably altered. She is no longer indiscriminately fertile, only selectively so; her bodily composition no longer serves as a nurturing place for femininity, but rather seems only hospitable to masculinity. Macbeth's observation indicates that even if Lady Macbeth has not succeeded in her plan to "unsex" herself, she has affected the perception of her sex in seizing power alongside her husband. She remains entrenched within a system of reproductive politics but uncertainly and uncomfortably so, with the difference rendered perceptible if not complete.

The tenuousness of this moment—the awareness of a shift, however momentary, in the role of the female body in the political system—captures the complexity of Elizabeth's legacy in the early years of the seventeenth century. Having proven the potential for women to rule outside of a system focused on marriage and reproduction, Elizabeth left in her wake a host of questions. What emerges in the absence of reproductive politics?[8] How is female corporeality conceptualized outside of the roles of mother and wife? How are we to regard the woman who refuses to reproduce, to allocate her power to another? To this last question, early modern responses were fairly clear, as Levin shows. In a description of Elizabeth that could just as easily refer to Lady Macbeth, she notes that in seventeenth-century England "to be successful a woman must move away from the expectations of her gender and 'act like a man.' But to do so makes her unwomanly, possibly even monstrous" (1). Detractors of Elizabeth would have seen their fears about female power embodied in the figure of Lady Macbeth—a woman rejecting her sex in order to exercise a tyrannical and violent power over others. But in a historical moment in which that fear was mingling with love and admiration, I want to suggest that we can also see these moments when Lady Macbeth rejects the practice of breastfeeding as moments in which a new model of female political agency was being formed. The recognition of a female figure of authority, rejecting reproductivity as her only means of asserting herself, could no doubt have called to mind not just the anxiety, but the peace and prosperity associated with Elizabeth.

Although the dynamics of feminine authority present in *Macbeth* are, as I have argued, grounded in the historically specific context of Elizabeth's shifting legacy, the implications of the play's commentaries on female corporeality and power are far reaching. Contemporary breastfeeding discourse has replaced sixteenth-century views on gendered ruling strategies with new arguments about the practice's inherently "natural" qualities. Such terminology, in addition to contributing to antivaccine and general antiscience sentiments, also engages in the same rhetoric of monstrosity that surrounds both Lady Macbeth and Elizabeth.[9] If breastfeeding is seen as natural, then the refusal or inability to do becomes framed as unnatural and deviant. Such language serves to reinscribe women within the power structures of reproductivity by demanding a model of motherhood dictated solely by the body. Looking to *Macbeth* and Elizabethan politics, we can see the transgressive value of divorcing feminine agency from female corporeality. Rejecting the rhetoric of naturalized breastfeeding helps to create a liberating and volitional model of parenting that amplifies female agency and privileges choice—including the choice to breastfeed—over obligation.

ENDNOTES

[1]I have silently modernized u/v distinctions; all remaining early modern spelling has been preserved.

[2] "Illness" in this context does not imply ailment but rather "wickedness" (*OED* def. 1).

[3]For more on this passage as a renunciation of menstruation, see La Belle, "'A Strange Infirmity': Lady Macbeth's Amenorrhea."

[4]Adelman argues that this line is more ambiguous than modern scholarship generally allows. Although most gloss the phrase as "take my milk in exchange for gall," it remains equally likely that "Lady Macbeth is asking the spirits to take her milk as gall, to nurse from her breasts and find in her milk their sustaining poison. Here the milk itself is the gall; no transformation is necessary" (134).

[5]For more on Hamlet's melancholy and on Shakespeare's use of Galenic language more broadly, see Paster, *Humoring the Body: Emotions and the Shakespearean Stage.*

[6]Many early projects questioned whether or not this line implied Lady Macbeth's motherhood in any tangible way. For a refutation of that line of thinking, see L.C. Knights essay, "How Many Children Had Lady Macbeth?"

[7]John King has argued that Elizabeth's chastity should not be seen as a single, life-long plan for virginity, but rather a series of careful decisions to respond to evolving political and personal scenarios.

[8]For a contemporary treatment of this same question in light of queer theory, see Edelman, *No Future.*

[9]For more on the risks of the term "natural" and the naturalization of breastfeeding, see: Martucci and Barnhill, "Unintended Consequences of Invoking the 'Natural' in Breastfeeding Promotion," and Wolf, *Is Breast Best?*

WORKS CITED

Adelman, Janet. *Suffocating Mothers: Fantasies of Maternal Origin in Shakespeare's Plays, Hamlet to The Tempest.* Routledge, 1992.

Alfar, Christina León. "'Blood Will Have Blood': Power, Performance, and Lady Macbeth's Gender Trouble." *Journal x,* vol. 2, no. 2, 1998, pp.179-207.

Chamberlain, Stephanie. "Fantasizing Infanticide: Lady Macbeth and the Murdering Mother in Early Modern England." *College Literature*, vol. 32, no. 3, 2005, pp. 72-91.

Edelman, Lee. *No Future: Queer Theory and the Death Drive.* Duke University Press, 2004.

Grosz, Elizabeth. *Volatile Bodies: Toward a Corporeal Feminism.* Indiana University Press, 1994.

King, John N. "Queen Elizabeth I: Representations of the Virgin Queen." *Renaissance Quarterly*, vol. 43, no. 1, 1990, pp. 30-74.

Knights, L.C. "How Many Children had Lady Macbeth?" *Explorations*, George W. Stewart, 1947, pp. 15-53.

La Belle, Jenijoy. "'A Strange Infirmity': Lady Macbeth's Amenorrhea." *Shakespeare Quarterly*, vol. 31, no. 3, 1980, pp. 381-386.

Martucci, Jessica, and Anne Barnhill. "Unintended Consequences of Invoking the 'Natural' in Breastfeeding Promotion." *Pediatrics*, vol. 137, no. 4, 2016, doi:10.1542/peds.2015-4154. Accessed 4 Nov. 2016.

Neale, J.E. *Queen Elizabeth I.* 1952. Academy Chicago Publishers, 1992.

Paster, Gail Kern. *Humoring the Body: Emotions and the Shakespearean Stage.* University of Chicago Press, 2010.

Rackin, Phillis. "Misogyny Is Everywhere." *A Feminist Companion to Shakespeare*, edited by Dympna Callaghan, Blackwell Publishers, 2000, pp. 42-56.

Roselin, Eucharius. *The Byrth of Mankynde, Otherwyse Named the Womans Booke.* Translated by Thomas Raynalde. London, 1598. STC 21160. *Early English Books Online*, eebo.chadwyck.com. Accessed 23 Sept. 2016.

Shakespeare, William. *Hamlet. The Norton Shakespeare*, edited by Stephen Greenblatt et al., W.W. Norton & Company, 2016, pp. 1751-2072.

Shakespeare, William. *Macbeth. The Norton Shakespeare*, edited by Stephen Greenblatt et al., W.W. Norton & Company, 2016, pp. 2709-774.

Sherlock, Peter. "The Monuments of Elizabeth Tudor and Mary Stuart: King James and the Manipulation of Memory." *The Journal of British Studies*, vol. 46, no. 2, 2007, pp. 263-89.

Somerset, Anne. *Elizabeth I.* St. Martin's Griffin, 1991.

Wolf, Joan B. *Is Breast Best? Taking on the Breastfeeding Experts and the New High Stakes of Motherhood.* New York University Press, 2011.

3.
Same-Sex Lactations in European Art and Literature (ca. 1300-1800)

Allegory, Melancholy, Loss

JUTTA SPERLING

In his *Memorable Doings and Sayings* (31 CE), Valerius Maximus illustrates the concept of "filial piety" through a variety of unusual anecdotes and historical examples—one of which centers on a young woman's breastfeeding of her mother who languishes in prison, condemned to death by starvation. According to this anecdote, the prison guard starts to wonder why the mother does not die after some time has passed, and watches the daughter when she comes to visit. What he sees is rather unsettling: "He noticed her putting out her breast and relieving her mother's hunger with the succor of her own milk" (499). After he reported this "novel and remarkable spectacle" to the judicial authorities, the mother's sentence was remitted. The prison guard, eager to find a moral in this story, takes the event as an illustration of piety—"whither does Piety not penetrate, what does she not devise?"—but not before wondering whether "this might be thought to be against nature, if to love one's parents were not Nature's first law." He concludes, "For what so extraordinary, so unheard of, as for a mother to be nourished by her daughters' breasts?" (499).

This "extraordinary" and "unheard of" act of breastfeeding one's own mother found considerable literary and artistic resonance in medieval and early modern Europe. Relying on medieval predecessors who took the story to illustrate Catholic "charity," Giovanni Boccaccio (1313-75) and Christine de Pizan (1364-1430) turned the allegory of the Roman daughter into a story of reciprocity in kinship relations. Boccaccio's fifteenth-century French translations of *Famous Women* were illustrated on several occasions with images of the mother-daughter breastfeeding scene. Hans Sachs (1494-1576) eroticized the scene in "Romana, the Suckling Daughter," whereas the anonymous playwright of *Moralité ou Histoire Rommaine* envisioned it as a drawn-out dialogue, in which the daughter argues with her mother before giving in to her demands. A century later, Nicolas Poussin (1594-1665) integrated the scene into his momentous painting *The Gathering of the Manna*, and Sibylle Schwarz von Greiffswald aus Pommern (1621-38) rewrote the story as a poem about egalitarian relationships among women. After Guercino (1591-1666) produced a startlingly intimate drawing of the daughter and her mother, the scene was no longer represented until the late eighteenth century, when several painters, among them Angelika Kauffmann (1741-1807), returned to it under the influence of the French Revolution.

These visual representations and literary works are difficult to consume and process for a modern viewer. The "mono-maternal" revolution—which was inaugurated in the eighteenth century, fuelled by Rousseau's Émile (1762) and his recommendation of exclusive maternal nursing—still prevents us from conceiving of mothers who share their milk with persons other than their own infants, much less adult men or women, with anything but disgust and embarrassment. Yet at the time of Rousseau, more parents than ever abandoned their infants to foundling homes (Sussman 21-22), hired wet nurses to feed their children (Fildes) and breast-suckers to help with engorgement (Sperling 276), or experimented with the medicinal use of breastmilk (Wunder 295-305). Also, the iconography of *Roman Charity*—which goes back to Valerius Maximus's twin anecdote about filial piety and features a daughter who breastfeeds her starving father—continued to enjoy great popularity in the eighteenth century, with works by Jean-Baptiste Greuze, Louis-Jean-François Lagrenée the Elder, Giuseppe Baldrighi, Jean-Baptiste Deshays, Noël-Nicolas Coypel, Jean-Jacques Bachelier, Jacques-Louis David, and others. Nonetheless, a profound change of sensibility was gradually taking place throughout Europe, such that by the early nineteenth century, the deeply layered allegorical meaning and erotic appeal of nonmaternal nursing were all but eradicated. The substitution of wet-nursing with formula in the early twentieth century added to the ongoing distancing from forms of milk-sharing, which is why present-day Western audiences find it hard to wrap their minds around the ubiquity of practices and depictions of breastfeeding "promiscuity" in the early modern age. If the cross-gendered lactation scene in *Roman Charity* seems perverse enough because it depicts—often in eroticized fashion—an old man's regressive fantasies, wants, and needs, and an incestuous exchange of body fluids in the form of second-order incest, in which the daughter assumes the position of her grandmother, the all-female breastfeeding scene adds yet another irritation. What if, as the prison guard who watches the "extraordinary spectacle" also remarks, this were an instance of same-sex desire instead of a daughter's love for her mother? Or, even worse, what if it were both simultaneously?

In order to make sense of the popularity of the story and its visual representations, I draw on Judith Butler's account of gendering and melancholia, in which she revises and complicates the Freudian story of how children internalize norms of heterosexuality. Butler explains that in order for the Oedipal incest taboo to work, a prior taboo on homosexuality needs to already be in place. Girls have to more thoroughly disavow their affection for their mothers than boys because of the need to replace them with a differently gendered object of desire, and it is this disavowal that produces melancholia (136). Melancholia, according to Freud, is an effect of the impossibility to grieve and results in the incorporation of the lost loved object. Butler sees melancholia as providing a space for interiority and constituting the ego as an archive of traces of disavowed love. She calls the "melancholic turn ... the mechanism by which the distinction between internal and external worlds is instituted" (171). Whereas mourning takes place in language "by declaring the object to be dead" (185), melancholia is governed by "unspeakability," or it expresses itself in "indirect or circuitous speech" (186).

The visual and literary representations of Maximus's all-female lactation scene resonate with Butler's concepts in uncanny ways because they seem to express a daughter's undifferentiated love for her mother prior to the process of disavowals and substitutions that patriarchy demands. Melancholia already dominates their encounter—purportedly because of the daughter's sadness at her mother's death sentence—but also, perhaps, because in "[giving] back to her mother in her old age what she had taken from her mother as an infant" the daughter realizes the exceptional quality and abject nature of her enactment of feminine reciprocity (Pizan 115). In fifteenth-century illuminations of Boccaccio's story of the "young Roman woman," both women look decidedly unhappy despite the intimacy and slight eroticism that also governs the scene. In both Figures 1 and 2, the daughter refuses to make eye contact with her mother and stares obliquely to the side, whereas in Figure 3, the mother's wrinkled forehead expresses great sorrow. It is as

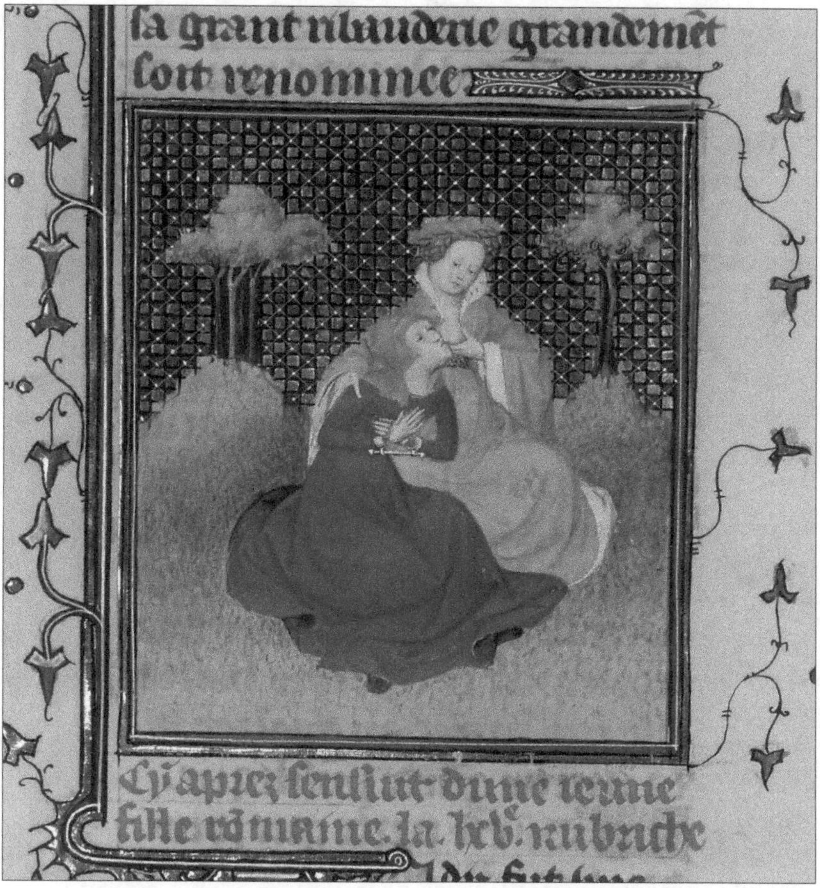

Figure 1. *Unnamed Roman Girl Feeds her Mother in Prison,* 1402, illumination, Giovanni Boccaccio, *De cleres et nobles femmes,* Paris, Bibliothèque nationale Fr. 12420, fol. 100 © Bibliothèque nationale de France.

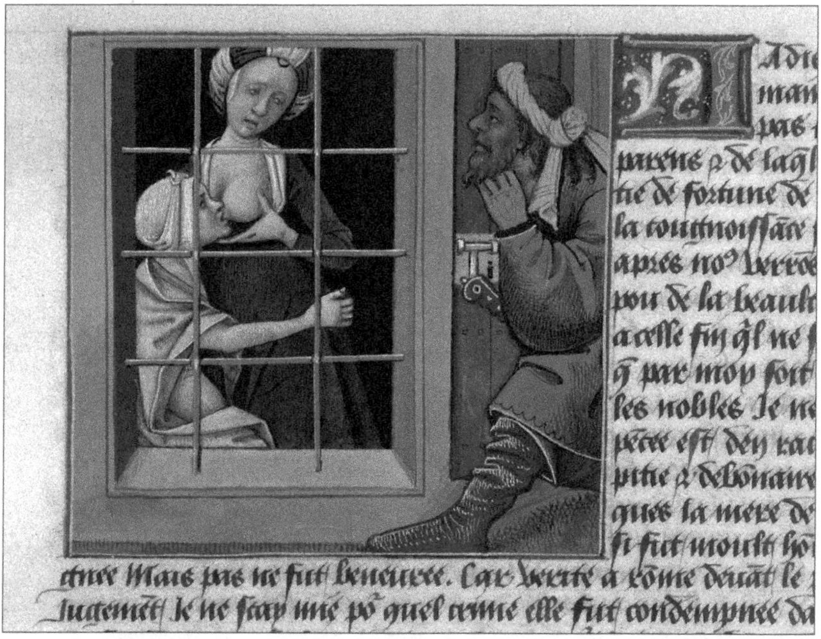

Figure 2 (right). *Mother and Daughter,* fifteen or sixteenth century, illumination, Giovanni Boccaccio, *De cleres et nobles femmes,* Paris, Bibliothèque nationale, Fr. 599, fol. 57v © Bibliothèque nationale de France.

if their performance of undoing the called-for disavowal of their love is hard to maintain, especially since it takes place under the condition of voyeurism—see the prison guard in Figure 2 scratching his beard in disbelief—and has the effect of subverting the imperial system of justice that condemned the mother in the first place.

In Maximus's anecdote as well as other subsequent retellings of the story, the daughter's maternal body language and non-verbal act of resistance against her mother's death sentence are juxtaposed to the multiple speech acts that relate "this novel and remarkable spectacle" among the various judicial authorities, ranging from the prison guard to the triumvir, praetor, and board of judges. The careful naming of the men's titles and competences contrasts greatly with the lack of specificity and differentiation the narrator employs when talking about the two women. Whereas Maximus carefully records the names of all other protagonists in his collection of anecdotes, the two heroic women remain anonymous. This bothered some medieval writers, who, such as the anonymous author

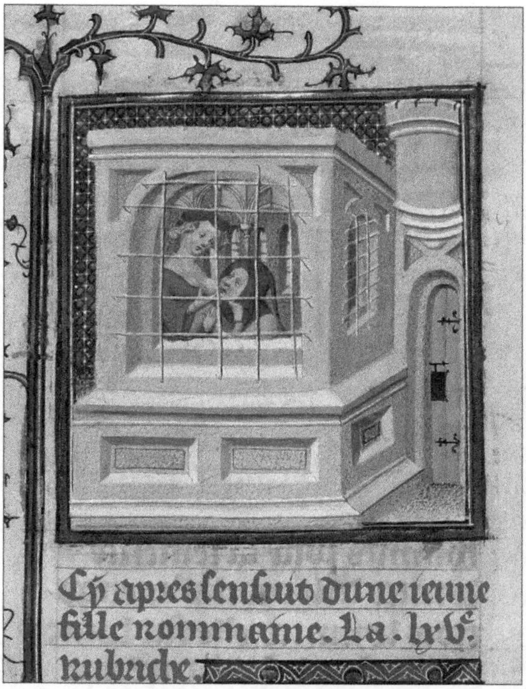

Figure 3. *Mother and Daughter,* early fifteenth century, illumination, Giovanni Boccaccio, *De cleres et nobles femmes,* Paris, Bibliothèque nationale, Fr. 598, fol. 99 © Bibliothèque nationale de France.

of *Girard de Rossillon,* invented a name for the daughter—"bone Berte"—and a noble lineage for the mother (196). In Maximus's account, by contrast, Butler's "unspeakability of melancholia" seems to emerge through the lack of specificity in narrating the daughter's act. Pliny the Elder notes that the unusual way in which she saved her mother was officially commemorated through the erection of a column devoted to Pietas in 192-91 BCE (VII.36), which confirms that the daughter's deed was regarded as a historical fact at the same time as it was allegorized as an expression of Piety personified. The omission of speech and specificity in relating the two women's experience suggests that not only was the event envisioned as having taken place in a remote past, but also that a certain pre- or extra-verbal quality governs their relationship. This extra-verbal quality that Maximus highlights as well as the spontaneous appearance of the women's sadness or melancholia in later retellings and visual representations confirms that a Butlerian reading of the scene may indeed be appropriate.

According to psychoanalytic theory, melancholia sets in as a result of the disavowal and incorporation of an object that is truly lost. The Roman daughter, however, prevents the loss from actually occurring. Rather than letting her mother die of starvation, she intervenes and keeps her mother alive, but her mode of doing so mirrors the process of incorporation and identification that according to Freud and Butler are the result of melancholia. The daughter, quite literally, becomes her mother by breastfeeding her. She erases the generational hierarchy that separates the two and performs an example of perfect reciprocity in kinship relations, which survives in Roman law as a regulatory ideal but is rarely realized due to the hierarchies and exclusions that govern patrilinearity. She also expresses a certain ego- and boundary-threatening love that continued to fascinate audiences for almost two millennia. She thus enacts, embodies, and literalizes in the exterior world the kind of psychic work that according to Butler ought to get performed internally, and, taking a historical perspective on psychological development, would have had to be performed internally by the time modern psychoanalytic theory emerged.

Of course, it is not reasonable to assume that same-sex adult lactations were ubiquitous and commonplace in ancient and pre-modern Europe, even though they did happen on occasion in medical practice. But the fact that Maximus's anecdote was retold many times and even entered visual culture suggests that audiences appreciated preserving it as a trace of alternative forms of affect and belonging at a time when patrilineal kinship systems denied mothers any legal recognition of their relationships with their children. Roman law was based on the fiction of paternal consanguinity, which assumed that only the father's blood was passed onto his children, whereas the mother provided an empty space for gestation (Pomata). By modelling "true" filial piety, thus, the daughter's act of breastfeeding her mother defies Roman law in multiple ways. For one, it expresses or enacts kinship by transferring milk up the generational ladder in a direct reversal of the paternal transmission of blood as sperm. Second, the daughter achieves, quite unexpectedly, the remittal of her mother's sentence because her "unheard of" and "extraordinary" display of piety astounds and confuses the legal establishment such that it suspends the workings of justice. And finally, in breastfeeding her mother, the daughter undoes the hierarchies and distinctions that govern patrilinearity and its far-reaching incest taboos. The regression and collapse of generational and gendered distinctions that she enacts confounds patriarchy at its core.

Although the incest taboos usually prohibit men's sexual access to their sisters', daughters', mothers', or nieces' bodies for the sake of exchanging women among strangers (Rubin), the daughter's milk exchange with her mother—and, in the case of Maximus's other example of filial piety, with her father—highlights the fact that no incest taboo prohibits the "pious" consumption of one's daughter's milk. Or does it? Perhaps it is precisely the transgression against an unspoken "law" that makes the viewer shudder and freeze in astonishment when they see depictions of Maximus's anecdotes? In addition to Judith Butler's claim for a pre-Oedipal taboo against homosexuality (135), a prohibition against sex with one's nurse or foster mother also would have had to be instituted before declaring sex with one's birth mother a crime—a rule that Oedipus notably and conspicuously did not transgress and of which only Islamic law bears traces in written form (Giladi). The case of the breastfeeding daughter confounds the very notion of an incest taboo, however, in that she does display physical love for her mother who presumably was also her nurse—but not in the form of genital sex. Her love finds expression in the exchange of a body fluid that women distributed quite widely before the modern age to the children of strangers, and to adult men and women on occasion in therapeutic settings (Sperling). Yet despite their familiarity with breastfeeding promiscuity, ancient and early modern audiences found the spectre of same-sex love that Maximus's anecdote evokes deeply unsettling, not only, we might speculate, because such love needed to be repressed in a patriarchal society (Park) but also because it presents mother-daughter relations at the origin of what we might call, with Adrienne Rich, a "lesbian continuum." Rich likens motherhood to the lesbian experience, which she says should encompass all forms of female bonding, and mentions breastfeeding in particular as one form of consummating this love:

> If we consider the possibility that all women – from the infant suckling her mother's breast, to the grown woman experiencing orgasmic sensations while suckling her own child, perhaps recalling her mother's milk-smell in her own; to two women—who share a laboratory; to the woman

> dying at ninety, touched and handled by women—exist on a lesbian continuum, we can see ourselves as moving in and out of this continuum, whether we identify ourselves as lesbian or not. ("Compulsory" 650-51)

It is thus noteworthy that most, but not all, of the literary renderings of Maximus's anecdote downplay or censor the "lesbian" threat it alludes to, whereas the visual representations find it hard to achieve such de-eroticization. Medieval authors typically do not report the prison guard's doubt that the daughter's breastfeeding of her mother "might be thought to be against nature" (Maximus 499), but focus on the "holiness" of filial love, which, according to Boccaccio, is even "superior to that natural instinct by which we are taught to raise our small children with milk" (271). Christine de Pizan, as already mentioned, interprets the event as an exercise in reciprocity (115), whereas the author of *Girard de Rossillon* calls it a story about "piety," "charity," and "sweet friendship" (196). Only Hans Sachs highlights that "the daughter suckles her mother with lust" (471), while Sibylle Schwarz von Greiffswald, possibly referring to Christine de Pizan's version, has the daughter pronounce "we shall both be daughters, and both mothers."

In his much-praised painting *The Gathering of the Manna* (1637), Nicolas Poussin took the unusual step of illustrating the Israelites' hunger in the desert through the pagan Roman icon of filial piety—the daughter-who-breastfed-her-mother (Figure 4). As a symbol of suffering, the suckling mother displays the abject state the Israelites found themselves in, while the breastfeeding daughter somewhat anachronistically competes for meaning with Catholic "charity." Since the fourteenth century, "charity" was allegorized as a breastfeeding woman or woman with children in her care to signify the indiscriminate love Christians were expected to practice vis-à-vis strangers. In Poussin's painting, the charity-group dressed in yellow and blue in the right half of the painting alludes to this iconographic tradition. Interestingly, the woman looks back to the breastfeeding daughter and points at her to signify that she embodies an earlier, pre-Christian, version of herself. The idea of having Maximus's allegory of "filial piety" prefigure Catholic "charity" in a painting about the Israelites' exodus meant that

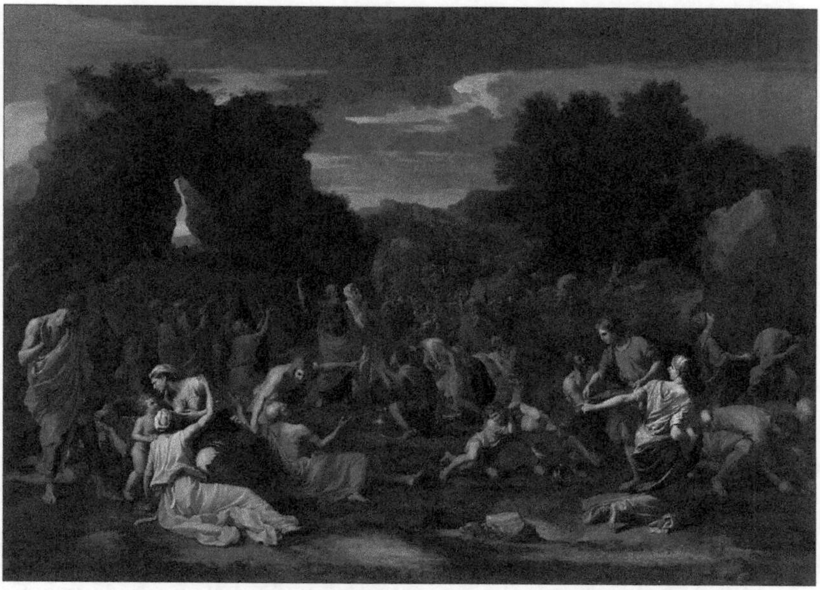

Figure 4. Nicolas Poussin, *The Gathering of the Manna,* 1639, oil on canvas, 149 × 200 cm, Paris, Musée du Louvre, inv. no. 7275 © Photo: Mathieu Rabeau, RMN-Grand Palais / Art Resource, NY ART490849.

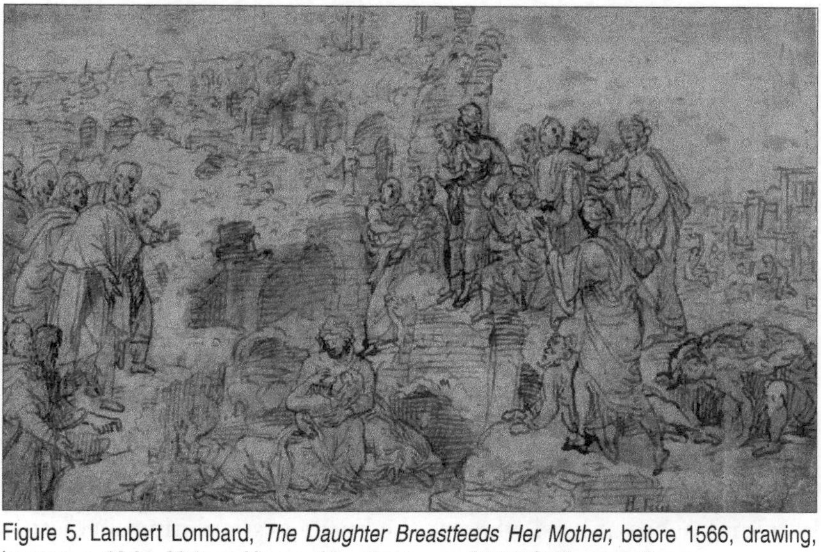

Figure 5. Lambert Lombard, *The Daughter Breastfeeds Her Mother,* before 1566, drawing, brown pen, 12.9 × 20.3 cm, Vienna, Albertina, inv. no. 35472 © Albertina, Vienna.

Jews and Romans already practised what counter-Reformation Catholics pronounced to be their superior virtue. In a letter to his friend Jacques Stella, Poussin worried that his audiences might not be able to read his painting correctly and thus misunderstand its complex, and provocative, political message. In another letter to the commissioner of the painting, Paul Fréart de Chantelou, he clarifies that the first seven persons in the left bottom corner "will tell you everything that is written there" (qtd. in Schlink 76). Charles le Brun—who declared Poussin's *Gathering of the Manna* to be the prime model of French history painting after the foundation of the Royal Academy of Painting and Sculpture in 1648—explains in great detail the important function of the man dressed in red to the left of the breastfeeding group. In oblique and circuitous language, Le Brun suggests that this man serves as observer and narrator of the breastfeeding scene, raising his hand to caution the audience against any undue misunderstandings. According to Le Brun, Poussin depicts this observer figure as a statuesque, heroic male, because a "rough and uneducated" man could not possibly have thought about all those things "that needed to be considered" when interpreting this "extraordinary act of charity" (qtd. in Schlink 38). What could have constituted such danger of misinterpretation other than the possibility of reading the scene as an act "against Nature," as already Maximus alluded to?

Again, the daughter's expression of sorrow in Poussin's painting collapses the pain of witnessing her mother's suffering with the psychic labour of melancholia in disavowing her love at the same time as she becomes her mother because of the impossibility of acknowledging her loss. According to Butler, such disavowal would have to be the first step toward the acquisition of compulsory heterosexuality, which is why the preclusion of any other same-sex object of desire adds to the daughter's sadness. Similar expressions of lesbian melancholia govern other representations of the breastfeeding daughter as well, for example in the drawing by Lambert Lombard (Figure 5). Here, we cannot discern the women's facial expressions, but the ruinous cityscape produces an almost romantic sense of loss, whereas the busily gesticulating spectators indicate the momentous nature of the event they are witnessing.

On a late fifteenth-century bronze medal (Figure 6), which inspired a ceiling fresco in an abbey in Cremona, the suckling mother assumes the pose of *Sleeping Ariadne* (117-138 CE), one of the

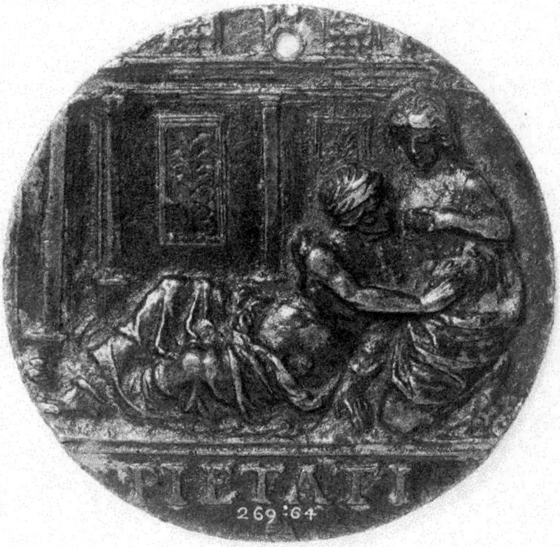

Figure 6. *Pietati,* early sixteenth century., bronze medal, London, Victoria and Albert Museum, inv. no. 269–1864 © Courtesy of the Victoria and Albert Museum.

most widely known ancient statues in the Renaissance. Abandoned by Theseus, Ariadne variously hangs herself, marries Dionysus, or dies in childbirth, and becomes one of the personifications of female melancholia in early modern art. The fact that the bronze maker adapted her pose for the representation of the starving mother cannot be an accident, especially since *Sleeping Ariadne*'s one bare breast already seems to invite fantasies of suckling. The most pitiful representation of the daughter's sorrowful love among all artistic renderings of Maximus's anecdote, however, might have been Guercino's drawing (Figure 7). Here, the poor daughter addresses the viewer with a half-opened mouth while the mother is hunched over to reach her daughter's breast. The daughter's gaze is startling because in looking at the beholder, she identifies him as a voyeur while also attempting to speak to him. The drawing reminds of Demetrius of Phalerum's third-century BCE treatise *On Style*, in which the author encourages his readers to imagine that personified abstract concepts, "assuming a woman's form, should address such and such reproaches to you" (qtd. in Paxson 12). Other ancient theorists of rhetoric such as Cicero and the anonymous author of *Rhetoric for Herennium* confirm that allegories or embodied figures of speech are usually women, children,

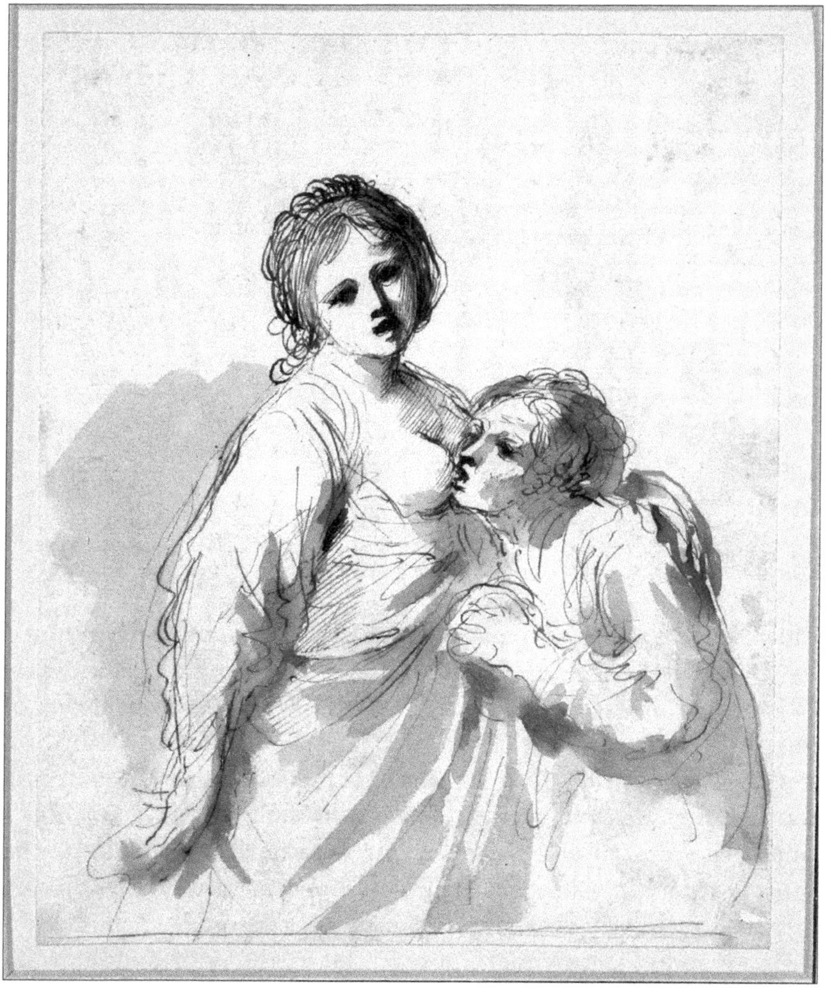

Figure 7. Guercino, *The Daughter Who Breastfeeds her Mother,* before 1661, drawing, London, Collection of Her Majesty the Queen at Windsor Castle, Royal Collection Trust, RCIN 902573 / © Her Majesty Queen Elizabeth II 2015.

or other "voiceless things" whose fictitious speeches are supposed to move their audiences to pity (qtd. in Paxson, 13-19). Female allegories can fulfill this function precisely because women are mute and absent in a male-dominated forum of public speech, which is why their ghostlike reappearance as figures of speech carries with it the trace of their exclusion and pitiful state. In this sense, the breastfeeding daughter functions as quintessential allegory, whose

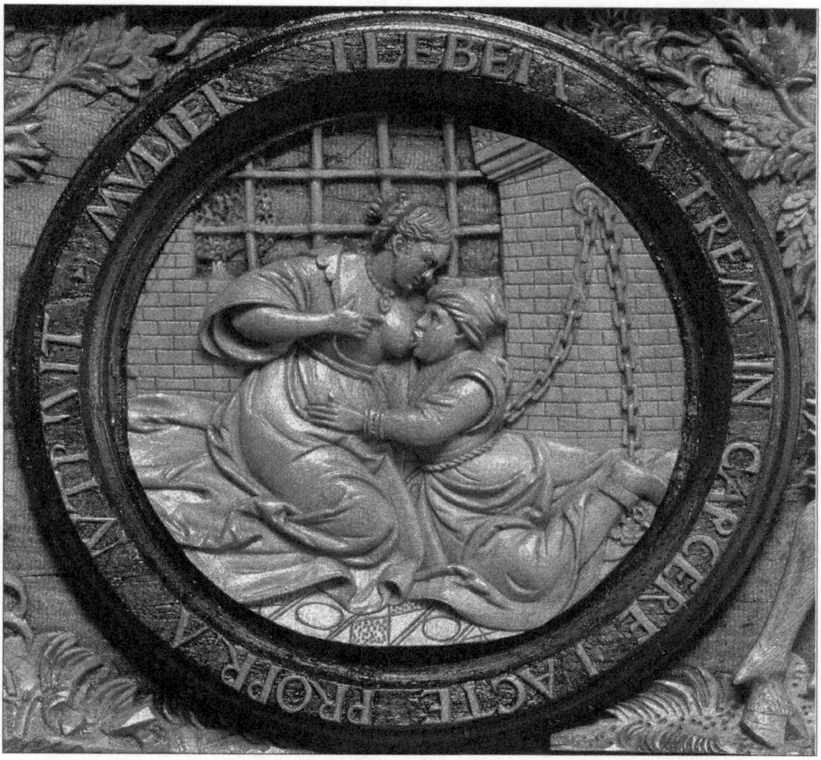

Figure 8. *Hans Kels the Elder, Daughter Breastfeeding her Mother,* 1537, detail, carved board game, Vienna, Kunsthistorisches Museum, KK 3419 © KHM- Museumsverband.

mute body language arouses pity among not only ancient judges but also early modern audiences. According to Joel Fineman, "the movement of allegory, like the dreamwork, enacts a wish" and ought to be studied more closely in conjunction with psychoanalysis, especially because allegories denote the (gendered) figurality of all language so important to theories of desire. Fineman also points out that allegories "regularly ... surface in critical or polemical atmospheres, when for political or metaphysical reasons there is something that cannot be said" (48). It thus seems that the unspeakability of melancholia accompanies and preconditions the work of allegory and that the disavowal of the mother may be looked at as the prime object of allegorization. That's why the daughter's truncated speech in Guercino's drawing is frightening: on the one hand, the viewer uneasily wonders what kind of reproaches she would utter if she could speak, and on the other, gets nervous at the danger of eruption into language of what can only be shown visually, and otherwise needs to be preserved in the preverbal realm of unconscious psychic structures. The drawing simply violates the rule of disavowal that later psychoanalysts identified as a vital part in the acquisition of heterosexuality.

Not all literary and visual representations of the breastfeeding daughter are steeped in melancholia or cast her as a voiceless being, but as always, the exception seems to confirm the rule. In *Moralité ou Histoire Rommaine*, a sixteenth-century French one-act, the daughter first pleads with the authorities to commute the death sentence of her mother into a shared punishment for them both such as amputating their legs and tongues (178). Once she has achieved the suspension of her mother's immediate decapitation and obtained visiting rights to her prison, she encourages her mother to endure her fate with greater poise before giving in to her demands for help (182-83). We can only speculate how the breastfeeding scene was staged, but chances are that it was quite graphic, if the director took inspiration from contemporary renderings of the iconography. Unlike the 1782 production of *The Grecian Daughter* by Arthur Murphy, in which the breastfeeding scene took place offstage (Sperling 255), the author of *Histoire Rommaine* conceived of two conversations happening simultaneously on stage—one in which the daughter offers her breast to her mother, and another one in which the prison guard wonders what could be sustaining the convict's life for so long. Although a certain amount of pathos and gravitas governs the play, Hans Sachs's contemporary short story of "Romana, the Suckling Daughter" is rather burlesque in tone. His mentioning of the "lüesten" (lust) with which the daughter nourishes her mother with "breasts full of milk" resonates with a detail on a contemporary carved chess board by Hans Kels the Elder, which shows how a well-nourished mother latches on to her smiling, beautiful daughter's exposed breast (Figure 8). By contrast, the classical architecture in Étienne Delaune's drawing fits into the French context of greater poise and elegance. Moreover, the daughter's transparent gown indicates a certain amount of eroticism heightened by the fact that the prison guard secretly watches the two women (Figure 9). Despite this interlude of more

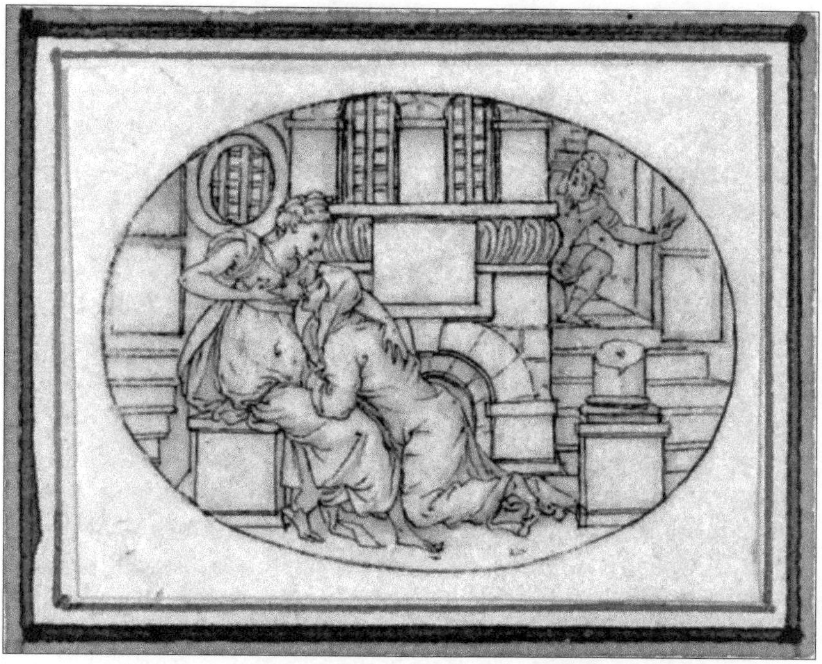

Figure 9. Étienne Delaune, *The Daughter Breastfeeds her Mother,* before 1583, ink on paper, 3.5 x 4.3 cm, Vienna, Albertina, inv. no. 11166 © Albertina, Vienna.

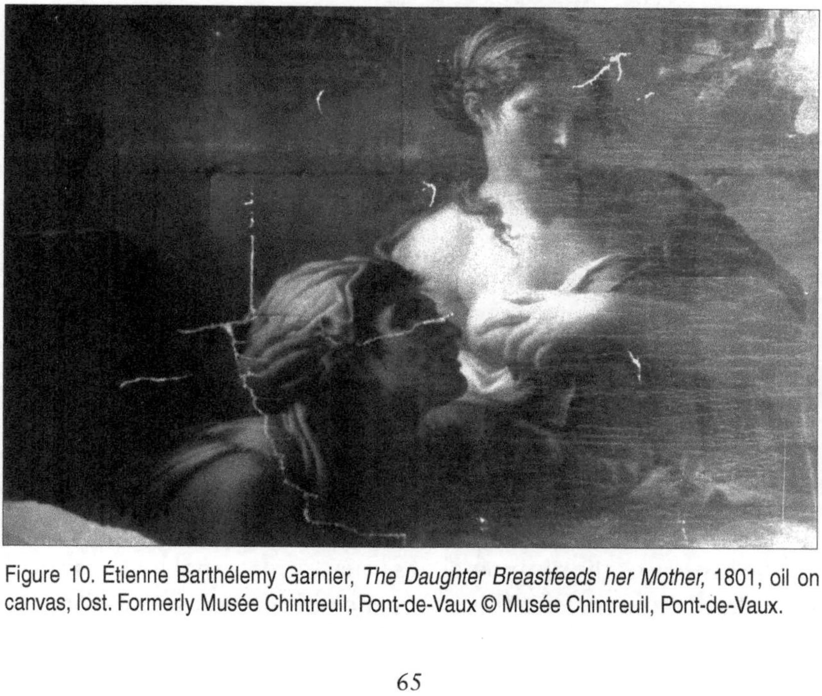

Figure 10. Étienne Barthélemy Garnier, *The Daughter Breastfeeds her Mother,* 1801, oil on canvas, lost. Formerly Musée Chintreuil, Pont-de-Vaux © Musée Chintreuil, Pont-de-Vaux.

lively, sexy, or verbal representations of the breastfeeding daughter toward the middle of the sixteenth century, melancholia emerges as prevalent mode and affect in all other known representations. The last one in this series is a lost painting by Étienne-Barthélemy Garnier from 1801, of which we have an old photograph (Figure 10). It shows the mother looking up at her daughter with big, sad eyes and a half-opened mouth, just moments before latching on, while the daughter modestly averts her eyes. She offers her beautiful breast with the typical V-hold to her mother in a tender, affectionate, and slightly erotic manner, but the usual sadness and abjection also pervade the scene.

In addition to Garnier's rendering, two other oil paintings of the mother-daughter breastfeeding scene are recorded for the revolutionary time period, one of which by Angelika Kauffmann (1794). This famous artist made women's sensibility and melancholia her signature themes in many paintings derived from Greek mythology (Rosenthal). It is, thus, reasonable to assume that similar affects dominated her rendering of Maximus's anecdote, which appeared in a series of four paintings depicting different types of love (Baumgärtel 108). The other scenes inspired by Greek and Roman history highlight the power of women as protectors of kings, temptresses of philosophers, and inspiration to artists (Manners). Kaufmann's pious daughter thus found herself in illustrious company—next to Phryne, Praxiteles's model, and the nymph Egeria. But the loss of the painting itself, as well as the loss of all other eighteenth-century renderings of the iconography, indicates how the depiction of an impending loss of a beloved mother and a daughter's ingenious way to prevent her death by "becoming her" would, on the threshold to modernity, no longer be regarded as intelligible, interesting, or even viewable. Paintings of its twin motif, the father-daughter breastfeeding scene alias *Roman Charity*, also suffered from systematic neglect since the early nineteenth century (Sperling 9), but the suppression of the all-female nursing scene was very thorough and suggests that modern sensibilities would not tolerate such queer and intimate depictions of milk-sharing among women.

The history of the disavowal of same-sex maternal love was now complete. Nonetheless, the resurgence of interest in the topic of mother-daughter love at the height of the revolutionary period and its aftermath suggests that during the process of de-differentiation that accompanied contemporary demands for "equality," the utopia of sisterhood entered the political imaginary in the form of visual representations of the breastfeeding daughter. In her book *Of Woman Born*, Adrienne Rich famously theorized the mutuality and reciprocity that govern relationships among and between women, which in her view emerge from the "quality of caring" and the "diffuse kinds of identification that exist between actual mothers and daughters" as well as nonmothers (*Of Women Born*, 253). The iconography and literary tradition of the breastfeeding daughter in medieval and early modern Europe—especially when rendered by female artists and writers—constitute historical traces of women's efforts "to accept and integrate and strengthen both the mother and the daughter in ... [themselves and each other]" (253). They are instances of a "radical vision[s] of sisterhood" that accompanied the onset of patriarchy itself.

WORKS CITED

Anon. "Girard de Rossillon." *Poème Bourguignon du XIVe siècle*, edited by Edward Billings Ham, Yale University Press, 1936.

Anon. "Moralité ou Histoire Rommaine." *Ancien théâtre françois,* vol. III, edited by Viollet Le Duc et al., P. Jannet, 1854-57, pp. 171-86.

Baumgärtel, Bettina. *Angelika Kauffmann (1741-1807)*. Beltz, 1990.

Boccaccio, Giovanni. *Famous Women.* Edited and translated by Virginia Brown, I Tatti Renaissance Library, 2001.

Butler, Judith. *The Psychic Life of Power*. Stanford University Press, 1997.

Fildes, Valerie. *Wet Nursing: A History from Antiquity to the Present*, Blackwell, 1988.

Fineman, Joel. "The Structure of Allegorical Desire." *October*, vol. 12, 1980, pp. 46-66.

Giladi, Avner. *Infants, Parents, and Wet Nurses: Medieval Islamic Views on Breastfeeding and Their Social Implications*. Brill, 1999.

Manners, Lady Victoria and Dr. G. C. Williamson. *Angelica Kauff-*

mann, R. A., Her Life and her Works. John Lane the Bodely Head Limited, 1924.

Maximus, Valerius. *Memorable Doings and Sayings*. Edited and translated by D.R. Shackleton Bailey, Harvard University Press, 2000.

Park, Katharine. "The Rediscovery of the Clitoris." *The Body in Parts: Fantasies of Corporeality in Early Modern England*, edited by David Hillman and Carla Mazzio, Routledge, 1997, pp. 170-91.

Paxson, James J. *The Poetics of Personification*. Cambridge University Press, 1994.

Pizan, Christine de. *Book of the City of Ladies*. Translated by Earl Jeff Richards, Persea Books, 1983.

Pliny the Elder. *Natural History*. Book VII. Edited by John Bostock, M.D. et al., 1855-57, http://www.perseus.tufts.edu/hopper/text?doc=Perseus%3Atext%3A1999.02.0137%3Abook%3D7%3Achapter%3D36. Accessed 27 July 2016.

Pomata, Gianna. "Blood Ties and Semen Ties: Consanguinity and Agnation in Roman Law." *Gender, Kinship, Power: A Comparative and Interdisciplinary History*, edited by Mary Jo Maynes et al., Routledge, 1996, pp. 43–64.

Rich, Adrienne. "Compulsory Heterosexuality and Lesbian Existence." *Signs*, vol. 5, no. 4, 1980, pp. 631-60.

Rich, Adrienne. *Of Woman Born: Motherhood as Experience and Institution*. W. W. Norton & Company, 1995.

Rosenthal, Angela. *Angelica Kauffmann: Art and Sensibility*. Yale University Press, 2006.

Rubin, Gayle. "The Traffic in Women: Notes on the 'Political Economy' of Sex." *Toward an Anthropology of Women*, edited by Rayna Reiter, Monthly Review Press, 1975, pp. 157-210.

Sachs, Hans. "Romana, die seugend dochter." *Hans Sachs*, edited by A. von Keller and E. Goetze, Literarischer Verein, 1895, pp. 470-71.

Schlink, Wilhelm. *Ein Bild ist kein Tatsachenbericht: Le Bruns Akademierede von 1667 über Poussins "Mannawunder."* Rombach Verlag, 1996.

Schwarzin vohn Greiffswald aus Pommern, Sibylle. *Sibyllen Schwarzin vohn Greiffswald aus Pommern Ander Theil Deut-*

scher Poëtischer Gedichten, vol. 2, edited by Helmut W. Ziefle, Peter Lang, 1980.

Sperling, Jutta Gisela. *Roman Charity: Queer Lactations in Early Modern Visual Culture*, transcript Verlag, 2016.

Sussman, George D. *Selling Mother's Milk: The Wet-Nursing Business in France 1715–1914*, University of Illinois Press, 1982.

Wunder, Heide. "Frauenmilch-Muttermilch. Eine Geschichte aus dem 18. Jahrhundert." *Geschichte in Geschichten: Ein historisches Lesebuch*, edited by Barbara Duden et al., Campus, 2003, pp. 295-305.

4.
Latch

The Object of the Breast Pump

ELAINE MCDEVITT

Humans are *Mammalia*, "of the breast." But are we? Or are we of the bottle, or the pump, or the tube? How has the proliferation of designed objects and material culture surrounding infant feeding changed the primal act of breastfeeding and its fundamental connection to our existence as a species? The contemporary experience of breastfeeding is significantly different from what it was even thirty years ago. However, contemporary mothers engage with an object that was either rarely or not available at all to previous generations—the breast pump. How can we trace this object in the context of material culture and design and social history? How have mothers actually encountered and used this object and how has this affected their infant feeding choices?

In conversation regarding the study of material culture, Amy Bentley advises,

> How to locate, and correctly interpret, the "culture" in material culture is important and complicated, and no doubt the answers and methods vary for different time periods ... historical context plays a great role, as does the means by which the object was created or circulated, the way in which the object was acquired, and the multivalent meanings that humans both bring to and inscribe upon the object. (Auslander et al 1367)

Issues surrounding infant feeding involve many fields of study and thinking—biological, feminist, psychological, historical, technological, cultural, medical, and commercial—but very little material exists regarding the infant-feeding objects themselves. Ian Wickes presents arguably the most comprehensive history of infant feeding, even six decades after its first publication, particularly in the context of childhood disease and infant mortality. Rima B. Apple, provides a comprehensive and oft-quoted history of many of the issues pertaining to this study in *Mothers & Medicine: A Social History of Infant Feeding 1890-1950*. Aligning the history of infant feeding with the concepts and trends of motherhood, she outlines the move from breastfeeding and motherhood as "the grand prerogative of woman," through eras of rational management and medical and scientific motherhood. Derrick Jelliffe and E.F. Patrice Jelliffe, meanwhile, approach breastfeeding from both a medical and anthropological perspective, and although their *Human Milk in the Modern World* is now somewhat dated, it does give a context to the practice of breastfeeding in traditional and tribal societies as well as allows us to consider breastmilk as object. Andrea Wiley's *Re-imagining Milk* is also useful in this regard. Naomi Baumslag and Dia Michels, Pam Carter, Bernice Hausman, Jessica Martucci, and Gabrielle Palmer have all produced extensive studies on the subject of infant feeding, and tend to approach the subject from a cultural, feminist, and sociological standpoint. Overall, their stance positions formula as controversial. Although there is significant crossover between these writers and Linda Blum, Shari Thurer, and Marylin Yalom, the latter position breastfeeding more fully in the context of discourse surrounding the breast and motherhood. In answer to the position of formula feeding as a controversial practice, Suzanne Barston, Madeleine Morris, and Courtney Jung, meanwhile, provide some counter-arguments to the established discourse and deal with the guilt faced by formula-feeding mothers. Rebecca Kukla, too, argues that mothering is an "embodied" process, regardless of feeding choice.

The briefest engagement with this topic quickly discloses what an emotive subject infant feeding is, with both breastfeeding and formula-feeding mothers sharing experiences of judgment and pressure regarding their feeding choices. The hashtags #bressure (breastfeeding pressure) and #fedisbest have even become commonplace on Twitter. As an object, the breast pump reflects, and sometimes contradicts, almost every argument surrounding infant feeding over the last two centuries and triggers many ethical, social, and cultural arguments of its own.

This chapter locates many of these issues in an Irish context and contextualizes them within international discourse. Although many of the infant-feeding patterns seen throughout the developed and industrialized world are common to one another and see a large-scale migration from breast- to bottle-feeding over the course of the twentieth century, this was particularly pronounced in Ireland (Clear). Breastfeeding rates in Ireland, though currently increasing, are still the lowest in the developed world (Growing Up in Ireland), and Ireland can, therefore, be seen as a microcosm of international trends. How has the material culture surrounding women as they embark upon feeding their infants influenced these changes? Many of my findings disclose great dichotomies in how infant feeding and the material culture of infant feeding are understood—all at once these things are loved and hated, luxurious and virtuous, embodied and disembodied, intimate and mechanically disentangled, useful and uncomfortable, private and public. In the material culture of infant feeding, many contradictions have emerged—it is certainly a more complex discourse than simply "bottle or breast."

In the past mothers chose to breastfeed or formula feed, but the availability of the breast pump has disrupted this dyad, making it a hugely significant object. As Maia Boswell-Penc and Kate Boyer acknowledge,

> The "bottle or breast" question has long been cast, at least partially, in terms of convenience, mobility, and the ability to integrate infant feeding with wage labor outside the home. In this context, generations of U.S. women have chosen infant formula over nursing. Over the last ten years, however, breast pumps designed for individual use have begun to hit the marketplace offering a "third alternative." (552)

The purveyors of public and private space, many women who choose to breastfeed do so with the aid of a pump. How does this intimate object enable the new mother to navigate her postpartum identity alongside that of her previous self? The breast pump affords us insight into the convergence of an ideal of motherhood born in the eighteenth century and a postmodern version of motherhood that negotiates complex cultural systems through individual experience. This chapter will trace a new experience of motherhood as manifested through the use of the breast pump and other breast-pumping products, an experience assessed in historically grounded terms of the distance created between mother and child, milk as commodity, and science over nature.

Although much of the contemporary academic discussion surrounding infant feeding centres on the United States, academics—such as Caitriona Clear, Tanya Cassidy, Pauline Dillon-Hurney, and Emma O'Toole—continue to engage in discourse surrounding infant feeding that is specific to Ireland. Studies, much like social commentary, often, but not exclusively, favour and advocate for breastfeeding, with such books as the La Leche League's *The Womanly Art of Breastfeeding*, the seventh edition of which, accredited to Diane Wiessinger, is referenced in this chapter, and Gabrielle Palmer's *The Politics of Breastfeeding*, achieving something of a cult status. Much of the academic discourse surrounding infant feeding is written from a medical or sociological perspective, and despite an understanding of the effects of the material culture of infant feeding as filtered through criticism of the formula industry, little attention is paid to the objects themselves. This chapter, deeply rooted in the contemporary experience, explores the influence and agency of the pivotal object of the breast pump, and argues that this object feeds into many of the concerns surrounding contemporary mothers as they navigate a mothering experience, which encourages breastfeeding while often dictating a return to the paid workforce.

RELIEVING THE BREAST

The breast pump originated as a medical device in order to "relieve" the breast, and has undergone dramatic changes, particularly in the last three decades. Martucci describes its historical origins as follows: "The modern electric breast pump is rooted in a far less complex ancestor. In the nineteenth-century medical world, swellings, stoppages, and inflammations often required the extraction of some offending obstruction through the administration of a purgative or emetic, or even bloodletting or cupping" (179). A *Book of Illustrations* (or catalogue) for S. Maw, Son & Thompsons, printed in London in 1869, illustrates some of the devices used, including a breast glass that in order to function as a pump required the user to suck on the mouth piece to create suction. It also shows a breast reliever comprising a funnel-shaped glass element, attached by a band to a rubber ball-shaped receptacle, with a similar mechanism to a contemporary nipple everter and referred to in The *Womanly Art of Breastfeeding* as a "bicycle horn" pump (119).

The basic components of this manual "bicycle horn" breast pump became a little more streamlined, as illustrated in a design manifestation used in a 1935 silent film made by the British Medical Association at Carnegie Welfare Centre, Shoreditch and made available online by the Wellcome Library. The fact that the film deals specifically with breastfeeding difficulties, including inverted nipples, is very telling, as the breast pump was largely used for medical reasons throughout the twentieth century—either for problems as described above, to express milk for a preterm or weak baby, or in some cases, to maintain supply in the absence of a baby or until an infection of the breast or nipple cleared up. For any of these purposes, manual pumping and hand expression were the standard options for women. Interestingly, Martucci explains that the first electric breast pump was patented in 1923 by dairy-machine engineer Edward Laskar, and was specifically considered a device for use under medical supervision only and not for "domestic technology" (183).

TOWARD SCIENTIFIC MOTHERHOOD

This role of medical supervision is key to understanding the changes to breastfeeding practices in the earlier parts of the twentieth century, and it is impossible to position the breast pump within breastfeeding discourse without acknowledging the rise of infant formula and artificial or bottle feeding. In her pivotal book *Mothers & Medicine: A Social History of Infant Feeding* 1890-1950, Apple explains how formula or "patent food" was first marketed as a safe alternative to breastfeeding in the late nineteenth century, and coupled with better bottles and an increased understanding of bacteria, it represented a huge improvement on previous artificial-feeding options. She describes how a highly managed medical practice of devising the best formula required individual physicians to "have on hand analyses of each mother's milk" (25) in order to tailor a substitute to the infant's digestion. Meanwhile, manufacturers advertised their infant foods to both the medical establishment and directly to the public. Whereas many babies were fed cow's milk directly, artificial food came in several powdered forms—a dried milk substitute that could be added to water and therefore avoid concerns over contaminated milk; or a food supplement to be mixed with cow's milk.

The bottle, which was to become the predominant vessel for infant formula during the twentieth century, was configured not to the ideal of the maternal breast but to a new ideal— science. Transparent, tall, cylindrical, or hexagonal-sided and with measurements furnishing the surface, either embossed onto the glass or transfer printed on the surface of the bottle—this basic bottle shape changed little over the course of the twentieth century. It was sleek, streamlined, and modern. This individual design represents, above all others, the commodification and scientific management of infant feeding.

Both Truby King and Christine Frederick were hugely influential in their promotion of strict feeding and sleeping schedules for babies. Whereas King promoted the advantages of breastfeeding, Frederick's focus was more purely on the schedule itself with no mention of breastfeeding, "9:00-10:00 Prepare baby's gruel, sterilized milk, etc. ; wash baby napkins while watching food (Baby naps 9:00-11:00)" (76). Irene Cieraad explains Frederick's belief that "when housekeeping was reformed according to the principles of efficiency it would turn a simple housewife into a respectable professional manager of household affairs" (264). Streamlined, transparent, and clean, the cylindrical bottle stands as a symbol for this highly managed and controlled method of feeding.

Throughout the twentieth century, innumerable brands produced versions of this bottle, first in glass and as the century wore on, in plastic. The number of associated products also grew—from insulating cases and pouches, bottle warmers, sterilizers, and sterilizing chemicals to the fluids and foods administered through the bottle. This cylindrical feeding bottle was to become so widely available and identifiable as a symbol of infant feeding that it was to challenge the cultural understanding and previous norms of breastfeeding. The bottle was quantifiable, regular, and wholly unlike the female breast.

"WHEN BREASTMILK FAILS"

In the 1920s, 1930s, and 1940s, we see not only an increase in the use of formula and bottle-feeding, but also the emergence of breastmilk as a subject within everyday discourse as separate from breastfeeding. In this same period, Lindsay Earner-Byrne describes how

> In Ireland, mothers became the target of health propaganda and mothercraft philosophies in a bid to improve infant mortality figures and family health.... Innate skills, or those passed down through the generations, were seen as dangerous as well as a source of suspicion or worse. The professional was meant to promote scientific rather than instinctive motherhood. (59-60)

Legitimate concerns over the welfare and nutrition of mothers and children, coinciding with the increased availability of formula, were reinterpreted to question mother's milk, both in the marketing of formula and in broader society and culture.

Although breastfeeding rates had been favourable at the turn of the century, and despite breastfeeding advocacy, slowly and subtly, suggestions were made over the course of the twentieth century that bottles were just like breasts, that formula feeding led to happy, cheerful babies, and that mother's milk, though still ideal, was somehow lacking. Formula companies offered solutions and alternatives. Glaxo, whose tagline reads "promotes breastfeeding," stated "Many of the mothers have a good quantity of milk but it is of poor quality"; the recommendation was for the mothers themselves to take Glaxo to "improve their milk" (7). Benger's

Food, meanwhile, encouraged mothers to partially feed with its product once "feeding begins to overtire" and to take it themselves while nursing (9). A 1937 advertisement for Sister Laura's Food presents a "laughing & growing" baby "when breast-milk fails" (5). The doubt over mother's milk established itself so strongly that even after the risks of widespread malnutrition had eased, a "Mother and Baby" advice column in a 1950 edition of *Model Housekeeping* proclaims, "Your breast food may not be adequate for his needs" and suggests supplementary feeding (732).

These advertisements and editorials give an Irish context to what Apple refers to as the accentuation of "the inadequacy of maternal instinct," as perpetuated through scientific motherhood. "Mothers did not 'just naturally' know how to care for infants and children; they needed instruction in paper childrearing techniques" (114). Breastfeeding advocacy too, by its very nature, assumes that mothers require instruction. "Gastro-Enteritis", a 1951 Irish Public Health Department notice published in *The Irish Times*, states, "The attention of mothers is earnestly called to the desirability of breast-feeding of infants as the best and safest method of feeding them" (3). By the end of the twentieth century, the pendulum of popular opinion had swung from the rigid parenting techniques advocated by King and Frederick to the more instinctive, mother- and child-centred approaches of the La Leche League and Dr. Spock's "Baby and Child Care" book and subsequent movement. Motherhood was becoming natural again, and the innate skills to which Lindsay Earner-Byrne referred were once more of value. However, the vastly changing attitudes toward infant feeding meant the skills that each generation could pass down to the next were now often at odds with the zeitgeist. Added to this, concerns over the quality and quantity of mother's milk were deeply embedded in the social environment in which the electric domestic breast pump emerged.

AN EMBODIMENT OF PROCESS

The breast pump, on the one hand, embodies the breastfeeding experience, and it becomes the location of the feeding process. Yet, the product is to be consumed elsewhere. In describing this dislocation, Rudzik states that "The medicalisation of breastmilk and its conceptual separation from the maternal body allows for it to be viewed as simply a product to be provided by any caregiver" (qtd. in Cassidy and El Tom 12). Attached to and removed from the body, the breast pump allows us to examine the product and process of breastfeeding removed from the maternal-infant dyad.

Kukla contests that "Nothing as self-standing and with such a specific function as a breast pump could ever possibly 'disembody' mothering" (*Mass Hysteria* 156). Certainly, it cannot be reasonably argued that a method of infant feeding disenfranchises the many other important aspects of motherhood. However, Chris Shilling contextualizes the body and technology in relation to embodiment: "The body may constitute a source of technology, yet history shows that technologies become embedded in customs, procedures and societal structures that seem to inscribe themselves on the actions and identities of embodied individuals and often appear fixed to new generations" (179). There are many reasons that a woman may wish to express, or extract, breastmilk, including the following: the need to maintain or boost milk supply; the need to feed a preterm infant; the inability of a baby to completely empty the breasts due to tongue-tie, ineffective suck, or latching problems; and even the induction of lactation when adopting a child. The widespread custom of expressing breastmilk is such a relatively new phenomenon that its effect on the embodied or disembodied individual is crucial to understanding contemporary motherhood. The idea of maternal guilt is not new and has manifested itself firmly within the material culture of breastfeeding. References to babies "full of life and energy," protected and nourished, have not been arbitrary; they have directly fed into the good mother/bad mother dichotomy. In their exploration of the dilemma of maternal guilt, K.T. Williams et al. reflect on how advocacy fails to address "negative emotions that mothers might experience as a result of the promotion of particular feeding practices as optimal" (342).

When considered in relation to the experience of guilt, the agency of the breast pump as an object becomes even more pronounced. It embodies the process of extracting breastmilk from the mother but renders the mother unnecessary in the feeding of milk directly to the child. In terms of material culture, this distance and disentanglement between mother and infant are well exemplified by the fact that the Medela Swing breast pump storage bag includes an inner pocket into which a mother can put a picture of her baby. The distance between mother and baby is poignantly designed into the object itself. Looking at an image of a baby in the absence of that baby can stimulate "let-down"—the release of milk that takes place during breastfeeding. It is worth remembering that whereas formula-feeding parents may choose this method of feeding from the start, mothers who express breastmilk have, most likely, chosen to breastfeed. The breast pump, in its simplest assessment, facilitates the administration of breastmilk to the baby in the absence of the mother. However, this absence and physical disentanglement may not be chosen. A mother expressing breastmilk may simply be doing so because it is the only way in which she can ensure her baby receives breastmilk, a substance she understands to be optimal.

LIQUID GOLD?

The classification of humans as *Mammalia*, a species that depends on the female producing milk to feed her offspring, coined by Carolus Linnaeus in 1758, literally meaning "of the breast" (Schiebinger 382). In considering the breast pump, Megan Garber describes "A device that allows for mother and milk to be mechanically de-entangled from each other—and that, in the process, helps breast milk to be transformed, essentially, from an intimacy to a commodity." In this way, the traditional baby and breast relationship—described by Baumslag and Michels as a "truly beautiful interactive process whereby both mother and child work together to produce a living biological substance that nourishes the infant" (xxi)—is altered by the breast pump.

Despite the reasonable nutritional balance provided by formula, breastmilk is a far more complex biological substance, which cannot be fully replicated and has no direct substitute. The trend toward milk expression, facilitated by the availability of the breast pump, objectifies the milk itself. It is still of the breast, but administered remotely, expressed human breastmilk (EBM) causes a shift in a deeply ingrained social understanding of breastfeeding. Through the consumption of the contemporary breast pump, the symbiosis of the mother-baby breastfeeding relationship is altered greatly. Breastmilk is extracted; it becomes EBM, and is deposited into storage bottles or breastmilk storage bags for later use. How does this manifest itself in the maternal experience?

Christine Cooper-Rompato's insightful 2013 study, "The Talking Breast Pump," describes the auditory illusion phenomenon where mothers hear their breast pumps speak (183). Often the comments heard are negative, and "Several mothers report hearing taunts about their insufficient milk production" (188). The quality of mother's milk, as we have already seen, has been consistently questioned within the breastfeeding narrative. In the United States, laboratories offer "breastmilk analysis" to the public, and mothers can even purchase alcohol test strips for their breastmilk. Jill Lepore describes the history of milk banks—companies or charities that collect, process, store and distribute breastmilk—the first of which was established in the U.S. in 1911. She further says, "Once milk banks replaced wet nurses, human milk came to be treated, more and more, as a medicine, something to be prescribed and researched, tested and measured, in flasks and beakers" (32).

The establishment of breastmilk as a commodity is exemplified most pertinently in relation to the sale of breastmilk, which has become something of a cottage industry in the U.S. (Bakalar). Websites specifically designed to accommodate breastmilk exchange are not subject to the same scrutiny as milk banks. Milk is not pasteurized and storage methods are not regulated. The milk is simply bought and sold. Unless the milk is analyzed, as described above, which can be an expensive process, there is no way to tell if the milk is free of alcohol, drugs, and other contaminants, or, indeed, if it is human milk at all. A 2013 study by Keim et al. examines samples from two large American human-milk-selling websites, and compares them to milk bank samples, which are pasteurized and subject to FDA governance. The study concludes the following: "Human milk purchased via the Internet exhibited high overall bacterial growth and frequent contamination with pathogenic bacteria, reflecting poor collection, storage, or shipping practices" (1227). Perhaps of most concern, Keim et al. comment on the presence of salmonella, which does not belong in milk. This contamination undermines the commonly held belief that breastmilk is better than formula and exposes another contradiction in infant-feeding dialogue.

BEHIND CLOSED DOORS

The breast pump, a private object, used sometimes in the public sphere, can be considered to "have special significance for understanding how gendered identities are shaped by a combination of public and private dimensions because they are both highly intimate, directly or indirectly contacting the body" (Turbin 47). It is used in bedrooms, lactation rooms, and with the help of a pumping bra, even in cars or at desks—as women try to make up some of the time lost to this activity. Both formula-feeding mothers and breastfeeding mothers claim a level of convenience relating to their infant-feeding choice. Convenience is rarely mentioned in relation to the breast pump. It demands all of the labour associated with both artificial feeding and breastfeeding—bottles must be sterilized, milk must be stored, and time must be allowed for a woman to extract the milk. There appear to be few, if any, positive testimonies regarding the experience of pumping breastmilk. Yet it is an experience with which many contemporary mothers engage. Thurer argues the following: "On a cultural level, if self-sacrifice is valued above all, one begins to understand how it becomes the collective goal or fantasy. That is, if the dominant culture wants mothers to be self-sacrificing, mothers want to be self-sacrificing. Mothers do not (or perhaps cannot) distinguish their own "want" from that which is imposed on them" (194). The breast pump's shift in position from a medical device to a standard breastfeeding object is reflected in its wide availability. Medela, the popular bottle manufacturers Tommee Tippee, and Phillips AVENT manufacture breast pumps that are stocked widely in Irish pharmacies and supermarkets, among many other brands. In fact, the trajectory of breast pump availability is not unlike that of infant-feeding bottles—the range of brands, shapes, and sizes has expanded exponentially, yet the basic engineering of the electrical breast pump remains relatively unchanged since its inception. Visually, as with the Medela designs, the average breast pump reflects a friendly but scientific approach. The colours used are generally yellow, blue, or white; edges are often rounded. Yet there is a sleekness and softness of shape that both echoes and belies its medical origins. It is trustworthy but homely.

The components, however, can be finicky in the extreme. The average baby bottle may consist of the bottle, a circular base for the teat that screws onto the bottle, the teat itself, and sometimes an inner component. An average breast pump, however, requires the bottle; a bottle lid to allow for storage; a valve; an inner connector; an outer connector; a breast shield; a tube; and the pump itself. Within breastfeeding discourse, all of this leads to a contradiction. The pump is used to extract mother's milk, or "liquid gold," but this method of expression is in direct contrast to "the image of breastfeeding that we regularly 'sell' in our culture—an image of a joyous and natural bonding practice" (Kukla, "Ethics and Ideology"163). The receptacle for the milk is not a human mouth but a complex mechanical construction of breast shield, tube, bottle, valve, and pump. By contrast, the object of the baby bottle is sleek, simple, and easy to use.

However, the supplemental nursing system (SNS), though similarly finicky to breast-pump components and nipple shields, allows us an opposite insight. When a baby is allowed out of its incubator, even for a limited time, a mother can begin the process of directly breastfeeding with the use of an SNS. This object allows for a baby who may not have well developed sucking reflexes to take milk at their mother's breast. A bag, which can be filled with formula, expressed, or donated milk, is worn around the mother's neck and connects to a tube taped against the breast. The opening of this tube is positioned at the nipple and held in place with a nipple shield so that the baby can ingest milk in the breastfeeding position. In doing so, the production of breastmilk is also stimulated. It exemplifies a connection between mother and baby that would otherwise not be possible. One of the contradictions emerging in the consideration of the breast pump and associated products is their simultaneous enablement, embodiment, and disentanglement of the process of breastfeeding.

IN THE WORKPLACE

The experience of breastfeeding is now often negotiated within and around the workplace. Hausman explains how "Breastfeeding represents a radical, alternative form of embodied subjectivity when compared to the idea of autonomous personhood held up as ideal in Western societies" ("The Feminist Politics" 276). This ideal of autonomous personhood is seen most clearly in the workplace; and more and more, the use of a breast pump facilitates the return of a breastfeeding mother to the workplace and, indeed, to a form of autonomous personhood. Barston attests that "We've turned into a nation of dairy queens, with political support for breastfeeding focusing primarily on achieving pumping right for working women rather than on fighting for better family leave policies that would allow parents—both male and female—to spend more time with their infants" (11). The increased use of the breast pump in the U.S. has been dramatic. This can be largely attributed to what Jung refers to as the "moral urgency" (11) surrounding "lactivism," the shortest maternity leave in the developed world Jung further explains, "pumping policies compel mothers to square the circle between the absence of maternity leave and the injunction to breastfeed exclusively for six months by pumping breast milk at work" (135). Both Barston and Jung hypothesize that much international breastfeeding advocacy is actually breastmilk and breast-pumping advocacy. Though longer maternity leave is established in Ireland, with a maternity benefit payable for a period of twenty-six weeks, the Irish law regarding breastfeeding in the workplace focuses on the substance of breastmilk more than the practice of breastfeeding: "The benefits of breastfeeding for both you and your baby are enormous. Breast milk provides all the nutrients your baby needs for growth and development, it contains anti-bodies which can help your baby's immune system and it assists the emotional well-being of both mother and baby" (*Citizens Information*). It also allows the employer to dictate the manner in which an infant receives breastmilk and whether or not the mother and infant actually physically connect. Policy states this how a mother 'chooses' to breastfeed her child in the workplace is "at the choice of her employer" and "the woman may therefore opt" for the choice her employer has made available. The lack of choice is further manifested in the fact that these options are available to women who have a baby aged six months or younger, when it is likely they would still be on statutory maternity leave. This means that if the woman wishes to continue breastfeeding her baby after returning to work in Ireland, she may have no legal choice but to physically interact with a breast pump. Her breastfeeding choice may, by necessity, be embodied by this technological object. The distinction between breastfeeding and the feeding of breastmilk is compounded.

In their exploration of "the extended self" in the workplace and the increasing crossover between work and home, public and private, Kelly Tian and Russell Belk explain that "As postmodern professional work makes increasing incursions into the home, it should not be surprising that the expression of self is increasingly evident in the workplace" (308). There can hardly be a better example for the incursion of home and family into the contemporary workplace than the use of the breast pump. Citing the work of Sidney M. Jourard and Susan L. Schieberg, Tian and Belk explain that the expression of self, made evident by "The process of self-disclosure through display of personal possessions," was also seen to reveal tender emotions and vulnerability (305). This understanding of self-disclosure through the incursion of personal possessions in the workplace highlights the vulnerability of a woman expressing milk, compounded by the literal disrobing of her professional self in order to fulfill a maternal function.

CONCLUSION

The subject of breastfeeding is a vast one but by locating the objects and their agency, several themes emerge—the disruption of the symbiotic nature of breastfeeding, the extended role of the mother, maternal guilt and the collision of technology and nature. We are afforded specific insights reflecting broader cultural developments, both internationally and in Ireland. The infant-feeding bottle becomes modern and scientific. The material culture of advocacy illustrates the desire to control and influence mother's feeding choices. The breast pump becomes an analogy for the complex contemporary cultural systems encountered through individual mother's experience. These objects, too, are inextricably linked to feminist discourse through their connection to the maternal role, reproductive rights, and the position of women in the workforce.

Jung attests that "The language of 'choice,' which figured so prominently in the struggle of second-wave feminists and still animates debates about abortion and other reproductive rights, is conspicuously absent then we discuss infant feeding" (55). On the surface, access to breast pumps and to a widened range of products reflects growing choices for contemporary mothers. However, as we have seen, the consumption of the breast pump is often indicative of a lack of choice in relation to the health of a baby, the necessity to return to work, or indeed physical problems in relation to breastfeeding. The breast pump is symbolic of the multifaceted levels of responsibility the modern mother undertakes in relation to family, home, and work. As Hausman explains,

> The discourses promoting breast pumping as the optimal practice for working mothers of infants is not merely a repetition of the moral injunctions for maternal nursing in the eighteenth century, but a new formulation of maternal responsibility that suggests that producing breast milk is only one function among many that she is obligated to continue as a modern woman. (*Mother's Milk* 230)

The perceived notion of choice has to be segregated from decision making. Infant-feeding objects, from baby bottles through to breast pumps, offer choice and limitation. Each is specific in function and can only aid infant feeding. It can only ever embody one aspect of the infant-feeding process.

Emily Martin claims that "Our focus on technology, its ever-changing needs and demands, diverts our attention from the social relationships of power and domination that are involved whenever humans use machines to produce goods in our society" (57). These social relationships are subverted by the use of the breast pump. It is the mother who is at once involved in the social relationships of power and domination and is the producer of goods. Likewise, the consideration of breastmilk as a commodity adds to its monetary value and questions its physical and biological value. Breastfeeding and breastmilk, once inextricably combined, are now separate and subject to individual examination. The breast pump embodies not only a new experience of motherhood but a shift in the process of breastfeeding. It provides both access and barrier; it is intimate, private, gendered, and highly complex in its cultural and feminist implications. As Dayan Sudjic attests, "Objects do not exist in a vacuum: they are part of a complex choreography of interactions" (54). The complex choreography of interactions negotiated by the breast pump and the experience of the breast pumping mother both encapsulate and fragment previous infant-feeding discourse.

WORKS CITED

Apple, Rima B. *Mothers & Medicine: A Social History of Infant Feeding 1890-1950*. The University of Wisconsin Press, 1987.

Auslander, Leora; Bentley, Amy; Halevi, Leor; Sebum, H. Otto and Witmore, Christopher. "AHR Conversation: Historians and the Study of Material Culture." *American Historical Review*, vol. 114, no. 5, 2009, pp. 1355-1404.

Bakalar, Nicholas. "Breast Milk Donated or Sold Online Is Often Tainted, Study." *The New York Times*, 2013, www.nytimes.com/2013/10/21/health/breast-milk-donated-or-sold-online-is-often-tainted-study-says.html. Accessed 21 Feb. 2018.

Barston, Suzanne. *Bottled Up: How the Way We Feed Babies Has Come to Define Motherhood, and Why It Shouldn't*. University of California Press, 2012.

Baumslag, Naomi, and Dia L. Michels. *Milk, Money, and Madness: The Culture and Politics of Breastfeeding*. Bergin & Garvey, 1995.

"Benger's Food Advertisement." *Cork Examiner*, Cork, Ireland, 6 Dec.1929, p.9.

"Book of Illustrations to S. Maw [and] Son's Quarterly Price-current: Maw (S.) [and] Son : Free Download & Streaming: Internet Archive." *Internet Archive*. archive.org/details/bookofillustrati00mawsuoft. Accessed 21 Feb. 2018.

Blum, Linda M. *At the Breast: Ideologies of Breastfeeding and Motherhood in the Contemporary United States*, Beacon, 1999.

Boswell-Penc, Maia, and Kate Boyer. "Expressing Anxiety? Breast Pump Usage in American Wage Workplaces." *Gender, Place & Culture,* vol. 14, no. 5, 2007, pp.551-67.

"Breastfeeding and Maternity Leave." *Citizens Information*, www.citizensinformation.ie. Accessed 21 Feb. 2018.

British Medical Association, Joint copyright *Wellcome Trust*, 2008, 1935. film.wellcome.ac.uk:15151/0055-0000-4137-0000-0-0000-0000-0-HI.mp4. Accessed 21 Feb. 2018.

Carter, Pam. *Feminism, Breasts and Breast-Feeding*. Palgrave Macmillan, 1995.

Cassidy, Tanya. "Historical Ethnography and the Meanings of Human Milk in Ireland." *Ethnographies of Breastfeeding: Cultural Contexts and Confrontations,* edited by Cassidy, Tanya, and Abdullahi Osman El- Tom. Bloomsbury Academic, 2015, pp. 45-57.

Cassidy, Tanya, and Abdullahi Osman El- Tom. *Ethnographies of Breastfeeding: Cultural Contexts and Confrontations*. Bloomsbury Academic, 2015.

Cieraad, Irene. "'Out of My Kitchen!' Architecture, Gender and Domestic Efficiency." *The Journal of Architecture*, vol. 7, no. 3, 2002, pp. 263-79.

Clear, Caitriona. "The Decline of Breast-feeding in Twentieth Century Ireland." *Irish Women's History*, edited by Alan Hayes and Diane Urquart, Irish Academic Press, 2004, pp. 187-98.

Cooper-Rompato, Christine. "The Talking Breast Pump." *Western Folklore*, vol. 12, no. 2, 2013, pp. 181-209.

Dillon-Hurney, Pauline. "Infant-feeding patterns". *Motherhood in Ireland: Creation and Context*, edited by Patricia Kennedy. Mercier Press, 2004.

Earner-Byrne, Lindsay. *Mother and Child: Maternity and Child Welfare in Dublin, 1922-1960*. Manchester University Press, 2007.

Frederick, Christina. *Household Engineering: Scientific Management in the Home, A Correspondence Course on the Application of the Principles of Efficiency Engineering and Scientific Management to the Every Day Tasks of Housekeeping*. American School of Home Economics, 1923.

Garber, Megan. "A Brief History of Breast Pumps: Debates about

Online Milk Exchanges Wouldn't Be possible without a Simple—yet Revolutionary—Machine." *The Atlantic*, 21 Oct 2013, www.theatlantic.com/technology/archive/2013/10/a-brief-history-of-breast-pumps/280728/. Accessed 21 Feb. 2018.

"Gastro-Enteritis." *The Irish Times*, 22 Feb.1951, p. 3.

"Glaxo Advertisement." *The Irish Times*, 17 Sept. 1920, p.7.

Hausman, Bernice, L. *Mother's Milk: Breastfeeding Controversies in American Culture*, Routledge, 2003.

Hausman, Bernice, L. "The Feminist Politics of Breastfeeding." *Australian Feminist Studies*, vol.19, no.45, 2004, pp.273-85.

"Innovation Center for Breast Milk Analysis. Explore Your Breast Milk." *MyMilk*, www.mymilklab.com/. Accessed 21 Feb. 2018.

Jelliffe, Derrick B., and E.F. Patrice Jelliffe. *Human Milk in the Modern World: Psychosocial, Nutritional and Economic Significance*. Oxford University Press, 1978.

Jung, Courtney. *Lactivism: How Feminists and Fundamentalists, Hippies and Yuppies, and Physicians and Politicians Made Breastfeeding Big Business and Bad Policy*. Basic Books, 2015.

Keim, S.A., et al. "Microbial Contamination of Human Milk Purchased Via the Internet." *Pediatrics,* vol. 132, no. 5, 2013, pp. 1227-235.

Kukla, Rebecca. "Ethics and Ideology in Breastfeeding Advocacy Campaigns." *Hypatia*, vol. 21, no. 1, 2006, pp. 157-80.

Kukla, Rebecca. *Mass Hysteria: Medicine, Culture, and Mothers' Bodies*. Rowman & Littlefield Publishers, Inc, 2005.

Layte, Richards, and Cathal McCrory. *Growing Up in Ireland: National Longitudinal Study of Children*. 2014.

Lepore, Jill. *The Mansion of Happiness: A History of Life and Death*. Alfred A. Knopf, 2012.

Martin, Emily. *The Woman in the Body: A Cultural Analysis of Reproduction*. Beacon Press, 1987.

Martucci, Jessica. *Back to the Breast: Natural Motherhood and Breastfeeding in America*. The University of Chicago Press. 2015.

Morris, Madeleine, *Guilt-Free Bottle Feeding: Why Your Formula-Fed Baby Can Be Happy, Healthy and Smart*. White Ladder Press, 2014.

"Mother and Baby." *Model Housekeeping,* vol. XXII, Sept. 1950, p. 732.

O'Toole, Emma. "'Toy guns, drums and swords': shopping for children's goods in eighteenth-century Dublin." *Material Culture and Consumption in Ireland.* Economic and Social History Society of Ireland Conference. Maynooth University, 25 and 26 November 2016.

Palmer, Gabrielle. *The Politics of Breastfeeding: When Breasts Are Bad for Business.* Pinter & Martin, 2009.

Schiebinger, Londa. "Why Mammals Are Called Mammals: Gender Politics in Eighteenth-Century Natural History." *The American Historical Review*, vol. 98, no. 2, 1993, pp. 382-411.

Shilling, Chris. *The Body in Culture, Technology and Society.* SAGE Publications, 2004.

"Sister Laura's Food Advertisement." *Irish Independent*, 6 Apr. 1937, p. 5.

Sudjic, Dayan. *The Language of Things.* Penguin Books, 2009.

Thurer, Shari. *The Myths of Motherhood: How Culture Reinvents the Good Mother.* Houghton Mifflin, 1994.

Tian, Kelly, and Russell W. Belk. "Extended Self and Possessions in the Workplace." *Journal of Consumer Research*, vol. 32, no. 2, 2005, pp. 297-310.

Turbin, Carole. "Refashioning the Concept of Public/Private: Lessons from Dress Studies." *Journal of Women's History*, vol. 15, no. 1, 2003, pp. 43-51.

Williams, K.T., et al. "Discursive Constructions of Infant Feeding: The Dilemma of Mothers' 'guilt.'" *Feminism & Psychology*, vol. 23, no. 3, 2012, pp.339-58.

Wickes, Ian G. "A History of Infant Feeding: Part IV—Nineteenth Century Continued", *Archives of Disease in Childhood*, vol. 28, no. 141, 1953, pp. 416-22.

Wickes, Ian G. "A History of Infant Feeding: Part V.—Nineteenth Century Concluded and Twentieth Century." *Archives of Disease in Childhood*, vol. 28, no.142, 1953, pp. 495-502.

Wiessinger, Diane. *The Womanly Art of Breastfeeding.* 7th ed. La Leche League International, 2004.

Wiley, Andrea S. *Re-imagining Milk: Cultural and Biological Perspectives.* Routledge Series for Creative, Teaching and Learning in Anthropology, Routledge, 2011.

Yalom, Marylin. *A History of the Breast.* Ballantine Books, 1997.

II.
Representations of Lactation and Breastfeeding in Contemporary Culture

5. "That's Not a Beer Bong; It's a Breast Pump!"

Representations of Breastfeeding in Prime-Time Fictional Television

KATHERINE A. FOSS

In the 2011 *Game of Thrones* episode "The Wolf and the Lion," noblewoman Lysa Arryn breastfeeds a school-age child. Online debates ensued, questioning whether the scene was appropriate given the age of the boy. The scarcity of extended breastfeeding representations, paired with this public reaction, illustrates media's narrow and problematic construction of breastfeeding—an issue that could significantly impede its normalization. Studies have established the problematic presentations of breastfeeding in advertisements, magazine articles, childrearing books, reality television, and media as a whole (Brown and Peuchaud; Foss and Southwell; Foss, "Perpetuating"; Foss, "Breastfeeding"; Frerichs et al.; Potter et al.; Young). Building on this work, I analyze depictions of breastfeeding in historical and contemporary fictional television programs, and demonstrate their implications for shaping cultural perceptions of breastfeeding. Through a qualitative textual analysis of fictional representations, I examine the so-called typical breastfeeding woman and experience, and overarching messages, and situate breastfeeding depictions within the American social and political context. A purposive sample was compiled through popular search engines, websites, input from social media participants, and a parenting community board; the sample totalled fifty-four representations from 1974 through 2012.

BREASTFEEDING ON FICTIONAL TELEVISION

Representations vary in genre and target audience, as crime and medical dramas, sitcoms, and animated programs have included breastfeeding references. Consistent with real-life rates, in recent years, breastfeeding representations in fictional shows have become more common—forty-eight of the identified portrayals appeared after 1998 ("Breastfeeding Report Card," p. 2). Multiple breastfeeding depictions were identified in the popular shows *ER*, *Friends*, *Two and a Half Men*, *The Big Bang Theory*, and *The Office*. Most programs presented breastfeeding as generally positive but limited.

THE BREASTFEEDING WOMAN AND EXPERIENCE

The breastfeeding woman in fictional television is professional, affluent, well educated, able-bodied, heterosexual, and usually Caucasian, as exemplified by the doctors in *ER*, Pam of *The Office*, Miranda in *Sex and the City*, and others. Similar to real-life statistics, in which 75 percent of this group attempt to breastfeed, it is assumed that female characters who fit this type will breastfeed ("Breastfeeding Report Card"). In a 2002 *Friends* episode, pregnant Rachel receives a breast pump as a baby shower gift. Upon receipt of the gift, she says, "Is that a beer bong for a baby?" Despite her lack of knowledge, Rachel goes on to successfully nurse Emma ("The One with the Baby Shower"). In both *The New Girl* and *The Office,* men make positive comments about pumping to their pregnant coworkers. Even childless women were perceived as future breastfeeders as demonstrated in another episode of *The Office*. In "Hot Girl" (2005), Dwight Schrute comments on the characteristics he finds attractive in a purse saleswoman: "The purse girl hits everything on my checklist: creamy skin, straight teeth, curly hair, amazing breasts—not for me, for my children. The Schrutes produce very thirsty babies."

Characters who breastfeed are Caucasian, with few exceptions—Asian American Dr. Jing-Mei Chen in *ER* (who then gives her baby up for adoption), African American Carla Espinosa on *Scrubs*, and a Hispanic mother in *ER*. Unfortunately, no additional women of colour are shown breastfeeding. Breastfeeding is also associated with being older and more established. For example, the detectives in *Bones* are surprised to discover that the victim, a poor, single mother, breastfed her baby. And in a 2009 *Secret Life of the American Teenager* episode, Amy, a fifteen-year-old with a newborn, only breastfeeds when her own mother forces her to try (which is not shown). None of these depictions include visuals of the mother breastfeeding, nor are they positive representations.

For the typical breastfeeding woman, the "learning to breastfeed" scene immediately follows the much-awaited delivery: The gown-clad mother closely holds her infant, as she expresses her breastfeeding uncertainty. Aided by a support person, she eventually succeeds, with peaceful music and soft lighting used to highlight her triumph. In the *ER* episode "Sailing Away" (2001), Dr. Elizabeth Corday attempts to latch on her baby as she says to her husband, "Mark, I don't think I can do this." Mark (also a physician) gently kisses his wife and reassures her, "It just takes patience." She then gets the latch and all is well. In the *ER* episode "Great Expectations" (1999), Nurse Abby Lockhart helps Nurse Carol Hathaway on how to nurse by telling her, "Wait until she opens her mouth really wide." Carol adjusts her breast over her gown, and Abby says, "That's it. Yeah, make sure her mouth covers the whole areola. Yes, see her little jaw moving." Likewise, a nurse in *Friends* helps a tearful Rachel latch baby Emma to the breast ("The One Where No One Proposes," 2002). In *Scrubs*, Turk takes his wife to see a team of lactation specialists, who help her succeed ("My Friend with Money," 2007). A 2010 episode of *The Office* adds a twist on the "typical" breastfeeding expert. In "The Delivery," a male lactation consultant helps new-mother Pam overcome her latch issues, as her husband, Jim, watches uncomfortably. The appearance of lactation experts primarily in the hospital suggests that problems with nursing end after the initial breastfeeding session, despite the ongoing struggles that most women face.

The limited diversity in breastfeeding women and experience is highly problematic, as it suggests that only one type of women breastfeeds, ignoring women of colour, adolescent mothers, and other women. More mothers of colour need to be shown; the absence of other representations could discourage other women from nursing by failing to present them as normal women who nurse. Many opportunities to promote breastfeeding for different women and with different experiences are missed, particularly with the "new baby" storylines of most comedies and dramas. It would be easy to expand representations to include breastfeeding twins, or premature babies, or nursing toddlers, and to insert positive storylines for diverse characters. In *ER*, several women of colour birth babies, but they are not shown breastfeeding. African American Dr. Peter Benton's ex-girlfriend gives birth to a premature baby in "Make a Wish" (1997). This storyline would have been an excellent opportunity to showcase an African American woman breastfeeding as well as the challenges of pumping and feeding a premature baby. More representations could help normalize and redefine the typical woman and experience.

THE BENEFITS OF BREASTFEEDING

Most representations offer little information as to why mothers should breastfeed. From these depictions, the correlation between intelligence and breastfeeding is conveyed through several exceptional characters. Viewers learn that top forensic anthropologist Dr. Temperance Brennan in *Bones* as well as the genius characters in *The Big Bang Theory* were all supposedly breastfed. Additional benefits conveyed in television include weight loss for the breastfeeding mother (*ER* and *Desperate Housewives*) and increased breast size (*The Secret Life of the American Teenager*).

Other health benefits of breastfeeding are only conveyed when for infants outside of the norm—a baby about to be adopted, a baby needing surgery for extreme birth defects, and nursing a much older child. In the *ER* episode "The Greatest of Gifts" (2000), Dr. Chen breastfeeds her son before giving him to the adoptive parents so that he can get the nourishment of colostrum, "which boosts their immune system." Also, in "Shari Noble" (2006) of *Nip/Tuck*, Sean McNamara encourages Julia to breastfeed: "We need to think about his surgeries, honey. His first one's in three months and breastfeeding helps him gain the weight he needs so that his immune system will be strong. Skin on skin contacts also make him secure so that he can handle the stress." And in the *Desperate Housewives* episode "Could I Leave You?" (2006), Veronica lists the benefits of extending breastfeeding her five-year-old, including immunity and IQ-boosting properties of breastmilk.

Long-term health benefits, such as reduced risks of breast cancer and osteoporosis, are absent from the representations studied. More information could help people understand the societal impact of increasing breastfeeding initiation and duration rates, including significant healthcare savings for the American public. Furthermore, programs could outline the lesser known health benefits for nursing mothers, such as lower risks of breast cancer and hip fractures (Cumming and Klineberg; Enger et al.). Knowledge about breastfeeding has been strongly correlated with a mother's confidence (Chezem et al.). If media representations conveyed positive impacts of breastfeeding on society, more people may be supportive of breastfeeding—for example, the productivity of nursing mothers in the workplace (because they take fewer sick days) or the billions of dollars saved in healthcare costs if the majority of the population breastfed (Bartick and Reinhold).

BREASTFEEDING OBSTACLES

On television, obstacles are limited to initial problems with nursing and are focused on individual problems. In the hospital and shortly after, characters face latch issues with their babies, which are easily resolved with a little coaching from a nurse, partner, or lactation consultant. Characters also complain of sore nipples in the early days of breastfeeding. In "The One Where Rachel Goes Back to Work" (2003) of *Friends*, Rachel visits her office and discovers her replacement, Gavin at her desk. He says, "Well, while you were on your baby vacation; I was doing your job." Rachel responds, "A vacation? My idea of a vacation does not involve something sucking on my nipples until they are raw." Gavin retorts, "Clearly you've never been to Sandals Paradise Island." In *Friends*, Carol (Ross's ex-wife) also states that breastfeeding hurt at first ("The One with the Breast Milk," 1995). And in *ER*, the character Chuck (using a supplemental nursing system) tells Dr. Carter about the pain of nursing ("Try Carter," 2004). No remedies, other than time and practice, are recommended to help with sore nipples.

Characters also become emotional and upset because of nursing. In *ER*, baby Ella wakes up Corday and Mark, who then complains that he has a shift in three hours ("The Longer You Stay," 2001).

Corday shouts, "What do you think I'll be doing in three hours? I'm the feeding trough!" Mark declares that he would nurse if he could. Elizabeth yells, "You take it! Take it all! The sore nipples, the rashes, the hemorrhoids, the leaking in your trauma gown, the public humiliation, the sleep deprivation, the incontinence, for goodness sake. Just take it. It's all yours!" Likewise, Carla, in *Scrubs*, weeps uncontrollably throughout the episode, even after her baby finally latches ("My Friend with Money," 2007).

In the *Nip/Tuck* episode "Shari Noble" (2006), the character Julia becomes emotional when she struggles to get her milk to let-down. A lactation consultant attempts to help her, which causes Julia more frustration. Several more times, Julia attempts to nurse, but she fails. In desperation, Julia contemplates using antidepressants so that she has to switch to formula. Finally, the help of the male nanny and some informal counselling, combined with a warm washcloth on her breasts, produce a milk let-down and her son is able to nurse (and does not switch to formula). This storyline highlights the connection between emotion and lactation, along with offering some practical advice on helping let-downs, and suggests that Julia's one milk let-down resolves all of her breastfeeding issues.

No storylines address breastfeeding a premature, jaundiced, or tongue-tied newborn, or address mastitis, thrush, clogged milk ducts, inverted nipples, or other issues that can impede success. And since these issues are not part of the storylines, remedies for these obstacles are also missing. Research has shown that women's concerns about lactation issues and the baby's nourishment are given as the most frequent reasons for weaning (Li et al.). These programs could help allay these fears—thus extending breastfeeding duration by counteracting myths about insufficient milk and offering solutions to typical problems. Furthermore, such depictions could reassure viewers these issues are normal and, therefore, not a reason to wean. Solutions could include dried breast milk for sore nipples, medication for mastitis and thrush, and pumping to boost supply.

Although breastfeeding a newborn in the hospital is conveyed as natural and fairly easy, it becomes restrictive and unprofessional once the women return to work—as illustrated in *Friends* with Rachel and her competitive replacement, Corday's leaking breasts during surgery in *ER* ("The Longer You Stay," 2001), and the awkward stares of coworkers for a woman pumping in *The Office* ("The Merger," 2006). Overall, although the individual women seem embarrassed by the need to pump, having a place to pump or concerns about job security are not issues, likely again because these women are in professional positions, not part of an assembly line.

Storylines about hospital practices hindering breastfeeding, breastfeeding policies and legislation, and lack of public support for breastfeeding could highlight problem areas and help to shape cultural attitudes (Koerber, "Rhetorical Agency;" Koerber, "Critical Perspectives; Wolf). More specifically, these messages help shift responsibility for breastfeeding success to the institutional level, highlighting the need for cultural change (and not simply an increase of individual women breastfeeding). Programs could also address strategies to help working women breastfeed—including onsite childcare, flexible working arrangements, sufficient pumping breaks, and extended maternity leave (Fein et al.; Wolf). Such representations could alert potential employers to the need of working mothers and garner public support for policies to protect them. Improving working conditions for breastfeeding is especially important given that working fulltime has been shown to decrease breastfeeding duration by an average of 8.6 weeks (Fein and Roe).

BREASTFEEDING: A PRIVATE ACTIVITY OR OBSCENE?

Most representations of breastfeeding consist of a mother calmly nursing her newborn, at home or in the hospital, covered by a blanket or clothing. No visual depictions of breastfeeding (even covered up) appeared until a 1994 episode of *ER*. The two representations before this episode are verbal references. In "The Lord is my Shepherd" (1974) of *Little House on the Prairie*, Dr. Baker advises Caroline to stop breastfeeding, which is not shown. And in "Hearts" (1983) of *St. Elsewhere*, a nurse asks a new mother if she will breastfeed. She does not and, ultimately, abandons the baby at the hospital.

Even with a cover, breastfeeding makes other characters visibly uncomfortable. In the *Friends* episode "The One with the Breast Milk" (1995), Carol nurses Ben, and Joey and Chandler become uncomfortable and walk over to the kitchen. Ross follows them, saying, "Look, will you guys grow up? This is the most natural, beautiful thing in the world." Joey replies, "Yeah, we know. But there's a baby sucking on it." Ross then explains, "This is my son having lunch, okay? It's gonna happen a lot so get used to it. Now if you have a problem with it, if you're uncomfortable, just ask questions. Carol's fine with it. C'mon." They return to the living room and began asking Carol bizarre questions, such as, "If he blows into one, does the other one get bigger?" At this point, Ross pushes them back into the kitchen. In *The O.C.*, characters Seth and Ryan also quickly leave when they learn Kristen is about to nurse ("The End's Not Near, It's Here," 2007). In *Gilmore Girls*, Lorelai complains about her friend Sookie breastfeeding at the dinner table, and argues that she and Luke should make Sookie and her husband feel equally uncomfortable ("The Prodigal Daughter Returns," 2005). And Carrie, of *Sex and the City*, becomes noticeably uneasy when Miranda unlatches her nursing bra in preparation to nurse ("Anchors Away," 2002).

Few representations actually show breastfeeding uncovered. In the *Sex and the City* episode "Anchors Away" (2002), Miranda's baby is visibly latched on, as he suckles her breast in her apartment. It should be noted that the naked breasts of two other characters, Samantha and Charlotte, also appear in this episode. *Two and a Half Men* also contains a less covered-up image of breastfeeding, when Alan's date nurses during dinner ("Castrating Sheep in Montana," 2007). And the animated *Family Guy* shows several breastfeeding sessions between Stewie and Lois in "I Take Thee Quagmire" (2006).

When women nurse in public onscreen, their actions are heavily criticized and conveyed as inappropriate. In the *Gilmore Girls* episode "Eight O'clock at the Oasis" (2002), Luke complains to Lorelai and Rory about a woman nursing in his diner: "Why? Why do they do this? It's a public place; people are eating here." Luke becomes uncomfortable and continues, "When did that become acceptable? In the old days, a woman would never consider doing that in public. They'd go find a barn or a cave or something. I mean, it's indecent. This is a diner, not a peepshow." At this point, Luke asks Lorelai to get rid of them. She refuses, although she does not defend the nursing mother. In *Two and a Half Men*, Alan dates a single mom. As they are having dinner, she begins to breastfeed her baby ("Castrating Sheep in Montana," 2007). He is surprised and then has trouble eating.

Many of the breastfeeding representations sexualize breasts, especially in programs geared toward men. The *Charmed* episode "The Bare Witch Project" (2004) begins with two of the main characters, Piper and Phoebe Halliwell, sitting at a café, while Piper nurses her son under an oversized blanket. Other customers snicker, which prompts the manager to ask Piper to leave. Throughout the episode, public breastfeeding becomes a symbol for female progress, as the sisters help a conjured Lady Godiva return to her historic time. At the end of the episode, inspired by Lady Godiva, Phoebe rides naked on horseback to the café, where she publicly declares the following: "[the manager believes women] should be ashamed of breastfeeding, the most natural thing in the world. Well, shame on him. I'm not ashamed and neither should you be. It's a shame women have to take off their clothes to be heard. We shouldn't have to be exploited like this. Right?" At this point, Phoebe's speech convinces the manager to take down the "right to refuse service" sign. Despite the declaration about nursing in public, after the initial scene, no images of breastfeeding appear. At the same time, Phoebe's actions reinforces the sexualization of breasts, as she rides naked on a horse to protest the ban, equating her nudity with breastfeeding.

In "Business Sucks" and "Business Still Sucks" (1994) of *Married with Children*, the character Al demands that a mother breastfeeding in his women's shoe store leave immediately. She later returns, accompanied by group of militant breastfeeding women. The leader, Al's neighbour, Marcie, challenges Al's actions: "How dare you deny her her God-given right to nurse her baby whenever Mother Nature calls! Breastfeeding is a natural, biological function." Al responds, "So's peeing, but you don't see me doing that in public." The studio audience cheers as Marcie says, "Well, the last time I looked, the side of my garage was in public." Although Al eventually allows breastfeeding in his store to please his boss, his initial refusal— backed by the studio audience's groans, laughs, and applause—frames public breastfeeding as absurd and obscene, even in a show that aims to be obscene. Furthermore, Al's disgust is contrasted to his attraction to women's breasts, as he comments to his (male) associate: "What is happening to this country when a woman of the opposite sex can just waddle into your place of business, your holy sanctuary, and bare her breasts. It's disgusting." The other employee replies, "It's repulsive." They reach down and pick up magazines with the titles *Big 'Uns* and *Black Big 'Uns*.

Other programs also blatantly sexualize breasts in connection to breastfeeding. In the same episode of *Sex and the City* that Miranda breastfeeds, Carrie accidentally sees Samantha and Charlotte flash their breasts to men at a party. Joey and Chandler (of *Friends*) mention feeling uncomfortable with breastfeeding because they view breasts as sexual. In *Two and a Half Men*, Charlie struggles with intimacy with Lisa after he sees her breastfeed ("Yes, Monsignor," 2004). Charlie says to Lisa, "I'm looking at the sexiest woman in the world and all I see is a thermos," implying that breastfeeding makes her less attractive to him. In another episode of this program, "It Never Rains in Hooterville," Charlie asks his brother to rewind a tape of a home movie so that he can see Alan's ex-wife breastfeeding. And in a *Family Guy* episode about weaning, the hypersexualized Quagmire becomes aroused by Lois's engorged breasts ("I Take Thee Quagmire, 2006). In another *Family Guy* episode, Peter returns from a Women's Sensitivity retreat ultra-feminine, which prompts him to breastfeed Stewie ("I am Peter, Here Me Roar," 2000). In the next scene, Lois tries to arouse Peter by shaking her breasts. *Beavis and Butthead* also sexualize breastfeeding in the episode "Holy Cornholio" (2011). While at the hospital, Butthead tries to peer into a delivery room, asking if the new mom is going to take out her "boob." He chuckles as she screams. The juxtaposition of breastfeeding with attraction reinforces the myth that breasts are sexual objects and, therefore, do not belong in the public eye.

Showing breastfeeding in episodes that also sexualize breasts may do little to change perceptions that breastfeeding differs from public nudity or indecent exposure. Although it may be difficult for actors to mimic breastfeeding, doing so would be a significant step toward normalizing breastfeeding, especially since mainstream media as a whole rarely include images of real breastfeeding. Bernice Hausman argues that media are more likely to show women in developing countries breastfeeding than so-called typical American women (i.e., Caucasian and middle-upper class). In other words, the women that we do see breastfeeding in images and videos are already marginalized and "othered"; these images present breastfeeding as something not done by regular women. The increase of diverse representations in television could then help broaden our definition of who breastfeeds and what the experience looks like.

Nursing in public is presented as negative and embarrassing, which suggests that the nursing mother may be ridiculed and asked to leave—not very encouraging for a new mother who would like to venture out in public. A mother would have a difficult time breastfeeding past a few months if she fears breastfeeding outside of her home. Although the *Charmed* and *Married with Children* episodes involve a protest of breastfeeding criticism, the storylines offer no practical advice on how to address concerns about nursing in public, such as support for lactation rooms or other facilities for nursing mothers (Li et al.). Positive depictions of public breastfeeding could help women become more comfortable with the notion, similar to the safe spaces that La Leche League provides for nursing mothers (Koerber, "Rhetorical Agency"). Repeated positive depictions could normalize public breastfeeding so that it no longer seems threatening to new mothers or offends onlookers.

BREASTFEEDING AS DEVIANT, SOCIALLY UNACCEPTABLE, OR HARMFUL

Fictional television clearly distinguishes between normal and abnormal breastfeeding activities. When mothers breastfeed their new babies covered up in their homes, it is presented as beautiful and natural, which suggests other breastfeeding activities are unacceptable or deviant. No programs visually portray women nursing multiples, even though *ER*'s Carol Hathaway gives birth to twins and breastfeeds ("Great Expectations," 1999). In the *Friends* episode "The One Where Rachel Has a Baby" (2002), Joey enters Rachel's hospital room and announces, "Hey, I just saw a woman breastfeeding both of her twins at the same time. It is like a freak show up here." In *7th Heaven*, Annie asks her daughter, Ruthie, for help in getting ready to breastfeed her twins ("It Happened One Night," 1999). Ruthie expresses disgust and quickly leaves the room. The babies' feeding is not shown.

A supplemental nursing system only appears in the *ER* episode "Try Carter" (2004), in which Dr. John Carter is surprised to see a man, Chuck, with a Lact-Aid system hooked up to his nipple and baby Cosmo in the cradle position. Carter exclaims, "Chuck, what are you doing?" Chuck responds, "Oh, it's a supplemental nursing device. What? You've never seen a father breastfeed his kid before?" Chuck adds, "These things are amazing. You know, it allows the father to bond with the child the same way that the mother does if you can get past the sore nipples. You want to give it a shot?" Carter looks puzzled and says "No" as he leaves the room. The absurdity of Chuck wearing the system, reinforced by Carter's reaction, emphasizes that this so-called abnormal situation serves as comic relief for the medical drama. The use of milk banks and supplemental nursing systems to relactate or nourish adopted children are not seriously explored. These tools could be viable options for women who adopt or have difficulty breastfeeding, especially if their babies are premature or suffer from chronic illness (Newman).

Older babies or toddlers are not shown breastfeeding. Instead, extended breastfeeding involves much older children and is presented as strange, inappropriate, and distracting. In *Desperate Housewives* "Could I Leave You?" (2006), employees discover a coworker, Veronica, breastfeeding her five-year-old in a conference room. Her coworkers agree that it is too "bizarre" and "distracting" for her to continue nursing, even if she breastfeeds in private. They insist that the only other female employee, Lynette, request Veronica to stop. In the end, Lynette tricks the child into weaning by offering him chocolate milk (so he no longer wants the breast). An episode of *30 Rock* also paints extended breastfeeding as deviant. In one episode, a strange and awkward man, named Donny, announces that he cannot be seduced by another woman's breasts because he was "breastfed until he was eleven" ("Rosemary's Baby," 2007). The television representations portray extended breastfeeding as deviant—an alarming finding considering that the health benefits for mother and child dramatically increase with duration (Cumming and Klineberg; Enger et al.; Gillman et al.; Von Kries et al.). Instead of highlighting the abnormality of nursing a school-age child, programing could include more portrayals of breastfeeding older babies and toddlers, which would reinforce recommendations of the World Health Organization (WHO) and the American Academy of Pediatrics.

Breastfeeding is also conveyed as dangerous or even deadly. In the 1974 *Little House on the Prairie* episodes "The Lord Is My Shepherd," parts one and two, Caroline Ingalls' newborn son, Charles Jr., becomes sickly and lethargic. The town physician, Dr. Baker, attributes the baby's condition to the quality of her breast milk; he states that it may not have the right "chemistry" for the baby's body and recommends cow's milk. Unfortunately, Charles Jr. continues to become sicker until he passes away. This storyline suggests that had Caroline not given the baby breast milk, thus initiating his weakened state, he might have survived.[1]

The *ER* episode "Under Control" (2000) conveys the dire consequences of drugs in breastmilk. In this storyline, a baby is rushed to the Emergency Room in cardiac arrest. The medical team desperately tries to revive the baby but cannot save her. Dr. Greene and Nurse Hathaway question the mother about the drugs.

> Mother: I work two jobs. Sometimes I get so tired; I take something to stay awake, but I never bring drugs home.
> Hathaway: Are you nursing the baby? [The woman nods.]
> Greene: The drugs are in the breast milk.
> Mother (cries): I love my baby. I would never hurt her. I didn't know. Really, I didn't know.

In this storyline, breastfeeding leads to the infant's unintentional death.

Finally, in a disturbing *Criminal Minds* storyline, a woman breastfeeds her victims because she believes each five-year-old boy is her infant son ("The Instincts," 2008). In this episode's context, breastfeeding is an act of torture, as the victims slowly starve to death on breastmilk. In the episode's climax, the SWAT team discovers the serial killer attempting to nurse her latest kidnap victim—a scene that emphasizes the woman's extreme psychosis. At the same time, the image of a woman breastfeeding a large child reinforces extended breastfeeding as deviant.

No positive representations of extended breastfeeding were identified, despite the known benefits of this practice (Gillman et al.; Von Kries et al.). These deviant storylines, which frame breastfeeding as dangerous, perpetuate what Hausman has called the "dead babies" media discourse. As breastfeeding promotion has become more prevalent, media backlash has highlighted extreme consequences of the "breast is best" message, with news stories of babies starving because their mothers refused to provide formula. Media stories, including fictional ones, that present breastfeeding as normal could help counter these sensationalized cases, especially images of women breastfeeding healthy babies.

CONCLUSION

This chapter highlighted the findings from a textual analysis of fictional television programs from 1974 through 2012. Representations consistently convey that for a certain group of women in a private place and for a newborn, breastfeeding is natural, beautiful, and easy. However, outside this narrow definition of "normal," breastfeeding is presented as absurd, unnecessary, socially unacceptable, or deviant. Benefits and obstacles largely focus on individual women, rather than macrolevel issues that impact success (i.e., hospital practices that interfere with breastfeeding). These findings are consistent with previous literature suggesting that contemporary media tend to present breastfeeding positively, but as a difficult endeavour for the individual woman (Foss, "Perpetuating"; Foss, "Breastfeeding"; Frerichs et al.; Potter et al.).

Although this study ended in 2012, television has continued to perpetuate many of these stereotypes of the breastfeeding experience—as a private activity, primarily for infants. One positive change has been the expansion of who breastfeeds. In the last few years, more women of colour have been shown breastfeeding in fictional television, including the Latina character Gloria in season four (2013) of *Modern Family*; Jasmine, who is African American, in season five of *Parenthood*; and Chinese American Angela in season seven of *Bones* (2012). Such depictions are a good start to normalizing breastfeeding for all women. In other words, the expansion and repetition of different women nursing presents breastfeeding as the means of feeding babies.

Since fictional programs can provide in-depth stories about breastfeeding, these fictional programs could be better used to provide detailed information about overcoming obstacles and to highlight many of the underlying macrolevel hindrances. For example, as Linda Blum has articulated, conceptions of motherhood and breastfeeding have contributed to guilt when mothers cannot breastfeed. Likewise, the hypersexualization of breasts has impeded cultural acceptance of breastfeeding (Hausman). This lack of cultural support for breastfeeding is reinforced by institutional barriers at work and in the community, highlighting the need for dramatic policy and legislative changes to create a society conducive to breastfeeding (Wolf). Furthermore, portraying breastfeeding as the cultural norm for all women would help create a breastfeeding-friendly society, with supportive restaurant managers, retail workers, and others workers in the community. Employers may be more willing to grant pumping time to working mothers if they realize that breastfed babies experience less illness, which would result in fewer absences for the mothers. Overall, general support would mean that more women would feel comfortable nursing, regardless of who may be watching. By presenting extended breastfeeding, public breastfeeding, and other so-called deviant behaviours as normal, media representations can help change attitudes. Moreover, they can help women feel more comfortable breastfeeding when and wherever their babies demand, without a fear of public scrutiny or police intervention. It is only when nearly all babies are breastfed in the United States that we can claim we are doing our best to protect our nation's health.

This chapter is based on the article: Foss, Katherine A. "That's Not a Beer Bong, It's a Breast Pump!" Representations of Breastfeeding in Prime-time Fictional Television," originally published in Health Communication *28.4 (2013): 329-340. Reprinted with permission.*

ENDNOTE

[1]In real life, the Ingalls family lost an infant son. However, most of this storyline was fictionalized for the show.

WORKS CITED

Television

"Anchors Away." *Sex and the City*, season 5, episode 1, HBO, 21 July 2002.
"And Unto Us a Child is Born," *The Secret Life of the American Teenager*, season 1, episode 23, ABC Family, 23 March 2009.
"Bad in Bed," *The New Girl*, season 1, episode 8, Fox, 6 Dec. 2011.
"Business Still Sucks," *Married with Children*, season 9, episode 6, Fox, 2 Oct. 1994.
"Business Sucks," *Married with Children*, season 9, episode 5, Fox, 2 Oct. 1994.
"Castrating Sheep in Montana," *Two and a Half Men*, season 4, episode 12, CBS, 8 Jan. 2007.
"Could I Leave You?," *Desperate Housewives*, season 2, episode 17, ABC, 26 Mar. 2006.
"Eight O'clock at the Oasis," *Gilmore Girls*, season 6, episode 9, Warner Brothers, 22 Oct. 2002.
"Great Expectations," *ER*, season 6, episode 8, NBC, 25 Nov. 1999.
"Holy Cornholio," *Beavis and Butthead*, season 1, episode 3, MTV, 10 Nov. 2011.
"Hearts," *St. Elsewhere*, season 1, episode 10, CBS, 11 Jan. 1983.
"I am Peter, Here Me Roar," *Family Guy*, season 2, episode 8, Fox, 28 Mar. 2000.
"I Take Thee Quagmire," *Family Guy*, season 4, episode 21, Fox, 12 Mar. 2006.
"It Happened One Night," *7th Heaven*, season 3, episode 15, WB, 15 Feb. 1999.
"Make a Wish." *ER*, season 3, episode 21, NBC, 8 May 1997.
"My Friend with Money," *Scrubs*, season 6, episode 5, NBC, 11 Jan. 2007.

"Rosemary's Baby," *30 Rock*, season 2, episode 4, NBC, 25 Oct. 2007.

"Sailing Away," *ER*, season 7, episode 19, NBC, 26 Apr. 2001.

"Shari Noble," *Nip/Tuck*, season 4, episode 4, FX, 26 Sept. 2006.

"The Bare Witch Project," *Charmed*, season 7, episode 2, WB, 19 Sept. 2004.

"The Delivery," *The Office*, season 6, episode 18, NBC, 4 Mar. 2010.

"The End's Not Near, It's Here." *The O.C.*, season 4, episode 16, Fox, 22 Feb. 2007.

"The Greatest of Gifts," *ER*, season 7, episode 9, NBC, 14 Dec. 2000.

"The Hot Girl," *The Office*, season 1, episode 6, NBC, 26 Apr. 2005.

"The Instincts," *Criminal Minds*, season 4, episode 6, CBS, 5 Nov. 2008.

"The Longer You Stay," *ER*, season 8, episode 2, NBC, 4 Oct. 2001.

"The Lord is my Shepherd," *Little House on the Prairie*, episode 114, NBC, 18 Dec. 1974.

"The Merger," *The Office*, season 3, episode 8, NBC, 16 Nov. 2006.

"The One Where No One Proposes," *Friends,* season 9, episode 1, NBC, 26 Sept. 2002.

"The One Where Rachel Goes Back to Work," *Friends,* season 9, episode 11, NBC, 9 Jan. 2003.

"The One Where Rachel Has a Baby," *Friends,* season 8, episode 24, NBC, 16 May 2002.

"The One with the Baby Shower," *Friends,* season 8, episode 20, NBC, 25 Apr. 2002.

"The One with the Breast Milk," *Friends,* season 2, episode 2, NBC, 28 Sept. 1995.

"The Prodigal Daughter Returns," *Gilmore Girls*, season 6, episode 9, Warner Brothers, 15 Nov. 2005.

"The Wolf and the Lion," *Game of Thrones*, season 1, episode 5, HBO, 15 May 2011.

"Try Carter," *ER,* season 11, episode 3, NBC, 14 Oct. 2004.

"Under Control," *ER,* season 6, episode 16, NBC, 23 Mar. 2000.

"Yes, Monsignor," *Two and a Half Men*, season 2, episode 9, CBS, 22 Nov. 2004.

Other Sources

Bartick, Melissa, and Arnold Reinhold. "The Burden of Suboptimal Breastfeeding in the United States: A Pediatric Cost Analysis." *Pediatrics*, vol. 125, no. 5, 2010, pp. e1048-e1056.

Blum, Linda M. *At the Breast: Ideologies of Breastfeeding and Motherhood in the Contemporary United States*. Beacon Press, 2000.

"Breastfeeding and the Use of Human Milk." American Academy of Pediatrics Section on Breastfeeding. *Pediatrics*, vol. 115, no. 2, 2005, pp. 496-506.

"Breastfeeding Report Card—United States, 2010." *Centers for Disease Control and Prevention*, 2010, www.cdc.gov/breastfeeding/pdf/breastfeedingreportcard2010.pdf. Accessed 13 July 2016.

"Breastfeeding." *World Health Organization*, 2010, www.who.int/topics/breastfeeding/en/. Accessed 12 July 2016.

Brown, Jane D., and Sheila Rose Peuchaud. "Media and Breastfeeding: Friend or Foe?." *International Breastfeeding Journal*, vol. 3, no. 1, 2008, pp. 1-3.

Chezem, JoCarol, et al. "Breastfeeding Knowledge, Breastfeeding Confidence, and Infant Feeding Plans: Effects on Actual Feeding Practices." *Journal of Obstetric, Gynecologic, & Neonatal Nursing*, vol. 32, no. 1, 2003, pp. 40-47.

Cumming, Robert G., and Robin J. Klineberg. "Breastfeeding and Other Reproductive Factors and the Risk of Hip Fractures in Elderly Women." *International Journal of Epidemiology*, vol. 22, no. 4, 1993, pp. 684-91.

Enger, Shelley, M. et al. "Breastfeeding History, Pregnancy Experience and Risk of Breast Cancer." *British Journal of Cancer*, vol. 76, no. 1, 1997, pp. 118-123.

Fein, Sara B., and Brian Roe. "The Effect of Work Status on Initiation and Duration of Breast-Feeding." *American Journal of Public Health*, vol. 88, no. 7, 1998, pp. 1042-46.

Foss, Katherine A., and Brian G. Southwell. "Infant Feeding and the Media: The Relationship Between *Parents* Magazine Content and Breastfeeding, 1972–2000." *International Breastfeeding Journal*, vol. 1, no. 10, 2006, pp. 1, /internationalbreastfeedingjournal.biomedcentral.com/articles/10.1186/1746-4358-1-10. Accessed 30 Jan. 2018.

Foss, Katherine A. "Perpetuating 'Scientific Motherhood': Infant Feeding Discourse in *Parents* Magazine, 1930–2007." *Women & Health*, no. 50, vol. 3, 2010, pp. 297-311.

Foss, Katherine. "Breastfeeding in the Baby Block: Using Reality Television to Effectively Promote Breastfeeding." *Beyond Health, Beyond Choice: Breastfeeding Constraints and Realities*, edited by Paige Hall Smith et al., Rutgers UP, 2012, pp. 226-35.

Frerichs, Leah, et al. "Framing Breastfeeding and Formula-feeding Messages in Popular U.S. Magazines." *Women & Health*, vol. 44, no. 1, 2006, pp. 95-118.

Gillman, Matthew, et al. "Risk of Overweight Among Adolescents Who were Breastfed as Infants." *JAMA*, vol. 285, no. 19, 2001, pp. 2461-467.

Hausman, Bernice L. *Mother's Milk: Breastfeeding Controversies in American Culture*. Psychology Press, 2003.

Koerber, Amy. "'You Just Don't See Enough Normal' Critical Perspectives on Infant-Feeding Discourse and Practice." *Journal of Business and Technical Communication*, vol. 19, no. 3, 2005, pp. 304-27.

Koerber, Amy. "Rhetorical Agency, Resistance, and the Disciplinary Rhetorics of Breastfeeding." *Technical Communication Quarterly*, vol. 15, no. 1, 2006, pp. 87-101.

Li, Ruowei, et al. "Public Beliefs about Breastfeeding Policies in Various Settings." *Journal of the American Dietetic Association*, vol. 104, no. 7, 2004, pp. 1162-168.

Newman, Jack. "Breastfeeding Your Adopted Baby." *Breastfeeding Online*, 2003, www.motherandchildhealth.com/breastfeeding/breastfeeding-your-adopted-baby. Accessed 30 Jan. 2018.

Potter, Beth, et al. "Content Analysis of Infant Feeding Messages in a Canadian Women's Magazine, 1945 to 1995." *Journal of Nutrition Education*, vol. 32, no. 4, 2000, pp. 196-203.

Wolf, Jacqueline H. "What Feminists Can Do for Breastfeeding and What Breastfeeding Can Do for Feminists." *Signs*, vol. 31, no. 2, 2006, pp. 397-424.

Young, Kathryn T. "American Conceptions of Infant Development From 1955 to 1984: What the Experts are Telling Parents." *Child Development*, vol. 61, no. 1, 1990, pp. 17-28.

6.
(Breast)Milking the Situation

Interracial Wet-Nursing in Sherley Anne Williams's *Dessa Rose*

ABIGAIL L. PALKO

"The baby was hungry and she fed him." (*Dessa Rose* 95)[1]

The basis of *Dessa Rose* (Sherley Anne Williams, 1986) is, like that of the contemporaneous novels *Beloved* (Toni Morrison, 1987) and *Moi, Tituba, sorcière noire de Salem* (Maryse Condé, 1986), the historical novelist's speculation about footnotes to history.[2] Williams's novel, again like Morrison's and Condé's, explores tensions between the maternal impulses of enslaved black women and the maternal norms espoused by the dominant white culture that abused its power to shape enslaved women's experience of motherhood; the result is, as Anne Goldman argues, that "her doubled oppression was carried out not so much via her womanhood as her motherhood" (315). *Dessa Rose* goes even further than the other novels, though, in its depiction of the only literary instance that I have found of a free white woman serving—voluntarily, no less—as a wet nurse for a black infant, the baby born to the runaway slave Dessa. The novel positions Rufel as an "othermother" to both Dessa's son Mony and Dessa herself through her acceptance of what Cindy Stearns terms "the embodied dimensions of mothering [in] *breastfeeding as body work*" (64; emphasis in the original).

The historical novel is an excellent genre for exploring cultural meanings of motherhood. As Dorothy Roberts points out, both echoing and anticipating numerous other scholars, "the meaning of motherhood in America ... is molded, on the basis of race as well as gender" (6). As a result, "Historically, motherhood has been a resilient site for a broad range of cultural and ideological work.

It has been used for the construction of racial and class-divisive notions of femininity, just as it has been an arena of cross-race and cross-class solidarity" (Schweitzer 122). In *Dessa Rose*, then, motherhood is intimately entwined with issues of race, as a quick summary of the narrative will reveal. Any attempt to summarize the plot necessarily revolves around Dessa's maternal status. After her master kills her husband, a pregnant Dessa strikes her mistress in response and is sold off as punishment. Fearful for her unborn child, Dessa runs away twice from the slave coffle transporting her west. She delivers her son in the woods and develops a fever. Her fellow runaways bring her to Rufel's plantation, Sutton Glen, rumoured to be a safe haven because of Rufel's incompetent management after her own husband's desertion. As Dessa and Rufel get to know each other, they develop a tentative mutual understanding of the impact of white Southern patriarchy on both of their lives. They reach an uneasy truce and, in a precarious partnership, undertake a slave-selling scam to raise funds to free both of them. This tentative collaboration, however, is always mediated through a structure of power that is really only mitigated—not erased—by their interactions.

Sherley Anne Williams was primarily known as a poet and an academic critic when she published *Dessa Rose*, her first, and only, novel in 1986. The first African American literature professor at the University of California, San Diego, Williams's abiding concern was the diversification of the faculty, the students, and the canon. As the daughter of cotton pickers, she identified with the struggles of lower income black women. Her hope for *Dessa Rose* was that it might heal wounds inflicted by postslavery racism. In "The Lion's History: The Ghetto writes B[l]ack," Williams explains:

> Slavery, however, is more scab than scar on the nation's body. It's a wound that has not healed and, until the scab is removed, the festered flesh cut away, it cannot heal cleanly and completely. African-American literary production is now a more or less accepted part of the historical record; we can thus be said to be writing history. I want, however, to make a distinction between inserting the Lion's history into the nation's chronicles and the writing of history itself.

> We now realize that the Lion, if he—or she—is to "write history," must tell not only his/her personal stories of exclusion and oppression; she/he must also tell the story of [white] men. (248-49)

Any consideration of Dessa Rose thus needs to situate its composition within the growth of Africana studies in the academy in the 1980s, as Williams herself does: "In the decade and more between the story's conception and the novel's inception, the history of black people in this country had become an accepted field of study on American college campuses" ("Lion's History" 255). Dessa Rose appeared at a moment that African American women's writing was flourishing, both in the publication of new texts and in the recuperation of earlier writings. In that vein, she notes of the fragments of Dessa's story that first spoke to her: "Here was a story worth telling, that focused not on slavery as an institution but on slaves as people, the major actors in their own stories, and I wanted desperately to tell them" (250).[3] This narrative move counters the double-bind felt at the intersection of slavery's essential assumptions that Roberts articulates: "the dehumanization of Africans on the basis of race, and the control of women's sexuality and reproduction" (7). In keeping with the corporeal quality which Williams ascribes to the wounds of slavery, it is through the body—and specifically the maternal body—that she explores the outcomes of ripping off the scab.

Writing within the tradition of neoslave narratives, Williams theorizes the gap between recorded history and lived history through her evocations of the feminine alliance made by Dessa with Rufel—depicting the confrontations that bell hooks has advocated as necessary components of revolutionary change. Thus, hooks's call in "Sisterhood: Political Solidarity between Women" for women to bond and develop political solidarity proves an important lens through which to understand the radical plot moves that drive this novel. The location of this political solidarity in domestic spaces heightens its radical potential; hooks theorizes the subversive value of homeplace as the "one site where one could freely confront the issue of humanization, where one could resist" ("Homeplace" 267). She explains that black women's actions to make a homeplace offering a safe haven in which to "heal many of the wounds inflicted by racist domination" should be read as explicitly coded resistance ("Homeplace" 267). Within this concept of "homeplace," maternity becomes radically subversive for hooks, and her description seems to imply a form of a black cult of motherhood:

> Black mother worship extols the virtue of self-sacrifice while simultaneously implying that such a gesture is not reflective of choice and will, rather the perfect embodiment of a woman's "natural" role.... Failure to recognize the realm of choice, and the remarkable re-visioning of both woman's role and the idea of "home" that black women consciously exercised in practice, obscures the political commitment to racial uplift, to eradicating racism, which was the philosophical core of dedication to community and home. ("Homeplace" 269-70)

For women of color, a crucial element of motherwork and their struggle for empowerment is the work undertaken to ensure their child's physical survival (Collins, "Shifting" 53-4). Patricia Hill Collins asserts that a rich theorization of African American women's experience of mothering (as opposed to feminist theorizations silently focused on white women's mothering) requires understanding "the importance of working for the physical survival of children and community, the dialectical nature of power and powerlessness in structuring mothering patterns, and the significance of self-definition in constructing individual and collective racial identity" ("Shifting" 49).

Culturally, the novel's publication coincided with the upsurge of media rhetoric about President Reagan's "welfare queens"—a term which became political code for a certain type of socially unacceptable mothering. Susan Douglas and Meredith Michaels capture the angst of this cultural moment, and highlight the media's role in stoking it and its aftereffects:

> If someone were to blurt out the words "welfare mother" right now, most Americans would immediately, without

> even thinking, picture an African American woman in some urban ghetto with six kids by six different men. This stereotype is so accessible, just waiting on the very surface of our minds to be evoked, because over the years, the newsmagazines and TV news have increasingly relied on images of black people, and more and more, black mothers with more than two kids to illustrate stories about welfare. (175-76)

Countering this popular rhetoric was the work of African American such theorists as Barbara Christian, Alice Walker, bell hooks, and Patricia Hill Collins; they analyze the differences between African-diasporic mothering practices and those of white middle-class feminists (Frampton 142). Patricia Hill Collins notes that media representations in the 1980s increasingly linked black women's maternal status with a perceived American decline, an anxiety which prompted efforts to control black women's fertility (*Black* 79-80). Barbara Christian similarly contends that the system of slavery clearly demonstrated the ways that antebellum society valued black women for only an animalistic role in the capitalistic system of labour and production, and not as human beings (219). Williams's narrative, thus, strategically maps out a bond between Dessa and Rufel that is dependent upon its corporeal embodiment through the act of wet-nursing[4]; in crucial ways, their relationship takes on elements of the othermothering tradition of African American culture. Collins defines "othermothers" as "women who assist bloodmothers by sharing mothering responsibilities" (*Black* 178). This is not solely biologically based, as "African-American community norms traditionally were such that neighbors cared for one another's children" (Collins, *Black* 179). It is a stretch to call Rufel Dessa's "neighbour"—but it is also a stretch to call her Dessa's "mistress." The novel's transformative power lies precisely in the liminality of the space that Rufel and Dessa share. The "cultural value placed on cooperative child care" (Collins, *Black* 179) justifies and compels Dessa's acceptance of Rufel's assistance.

The novel—its narrative structure, the narrative voice, and the characters themselves— repeatedly insists upon the multitude of similarities that bind Dessa and Rufel together, and acknowledges the difficulties these connections engender. After a particularly painful fight between Dessa and Rufel, for instance, Nathan (another runaway slave) observes:

> "Mis'ess?" She looked up. "I wouldn't take what Dessa say much to heart. She been through a hard time. You know you been through a hard time, too—your man gone, Dorcas dying."
>
> It was what her own common sense told her but she was outraged to hear herself compared to the wench. (137)

As a result, several critics usefully turn to Mikhail Bakhtin's notion of dialogism to interrogate the novel.[5] In considering the role of breastfeeding, however, his theorizations of the carnivalesque and the grotesque also offer fruitful insight into the symbolism evoked by Rufel's wet-nursing of Mony. Williams uses moments of the Bakhtinian grotesque to provide a catalyst for a narrative shift, (most notably, for my purposes here, in Rufel's nursing of Mony). Each "grotesque" event produces a moment of clarity and change for Dessa. It is the centrality of bodily functions in the scene that creates the grotesque element according to Bakhtin, as "confines between bodies and between the body and the world are overcome" (317). As a result, in *Dessa Rose*, the humour of the novel combines with the carnivalesque to move the narrative beyond the impasse imposed by the power differential between Rufel as a white land-owning woman in the antebellum South and Dessa as a black runaway slave.

The relationship between Rufel and Dessa is, as Gretchen Michlitsch notes and I concur, specifically nurtured and embodied by the particular role of Rufel as wet nurse and Dessa's particular role as birth and cultural mother; Michlitsch asserts in her analysis of the development of this bond that "The specific situation of the hungry newborn and the lactating white woman—the symbiotic relationship between Dessa's son and Rufel, the crazy white woman—challenges stereotypes and instigates ultimately revealing interactions between blacks and whites" (337).[6] I would like to push this assertion further and examine the impact on Dessa specifically as a mother that is a direct result of her particular role in the relationship—as well as the influence of 1980s cultural rhetoric on the novel. Whereas Michlitsch argues that the significance of the novel lies in its ability to demonstrate "the potential for one infant's need and one woman's response to challenge social construction of race and class, [to] imagine an instance in which class and race become subsumed to practical human needs" (329), I would argue that Rufel's nursing of Dessa's child functions in a much more complex manner in the women's respective intimate processes of developing and asserting their individual identities within the antebellum ideals of motherhood and the cult of true womanhood. Given that Dessa's engagement with these social ideals is mediated through her maternal status, it is significant that she has a son. By providing Kaine with a son (albeit posthumously), she has fulfilled the patriarchal imperative of providing an heir. It is also significant that Dessa does not have a daughter: as Patricia Hill Collins theorizes, mothering a black daughter poses particular challenges, as the mother must simultaneously ensure her daughter's physical survival and emotional wholeness (*Black* 102, 185-86). Consequently, within the highly charged atmosphere of the 1980s, these characters suggest impossibly idealistic versions of maternal femininity.

Collins has argued that "Black women's failure to conform to the cult of true womanhood can [...] be identified as one fundamental source of Black cultural deficiency" (*Black* 77). In *Dessa Rose*, however, both Rufel and Dessa engage with the cult of true womanhood. As Michlitsch points out,

> Whites have compromised Dessa's capacity as a mother to breastfeed her son. Not only was her illness the result of her treatment by the whites and her perilous escape from them, but the white woman takes over the feeding of Dessa's son while Dessa is unconscious and recovering. That very act which makes Rufel "a human being" precludes Dessa's own breastfeeding relationship with her son, leaving her feeling like "less than a woman." (336)

It is precisely because of the mistreatment Dessa suffers at the hands of the white slave owners that she cannot fulfill either traditional role of Mammy or Matriarch; rather, she interacts with her son in a manner reminiscent in several ways of that of the white plantation mother and her children. That is, Dessa has in some ways entered the cult of true womanhood, as she is pressured to enact aspects of white womanhood—but at what cost? Rufel steps down from the cult's pedestal at the same time, as Suzan Harrison points out: "In an inversion of the mammy stereotype, Rufel, a white woman, nurses Dessa's child while Dessa lies in a feather bed with linen sheets, recovering from childbirth and imprisonment" (18-19). In this reversal, Rufel starts to serves as an othermother to both Mony and Dessa: she offers Dessa the physical respite and comfort that a plantation Mammy often offered her female charge beyond childhood into adulthood (here, Rufel is imitating Dorcas' care of her); her example will also influence and facilitate Dessa's mothering of her son in freedom.

Through Rufel's wet-nursing of Dessa's son, the two women create a relationship characterized by bodily intimacy and power to force a reversal of roles on the women; their relationship is further complicated by the cultural norms and racially imposed differences that mark it. Jennifer Fleischner highlights the "web of feeling between masters and slaves" engendered by the formulation of "family" on the plantation in her study of enslaved women's narratives (30). The blurring of boundaries that happened when enslaved children played with the mistress's children under the mistress's supervision so that the enslaved mothers could work in the field initiates a form of othermothering that is simultaneously saving and devastating: "however necessary 'family' was for the psychological and physical well-being of slave narrators as children, it was a tainted wellspring for nourishing the self" (Fleischner 31). The shock that Dessa feels at the sight of Rufel nursing her child—a shock that mirrors Rufel's own surprise that she unthinkingly began and consciously continues to nurse an enslaved woman's baby—signals the complete lack of any frame of reference within which she can make sense of Rufel's actions:

> And the white woman let them stay, nursed—Dessa knew

> the white woman nursed her baby; she had seen her do it. It went against everything she had been taught to think about white women but to inspect that fact too closely was almost to deny her own existence. That the white woman had let them stay— Even that was almost too big to think about. (117)

As the product of a culture that has defined Dessa against white womanhood—Dessa being everything that Rufel is not, or not being anything that Rufel is—she is incapable of reconciling Rufel's actions with her own understanding of the antebellum South's patriarchal order. The important phrase in Dessa's thoughts is her acknowledgement that "to inspect that fact too closely was almost to deny her own existence." For in her world, nursing—the physical act of nurturing a helpless baby—is the only aspect of mothering that has been reserved as the sole province of black women. Rufel usurps not only Dessa's position with her own son but Dessa's position on the plantation; Dessa should nurse Clara, Rufel's daughter, rather than Rufel nurse Mony.

Similarly, Rufel has no frame of reference within which to begin to comprehend Dessa's world. So Rufel chatters on to the now-dead Dorcas, whom she calls "Mammy," about sleeves and bonnets while nursing the children. Dessa, recuperating in the same room, hears "Mammy" and thinks of her own mother and her mother's lost children. Or, as Ashraf Rushdy observes, "whereas Rufel thinks of Dorcas as a supplement to selfhood, Dessa thinks of her mother as a source of selfhood" (376). The incongruence of Rufel's prattling (the slightly omniscient narrator implies a child-like quality to Rufel's words) and the reality of her own mother's existence drive Dessa to push back against Rufel's memories:

> "Wasn't no 'mammy' to it." The words burst from Dessa. She knew even as she said it what the white woman meant. "Mammy" was a servant, a slave (Dorcas?) who had nursed the white woman as Carrie had nursed Young Mistress's baby before it died. But, goaded by the white woman's open-mouthed stare, she continued, "Mammy ain't made you nothing!" (118)

Rufel's attempt to clarify with the possessive adjective "my" only angers Dessa more:

> The words exploded inside Dessa. "*Your* 'mammy'—" Never, never had that white baby taken Jessup's place with Carrie. "Your 'mammy'!" No *white* girl could ever have taken *her* place in mammy's bosom; no one. "You ain't got no 'mammy,'" she snapped. (118; emphasis in the original)

The core truth that Dessa's words reveal is the double meaning inherent in the word "Mammy" itself. For Dessa, it signifies an emotional relationship, the intimate mother-child bond that she locates "in mammy's bosom." She comes to understand that for Rufel, it indicates an economic relationship, of childcare purchased, even if Rufel does not recognize this aspect of it.

For Rufel, the word signifies the complicated inferior-yet-superior surrogate mothering that Dorcas offered, which the cult of true womanhood inhibited her own mother, Mrs. Carson, from providing: "She praised where Mrs. Carson had criticized, hugged where Rufel's own mother had scolded. Whatever Rufel had not taken to the pillowy bosom seemed insignificant to her now; and she had been taken to that cushiony bosom, been named there 'Fel, Rufel. To hear the names on Mammy's lips was to hear, to know herself loved" (124). Whereas Dessa locates this relationship "in mammy's bosom," it is merely symbolized by Mammy's bosom for Rufel.[7] And Dessa must push back against Rufel's memory in order to assert her own rightful place in her mother Rose's life. Dessa's double assertion that neither Young Mistress's baby nor any white girl had replaced their birth children in her sister's and her mother's affections is driven by her need to protect her own existence. Dessa's confusion at the thought of Rufel nursing her son—her inability to contemplate the implications of this action—derives directly from this need to distinguish between kinds of nursing and the emotional bonds carried and sustained by each.

The narrative, thus, must tease out the tangled implications of what it means to nurse a child. Dessa is distraught at the thought that she cannot nurse her child: "It hurt me to my deepest heart not to nurse my baby. Made me shamed, like I was less than a woman.

And to have him nursing on her … oh, I accepted it. Wasn't no choice; but I never did like to see it. And she act like it wasn't no more to her than nursing her own child" (170). For Dessa, nursing is a multifaceted act that defines several elements of her identity. As Farah Jasmine Griffin claims, "for Dessa Rose, giving birth to a free child and nursing him are acts of agency" (535); the fact that Dessa never successfully nurses Mony, however, troubles this assertion. Although she highly valorizes nursing, circumstances force Dessa to find other ways of asserting her maternal agency. Dessa's recognition of the connections between the way black men look at enslaved women and the way that slavery has circumscribed their mothering is therefore all the more poignant:

> Was that what they thought of us? Mules. I was so choked I couldn't speak.… Mules. Milly who had birthed seventeen children in eighteen years and seen them all taken from her as she weaned them, been put outsides herself when she went two years without starting another child. They had taken Flora's baby from her, put her out to nurse with someone else because Flora could do as much as any man in the fields. This is what broke Flora from slavery; this why she runned, so she could keep her babies for herself. Janet was mistreated because she was barren; Ada's master had belly-rubbed with her then wanted to use her daughter. I had been spared death till I could birth a baby white folks would keep slaved. Oh, we was mules all right. What else could peoples use like they used us? (183)

The evocation of mules symbolically erases enslaved women's maternity, of course, since mule pregnancies are rare (though not impossible); similarly Dessa comes up against the presumption that enslaved mothers are not emotionally attached to their children.

When Harker and Nathan propose the slave-selling scam to Dessa, the unspoken—as well as unseen and unacknowledged by the men—cost of her participation is the nurturing of her bond with Mony. Griffin suggests that Dessa refuses to participate in the slave-selling scam because she believes "that all black men desire white women, and feel[s] rejected by them" (530). Dessa is certainly motivated by the pain that seeing Nathan willingly engage sexually with Rufel causes her. But the almost unacknowledged larger force driving her here is her desire to stay with her child. Mae Henderson's extortion that we read *Dessa Rose* through a theoretical "model that seeks to account for racial difference within gender identity and gender difference with racial identity" (2) highlights the gendered approaches to the slave-selling scam. Nathan and Harker cannot understand the anguish that Dessa feels at either the idea of Nathan and Rufel becoming lovers or at the thought of leaving her son behind on a strange plantation whose owner may return before she does and claim Mony as his own property. In initially refusing to participate in the slave-selling scam, Dessa tries to assert herself against the masculine forces that would deny her both her femininity and her son:

> Harker was speaking to me. He'd sent Red back down to Dallas county to bring out Red's wife, Debra, and they baby; she was still nursing and could nurse Mony while we was gone. All they needed now was for me and Miz Lady to come on in. I swallowed down; that bloodhound was still at my throat and my voice was rough. "Get another mule," I told him; "this one don't know how to be no maid." (184)

The two passages above, with their references to "mules,"[8] encapsulate the complicated role that nursing plays in the novel, where it is alternately represented as an animalistic way of feeding children (when Flora's child is taken from her) and as a humanizing, feminizing force. (Dessa feels "less than a woman" because she cannot nurse.) It is a method of bonding between mother and child—but not the only one. Numerous scenes tenderly capture the way Dessa cuddles with Mony in bed, and when she does acquiesce to the plan, the narrative implies that she is much more upset about having to leave Mony behind than she is about the concessions she must make in order for her and Rufel to work together; she tells us, "I didn't want to leave Mony; he already knowed me and smiled when he seed me, and, oh, I didn't want to go nowhere without him" (195).

Simultaneously, Dessa's inability to nurse Mony becomes the vehicle for freeing Debra and her child from slavery: because Debra is still nursing and can feed Mony while Dessa and Rufel are gone, the men take the chance on freeing her before they begin the confidence trip. Nursing is, thus, the physical claim of an enslaved woman on her child, but also of enslaved women on their community's children. The act of nursing enables them to recreate the physical bond they had had with their own mother before slavery broke it.

For Rufel, too, the link between her sense of herself as a (surrogate) daughter to Dorcas and her ability to nurse Mony are intricately linked: "'She treated me just like, just like—' She stuttered and could have wept again, seeing with an almost palpable lucidity how absurd it was to think of herself as Mammy's child, a darky's child. And shuddered. A pickaninny" (125). The very next time that Mony needs to be nursed, Rufel "shrank from the thought of nursing him, a *pickaninny*, seeing this for the first time as neighbors might—*would*—see it" (127; emphasis in the original). Rufel's thoughts here seem to imply that her own racial purity has been compromised (Roberts 8). So long as Rufel can claim the nurturance that Dorcas bestowed on her as a form of othermothering, she can in turn take care of Dessa's child; forced to acknowledge that Dorcas's care was not freely given, Rufel remembers the racial lens through which she is supposed to filter her responses to Dessa and Mony.

Both Dessa and Rufel have been prepared for their relationship by earlier encounters with Kaine and Dorcas. Kaine has prepared Dessa for her encounter with Rufel through his (to her) daring and almost disrespectful view of the white people among whom they live. The narrator describes Kaine's way of speaking: "He wanted, she knew, to shock her, to make her see that white people, except for their skin color, were no different from her, from him—from any of the people" (47). Similarly, interacting with Dorcas shows Rufel that both black and white people are human. When Dorcas is dying, Rufel has Dorcas's mattress moved into the parlour, where she nurses her. The narrator notes, "Both of them enjoyed the brief reversal—though Mammy only let Rufel do so much and no more—neither believing that Mammy could come to harm over such a little cold" (129). The omniscient voice here equalizes the two women—attributing the same emotions to each and entrusting power over the relationship to the enslaved woman. The grief that overwhelms Rufel at Dorcas's death stems in large part from her belated realization of just how little she knew of Dorcas's life, of just what distance she (and society) had maintained between them: enumerating five facts about Dorcas and five physical traits, Rufel thought, "That much and no more ... eleven years and only then to know the feel of a loved one's hair under a loving hand" (129). Her sense of shame over knowing so little of the woman who played such a formative role in her own life hints at a developing understanding of the ways that her acquiescence to the institution of slavery blinded her to Dorcas's humanity.

The relationship that Dessa forges with Rufel ultimately provides her with the resources to save Kaine's child—the child of their love and whom Dessa fought so strenuously to keep—from his father's fate. Dessa has been indelibly marked by Kaine's teaching:

> "Niggas," Kaine tell me, "niggas just only belongs to white folks and that be's all. They don't be belonging to they mammas and daddies; not they sister, not they brother." Kaine mamma be sold when he little bit and he never know her face. And some time he think maybe his first masa or the driver or maybe just some white man passing through be his daddy. (38)

Adam McKible characterizes the role that Mony plays in Dessa's mourning for Kaine and her efforts to create a new life: "[Kaine's] child's very existence embodies Dessa's resistance and the possibility of future redemption" (229). Although Dessa pays a very high emotional price for the action, Rufel's spontaneous decision to nurse Mony in the end preserves his life, and more important to Dessa, the ties binding him to his mother and his father's memory, and, ultimately, Dessa's own life.

In an autoethnographic study, food studies scholar Psyche Williams-Forson analyzes the ramifications of allowing other women the intimate access to her household (particularly her marriage) by allowing them to cook traditional food for her Ghanaian-born husband. Given the contextual similarities—the intimacy of the relationship in question (mother-child, wife-husband), the cross-cultural provisioning of food—Williams-Forson's observation that "Primary food providers engage in survivalist techniques and strategies that assist in humanizing multiple environments" offers an important lens through which to view Dessa's acceptance of Rufel's assistance (451). For Dessa, accepting—without liking it—the fact that Rufel must feed her son ensures his survival; her decision to accept it reflects maternal agency on her part that humanizes the experience of enslaved maternity. It also reflects an interracial alliance that, positioned within the framework of motherhood, complicates institutionalized assumptions of (white) second-wave feminism. This agency then drives her to move from the Big House to the Quarters in order to control her domestic space when she realizes that Rufel and Nathan are lovers; Rufel, in turn, acknowledges Dessa's autonomy within Sutton Place. Crossing racial barriers forces Dessa and Rufel to confront their respective prejudices about the other; each must fulfill the role she is best suited for (which is not the role society sanctions for her) in order for them to be able to raise their children free from the patriarchal hegemony that subordinates them. Resisting the urge to offer a utopian ending, *Dessa Rose*, through its realistic evocation of women's interracial alliances, highlights the political potential of feminine friendships and motherhood, and underscores the importance of bloodmothers and othermothers to the development of African American children outside of slavery. Ultimately, nursing becomes the medium of reconciliation between Dessa and Rufel precisely because it facilitates the recreation of the act that threatens to divide enslaved women from their children—the practice of wet-nursing.

Amy Kaplan's concept of "manifest domesticity"—by which she characterizes mid-nineteenth-century America, when "domesticity dominated middle-class women's writing and culture" and when *Dessa Rose* is set—enables us to see why this inversion of roles is so threatening to the social order (584). Kaplan argues that "through the process of domestication, the home contains within itself those wild or foreign elements that must be tamed;

domesticity not only monitors the borders between the civilized and the savage but also regulates traces of the savage within itself" (582). Since Rufel's actions in embracing elements of the othermother role explicitly invite the foreign into the home, she seemingly is fulfilling her maternal obligation "to conquer and domesticate the foreign, thus incorporating and controlling a threatening foreignness within the borders of the home and the nation" (Kaplan 591). But only seemingly, as Rufel's actions are prompted by empathy and a desire to prove her own strength, not out of a sense of duty to uphold the patriarchal norm: "The girl's desolate face, the baby's thin crying—as though it had given up all hope—had grated at her; she was a little crazy, she supposed. But she could do something about this, about the baby who continued to cry" (95). In this moment, Rufel sees and hears what she is supposed to be oblivious to: the proof of Dessa and Mony's humanity. The focus of these actions on the realm of the family heightens their subversive power: "Under slavery, blacks' attempts to maintain the integrity of family life amounted to a political act of protest" (Jones 237).[9] Both Dessa and Rufel offer political protest, as Dessa accepts Rufel as Mony's othermother in order to preserve her family and as Rufel offers Dessa a valuable commodity for free.

The othermothering relationship begins in the moment that Rufel assumes an "ally identity," to use social psychology's term for her position. As an ally, she necessarily positions herself liminally: "Allies are trapped between not fully belonging to the group they chose and not fully belonging to the mainstream group they left" (Myers 170). It is solidified during their travel on the slave-selling scam when Dessa realizes that Rufel is also vulnerable to a white man's predation. Thus, whereas Rufel comes to understand herself as an ally, Dessa begins to see them as sharing commonalities; this new understanding deeply challenges Dessa to reconcile her "acute aware[ness] of the power of these controlling images" of black womanhood that Collins identifies with a more empowered self-perception (114). Collins cites an anecdote that demonstrates how the difference between the controlling images applied to African-American and white women is one of degree, not of kind:

> My mother used to say that the black woman is the white man's mule and the white woman is his dog. Now, she said that to say this: we do the heavy work and get beat whether we do it well or not. But the white woman is closer to the master and he pats them on the head and lets them sleep in the house, but he ain't gon' treat neither one like he was dealing with a person" (p. 148). Although both groups are objectified, albeit in different ways, the images function to dehumanize and control both groups. (114)[10]

The bonds created by Rufel's wet-nursing of Dessa's child, through which she "shar[es] black experience" (Byerman 62), facilitate mutual recognition of the other's humanity. Prompted by this experience, each of them chooses to undertake the journey toward self-definition, which challenges the roles white patriarchy works to force them into.

The costs of this decision are most fully realized in the novel's conclusion, when Rufel goes to "Philly-me-York—some city didn't allow no slaves" (236) rather than west with Nathan as she wishes or home to her family in Charleston. The novel frustratingly leaves us with only Dessa's conjectures about Rufel: "Miss her in and out of trouble—(Do she call my name to Clara?" (236). Both Rufel and Dessa, the text implies, are the richer for having known each other, but the poorer for having been born in a world where "We couldn't hug each other, not on the streets, not in Arcopolis, not even after dark" (233). Ultimately, Dessa's hope that "they never have to pay what it cost us to own ourselves.... Oh, we have paid for our children's place in the world again, and again" (236) applies equally to herself and to Rufel.

Yet while the ending seems to eschew utopian impossibilities, the novel's very attempt to construct a meditation on interracial mothering practices creates an idealistic reconfiguring of history that is ultimately completely dependent upon the fairytale ending it claims to reject. *Dessa Rose*'s appearance at the particular moment of the mid-1980s demands critical attention. Its position within the trajectory of the neoslave narrative has rightfully been well documented, as has its contribution to the flourishing of African American women's writing. But the larger American cultural context—that of the neoconservative war against the women they labelled "welfare queens"—as well as the difficulties created by the racial tensions that plagued second wave feminism in the 1980s have been largely overlooked, despite the fact that their influence on the novel is palpable. Both of these latent tensions are almost too neatly resolved in the novel by the very optimistic ending, wherein Rufel helps Dessa and the other runaways escape to the west where Dessa will marry Harker and be able to provide for her son—thereby escaping the stereotypes of the unwed welfare mother that have long plagued so many African American women. As a result of the influence exerted on the novel by this larger cultural context, *Dessa Rose* ultimately cannot escape devolving into a utopian vision, despite its very best efforts to do so. The novel offers a rich view of black mothering in which maternal bonding is facilitated by, but not dependent on, breastfeeding. The complexity lies in the fact that this breastfeeding work is undertaken not as expected by the enslaved woman for the plantation owner but by the plantation owner for the enslaved woman in the utopian model of interracial friendship that Williams offers in *Dessa Rose*. Thus, I would argue, one of Williams's greatest literary contributions is her depiction of a multifaceted and successful black mothering practice. In the end, it is as simple—and as richly evocative and complex—as feeding a baby: "The baby was hungry and she fed him" (95).

ENDNOTES

[1]I have been engaged with *Dessa Rose* since I first read it for Anne Goodwyn Jones's NEH Seminar at the Virginia Foundation for the Humanities in 2002. This essay began as a MIRCI conference presentation (October 2010); I also presented it to Notre Dame's Gender Studies Program's Research Workshop (March 2012). I would like to thank the audience members in both settings whose feedback was so helpful to me. I am also very grateful to Jeanne Ewert, April Lidinsky, and Genevieve Brackins who generously read and commented on it at various stages of the writing process, and my co-editor Ann Marie Short, who encouraged me throughout the process of compiling this book.

[2] See the Author's Note in *Dessa Rose* for Williams's explanation of her inspiration (5-6).
[3]*Dessa Rose* began as a short story, which Williams expanded into the novel.
[4]As a result, when Biman Basu reads *Dessa Rose* through a lens of Foucauldian masochism, his insightful claim that they share a form of intimacy marked by displacements in which "interracial heterosexual desire serves as an alibi for interracial lesbian desire" (393), nevertheless, misses the crucial element of their shared maternal status that bonds Dessa and Rufel in complicated ways.
[5]See, for instance, Mae Henderson's classic analysis of *Dessa Rose*, "Speaking in Tongues: Dialogics, Dialectics, and the Black Woman Writer's Literary Tradition."
[6]Ashraf Rushdy attributes their relationship to a different, yet still maternal, foundation:

> She represents their meeting in terms of what we may call a "subject of relation." The "subject," in this case, is truly an absence in the novel—she is Dorcas, Rufel's slave "Mammy" ... She exists only as a mental presence in Rufel's mind.... The figure of the "Mammy," then, and a "mammy" who is a virtual absence in the action of the novel, provides Williams with a way of exploring the meeting of two women working towards a definition of how to read other people in the hope of achieving dialogue and managing a sense of supportive community. (368)

[7]For a discussion of the racialized differences between white and black mothers in slavery, see Ivy Schweitzer, "The Mammy and the Mummy: Cultural Imaginary and Interracial Coalition."
[8]The word "mule" significantly evokes Zora Neale Hurston's *Their Eyes Are Watching God*, strengthening the intergenerational literary links Williams aspires to in writing *Dessa Rose*.
[9] See Jacqueline Jones, "'My Mother Was Much of a Woman': Black Women, Work, and the Family under Slavery" for an historical exploration of maternity under slavery.
[10] I am grateful to the anonymous reviewer who called my attention to this anecdote.

WORKS CITED

Bakhtin, Mikhail. *Rabelais and His World.* Translated by Helene Iswolsky, Massachusetts Institute of Technology, 1968.

Basu, Bisan. "Hybrid Identity and an Ethics of Masochism: Nella Larsen's *Passing* and Sherley Anne Williams's *Dessa Rose.*" *African American Review*, vol. 36, no. 3, 2002, pp. 383-401.

Byerman, Keith. *Remembering the Past in Contemporary African American Literature.* University of North Carolina Press, 2006.

Christian, Barbara. *Black Feminist Criticism: Perspectives on Black Women Writers.* Pergamon, 1985.

Collins, Patricia Hill. *Black Feminist Thought: Knowledge, Consciousness, and the Politics of Empowerment.* Routledge, 2000.

Collins, Patricia Hill. "Shifting the Center: Race, Class, and Feminist Theorizing about Motherhood." *Mothering: Ideology, Experience, and Agency,* edited by Evelyn Nakano Glenn, Grace Chang, and Linda Rennie Forcey, Routledge, 1994, pp. 45-65.

Douglas, Susan. J., and Meredith W. Michaels. *The Mommy Myth: The Idealization of Motherhood and How It Has Undermined All Women.* Free Press, 2005.

Fleischner, Jennifer. *Mastering Slavery: Memory, Family, and Identity in Women's Slave Narratives.* New York University, 1996.

Frampton, Edith. "'You just can't fly off and leave a body': The Intercorporeal Breastfeeding Subject of Toni Morrison's Fiction." *Women: A Cultural Review*, vol. 16, no. 2, 2005, 141-63.

Goldman, Anne E. "'I Made the Ink': (Literary) Production and Reproduction in *Dessa Rose* and *Beloved.*" *Speaking for Others/ Speaking for Self: Women of Color*, special issue of *Feminist Studies*, vol. 16, no. 2, 1990, pp. 313-30.

Griffin, Farah Jasmine. "Textual Healing: Claiming Black Women's Bodies, the Erotic and Resistance in Contemporary Novels of Slavery." *Emerging Women Writers: A Special Issue*, special issue of *Callaloo*, vol. 19, no. 2, 1996, pp. 519-36.

Harrison, Suzan. "Mastering Narratives/Subverting Masters: Rhetorics of Race in *The Confessions of Nat Turner, Dessa Rose,* and *Celia, A Slave.*" *Southern Quarterly*, vol. 35, no. 3, 1997, pp. 13-28.

Henderson, Mae G. "Speaking in Tongues: Dialogics, Dialectics, and the Black Woman Writer's Literary Tradition." Reprinted in *The Scholar & Feminist XXX: Past Controversies, Present Challenges, Future Feminisms*, vol 3, no. 3 and vol. 4, no. 1.

hooks, bell. "Homeplace: A Site of Resistance." *Maternal Theory: Essential Readings*, Edited by Andrea O'Reilly, Demeter, 2007, pp. 266-73. hooks, bell. "Sisterhood: Political Solidarity between Women." *Dangerous Liaisons: Gender, Nation, and Postcolonial Perspectives*, edited by Anne McClintock et al., University of Minnesota, 1997, pp. 396-411.

Hurston, Zora Neale. *Their Eyes Were Watching God*. 1937. Harper & Row, 1990.

Jones, Jacqueline. "'My Mother Was Much of a Woman': Black Women, Work, and the Family under Slavery." *Feminist Studies*, vol. 8, no. 2, 1982, pp. 235-69.

Kaplan, Amy. "Manifest Domesticity." *No More Separate Spheres!* Special issue of *American Literature*, vol. 70, no. 3, 1998, pp. 581-606.

McKible, Adam. "'These Are the Facts of the Darky's History': Thinking History and Reading Names in Four African American Texts." *Black Women's Culture Issue*, special issue of *African American Review*, vol. 28, no. 2, 1994, pp. 223-35.

Michlitsch, Gretchen. "Dessa and the Crazy White Woman: Cross-racial Breastfeeding in Sherley Anne Williams's *Dessa Rose*." *Australian Feminist Studies*, vol. 19, no. 45, 2004, pp. 329-39.

Myers, Daniel J. "Ally Identity: The Politically Gay." *Identity Work in Social Movements*, edited by Jo Reger et al., University of Minnesota, 2008, pp. 167-87.

Roberts, Dorothy E. "Racism and Patriarchy in the Meaning of Motherhood." *Journal of Gender and the Law*, vol. 1, no. 1, 1993, pp. 1-38.

Rushdy, Ashraf. "Reading Mammy: The Subject of Relation in Sherley Anne Williams' *Dessa Rose*." *Women's Culture Issue*, special issue of *African American Review*, vol. 27, no. 3, 1993, pp. 365-89.

Schweitzer, Ivy. "The Mammy and the Mummy: Cultural Imaginary and Interracial Coalition." *Mothers and Daughters: Connection, Empowerment, and Transformation*, edited by Andrea O'Reilly and Sharon Abbey, Rowman & Littlefield Publishers, 2000, pp. 121-39.

Stearns, Cindy A. "The Work of Breastfeeding." *Mother*, special issue of *WSQ: Women's Studies Quarterly*, vol. 37, no. 3-4, 2009, pp. 63-80.

Williams, Sherley Anne. *Dessa Rose*. 1986. Harper Collins-Quill, 1999.

Williams, Sherley Anne. "The Lion's History: The Ghetto Writes B[l]ack." *Soundings: An Interdisciplinary Journal*, vol. 76, no. 2-3, 1993, pp. 245-60.

Williams-Forson, Psyche. "Other Women Cooked for My Husband: Negotiating Gender, Food, and Identities in an African American/Ghanaian Household." *Feminist Studies*, vol. 36, no. 2, 2010, pp. 435-61.

7.
Gender, Psychology, and Breastfeeding as "Preverse"

From *A Clockwork Orange* to *Game of Thrones*

TATIANA PROROKOVA

THE CULTURE OF LACTATION: CINEMATIC EXPLOITATIONS OF BREASTFEEDING

The mother, as Sara Ruddick explains, plays a substantial role in the life of her child (17). A mother's care during the first years of a child's life is especially significant. Not only because her presence creates the sense of psychological calmness and security in the baby's mind, but also because the woman fulfills a vital function—she feeds the baby. The only possible ways of nourishing the baby at such an early age are breastfeeding and formula feeding. Depending on medical, sociocultural, geographical, and temporal factors, mothers choose either of the options. Breastmilk is considered a healthier option for a baby (and in some settings, it is), and from a biological perspective, it is the only natural food that mammals can provide their infants with. Therefore, from a biological viewpoint, breastfeeding is a natural practice. Sherry B. Ortner's discussion of the "nature-culture dichotomy" that the woman embodies, however, highlights the ways breastfeeding becomes a point of contention. Ortner argues the following: "Her 'natural' association with the domestic context (motivated by her natural lactation functions) tends to compound her potential for being viewed as closer to nature, because of the animal-like nature of children, and because of the infrasocial connotation of the domestic group as against the rest of society" (34). Thus, although biologically speaking it is a natural practice, breastfeeding also has profound cultural implications.

Cultural representations of breastfeeding are not always supportive of breastfeeding. Although some examples promote nursing, many others explicitly or implicitly challenge the positive nature of this practice. This chapter focuses on the latter and contends that recent film and television display nursing either as an act of cannibalism or as a gendered phenomenon that can turn into a perverse act once it is used to nourish grownup boys. Portraying breastfeeding as a perversity, film reveals the cultural anxieties surrounding nursing and comments on the strong social and cultural tendency to equate breastfeeding to good motherhood. To specify, film attempts to refute the argument for breastfeeding as a major signifier of being a good mother. Providing multiple portrayals of breastfeeding being either overused or misused, film, on the one hand, demonstrates the cultural and social pressure on women to breastfeed, while, on the other hand, it acknowledges the existence of negative views on breastfeeding, and displays these anxieties in, perhaps, an exaggerated yet more tangible form.

As a traditional part of the mother-infant relationship—the relationship that, according to Ortner, "may be seen as a challenge to culture and society 'from below,' insofar as it represents the fragmentary potential of individual loyalties vis-à-vis the solidarity of the group" (37)—breastfeeding has become a cultural phenomenon. Consider, for example, the scenes that depict the woman breastfeeding her baby in film and television. The purpose of their inclusion can vary—from teaching female sexuality, to celebrating or making fun of femininity, and beyond. The initial reading of such scenes is usually dictated by the film or series genre. The reason why film turns to exploring such deeply intimate female practices as menstruation, pregnancy, and breastfeeding is both perverse and empowering. In their nature, cultural depictions of the biological changes that the female body experiences potentially emancipate women, as they can shatter the idea of male dominance and demonstrate that there is nothing shameful about the changes the female body undergoes. On the other hand, these portrayals are largely diminishing because, whether intentionally or not, they strongly reinforce the idea of a woman as a vulnerable object. This problem is thoroughly elucidated by Iris Marion Young, who claims the following:

> Patriarchal society defines woman as object, as a mere body ... in sexist society women are in fact frequently regarded by others as objects and mere bodies. An essential part of the situation of being a woman is that of living the ever present possibility that one will be gazed upon as a mere body, as shape and flesh that presents itself as the potential object of another subject's intentions and manipulations, rather than as a living manifestation of action and intention. (154)

The culturally and socially created image of the woman as a "mere body" prompts some of the anxieties surrounding breastfeeding and, even more importantly, has made nursing an obligatory task for a woman, who—because of her anatomic features—is biologically responsible to be a "living bottle" for her progeny. Female breasts are potentially viewed either as a sexual object for heterosexual men or as an "equipment" to be used to feed infants, which, indeed, reduces the woman to an object. Although menstruation, pregnancy, and breastfeeding are also associated with the changes that potentially make the woman stronger than the man—because her body can transform to bear a child and, thus, secure the existence of the human race—film frequently treats these transformations rather inadequately. To be more precise, film either positions them as horrific (the transformations include menstruation and pregnancy, as one can observe in the films *Carrie* [2013], *Devil's Due* [2014], and the mini-series *Rosemary's Baby* [2014]) or humorous (these are usually breastfeeding scenes, as depicted in the series *Friends* [1994-2004], the films *Flirting with Disaster* [1996], *Meet the Focker's* [2004], *The Hangover* [2009], and even in the animated sitcom *Family Guy* [1999-]).

Portraying breastfeeding as a comical process, film and television usually resort to two main issues. First, breastfeeding is an intimate practice during which a woman uncovers her breast. Therefore, although a naked breast is an overt symbol of female sexuality that draws attention of heterosexual men, its usage as a "living bottle of milk" provokes men's hesitation and eventual repulsion. The paradox of the sexualized breast with its biological and non-sexual function has been artificially created by patriarchy, which vehemently diminished the role of a woman to a biological and sexual object only. It is, however, pivotal, that though imposing both functions on the woman, patriarchy draws an explicit line between the two, as the two can manifest each other only separately and never simultaneously. Moreover, the agents that participate in the act of using female breasts can never meet: breasts as a sexual object are meant for men, whereas breasts as food containers are only for infants. Breaking these rules leads to social and cultural confusion, and is, evidently, exploited by the genre of comedy to make the viewer laugh (or, by the horror genre, to make the viewer uncomfortable).

Second, breastfeeding can at first be complicated for women. The awkwardness, lack of experience, and, as a result, the questions the woman asks are often used to generate a comedic effect. In this case, film, by no means, undercuts new mothers; instead, it censures the function of a "living bottle" that society has imposed on mothers, attempting to argue that the woman is not an object biologically programmed to be a food provider, but someone victimized by male-dominated society and reduced to an image of a "living bottle"—as her inexperience and clumsiness provoke laughter rather than empathy from the audience.

Despite the directors' interpretation of breastfeeding as an uncomfortable and ultimately humorous action, there is another persistent connotation that nursing has gained in film, namely a perversion. This depiction of breastfeeding reveals the paradox of the existing pressure on women to breastfeed to be good mothers and the existing cultural discomfort with nursing. Breastfeeding as an abnormal act has been exploited both by the comedy and horror genres. By portraying breastfeeding as an almost ritual practice, the horror genre has investigated the problematic nature of nursing as a socially imposed practice; in other instances, by depicting it as a precarious act, horror films have scrutinized the dark side of breastfeeding, symbolically hinting at the social discomfort with nursing. Horror films comment on the perversity of the act and its inherent danger, and depict breastfeeding as a form of cannibalism: sucking its mother's breast, the baby is metaphorically turned into a vampire that feeds from its victim. And although breastmilk is not blood, it is, indeed, the liquid produced by the human body. Hence, eating the product of its mother's body, the baby turns into a cannibal. This idea is developed even further in the horror film *Grace* (2009), which this chapter extensively focuses on. In it, the baby rejects milk and demands blood instead, and, in the end, eats her mother's breast because she needs human flesh in order to survive. The connection of breastfeeding to cannibalism or, generally, to human violence has also been widely used in film to explain abnormal behaviour and, frequently, the brutality of mothers who breastfeed as well as of their babies who feed. This is vividly demonstrated in the film *A Clockwork Orange* (1971) and the HBO series Game *of Thrones* (2011-).

Similarly, although from a different perspective, the comedy film has commented on the perversity of breastfeeding. In comedy, this perversity is often discussed through the prism of sexualization. Breastfeeding can arguably be sexualized from two perspectives. The first one is revealed through the reaction of heterosexual men, who usually consider female breasts an explicit symbol of female sexuality. When female breasts are, however, used to provide food to the infant (but not to pleasure the man), this act is viewed—significantly, again, through the eyes of the heterosexual man—as a perversity. The second one is stipulated, to a larger degree, by the relationship of the mother and her infant. The feminist film scholar Linda Williams characterizes breastfeeding as the act "in which one erotogenic zone—the mother's nipple—excites another—the infant's mouth" (312). An even more horrifying factor about breastfeeding in this case is the mother's subjective enjoyment of it. That is, the breast is not just an object but is also a site of women's subjective pleasure. Although none of the films analyzed in this chapter explicitly comments on this problem, one can speculate that the mother's literal obsession with breastfeeding depicted in these examples may ambiguously hint at the issue of pleasure involved in the process. Whereas the sexual implication of exciting the child's mouth is not specifically dangerous when the child is an infant, it can be when the mother breastfeeds older children. As the comedy film *Grown Ups* (2010) illustrates, breastfeeding at later stages can make both the mother and the child appear crazy and abnormal in the eyes of the others, and it ultimately provokes either laughter (as in *Grown Ups*) or repulsion (as in *Game of Thrones*).

The examples that explicitly deal with the problem of breastfeeding as a perverse act, on which this chapter focuses, include the films *A Clockwork Orange* (1971), *Grace* (2009), *Grown Ups* (2010), as well as the HBO series *Game of Thrones* (2011-). Adopting the genres of fantasy, horror, and comedy, these films and series reveal a unique understanding of breastfeeding as a practice with specific boundaries. Highlighting families where mothers breastfeed older sons, the selected examples overtly deal with breastfeeding as a gendered and heteronormative issue. These films and the series suggest that allowing grown-up boys and men to see and suck their mothers' breasts is abnormal, thus reinforcing the dichotomy characterizing female breasts as either an object of sexual desire or the part of female body that is used to feed babies. According to *A Clockwork Orange*, *Grown Ups*, and *Game of Thrones*, breastfeeding grownup boys is a manifestation of a social and cultural malfunctioning of female breasts. The selected examples seem to criticize protracted breastfeeding, and view it as a ramification of the social pressure that mothers experience, according to which, breastfeeding is the key to being a good mother (i.e., the longer the mother breastfeeds, the better mother she is). To illustrate this point in the most comprehensible way, the films and the series resort to exaggeration, displaying mothers nursing their grownup children, teenagers, and even adults. Predominantly focusing on male children, these examples reveals the cultural and patriarchal horror of women infantilizing men by prolonged breastfeeding; but they also remind men that men were once dependent on the woman, thus celebrating the ability of the woman to be a birth giver, a nurturer, and a mother. The perversion of breastfeeding is strengthened further and manifested in *Grace*. There the grandmother wants to breastfeed her grandchild; yet the baby eventually turns into a cannibal, and literally eats her mother's breast. Adopting this rather horrific stance on the breastfeeding practice, this film attempts to raise the issue of breastfeeding as a serious one. Unlike the numerous comedies that tend to make fun of breastfeeding, *Grace* claims that this process is a natural right of the mother and her baby. Yet all films and the series selected for analysis here insist that breastfeeding can lead to serious and even critical consequences, harming, first and foremost, the mother and her baby. The reason for that, however, is the inadequate social reaction to nursing in general that manifests itself either in the form of an overwhelming support or in the form of strong condemnation and/or anxiety—none of which allows the woman to make a personal decision concerning breastfeeding.

ABNORMAL BREASTFEEDING IN *A CLOCKWORK ORANGE* AND *GRACE*

All the films and series examined in this chapter suggest that breastfeeding a grownup child (i.e., the child is well aware of his or her gender identity) is a perverse practice. It is perverse—as in deviating from a largely established norm—both because the child still consumes the milk meant for babies and because the mother allows the child to see and touch her breast. Both the mother's willingness to nurse (exposing her breast to her child) and the child's desire to drink breastmilk are abnormal at a certain stage. *A Clockwork Orange* (1971) and *Grace* (2009) are two cinematic examples that comment on these problems most overtly.

A Clockwork Orange is primarily concerned with the issue of violence, yet it arguably also implicitly deals with the problem of breastfeeding. The film narrates the story of a young man, Alex, and his small gang who spend their lives fighting, killing, and raping. The film's focus on violence is, therefore, very explicit. Yet already by the first scene in *A Clockwork Orange*, the film explains what makes the young men so aggressive. It opens with a close-up of Alex's face; he stares arrogantly at the viewer, holding a glass of milk in his hand. As soon as he takes a sip of the milk, the camera is slowly pulled back and the other members of the gang are displayed in the shot. Each of them holds a glass of milk and stares rather absently in front of himself. The camera reveals the statues of naked women that serve as furniture, specifically tables, where the men can place their glasses and feet. Indeed, to borrow from Vivian C. Sobchack, "the decor with its particular emphasis on painting and sculpture is a significant element of *A Clockwork Orange*" (93). It is also important in the portrayal of, as I term them, "the breastfeeding scenes." The women-shaped furniture is mostly placed in such a way that the viewer can observe the exposed female genitals, which, to some extent, imitates the act of giving birth. The other statues explicitly show female breasts and serve as milk machines. Later in the film, a gang member approaches one of these statues and pours milk right from her nipple. Although this is not human milk that the men drink, the act of consuming this milk implicitly stands for breastfeeding. Significantly, when they drink milk and eventually commit violence, the men are always dressed in tight white clothes reminiscent of swaddling clothes. The pad they wear, on the one hand, accentuates their genitals and makes them visually look bigger, thus underscoring their maleness; yet, on the other hand, due to its shape, the pad can be interpreted as a baby diaper. Thus, the main characters are portrayed as newborn boys, both through the way they look and the way they feed.

Nevertheless, the inclusion of acts of violence and sex performed by the young men from the Korova Milk Bar does not allow one to view these men as innocent children. On the contrary, they are fully aware of what is going on; thus, breastfeeding grown men is understood to be perverse. The film insists on the perversity of breastfeeding, claiming that nursing results in children's aggressive behavior. As Alex states, "The Korova Milk Bar sold milk plus, milk plus vellocet or synthemesc or drencrom which is what we were drinking. This would sharpen you up and make you ready for a bit of the old ultra-violence." Breastmilk is, hence, compared to alcohol or drugs, which provoke deviant behaviour. The process of milk drinking in *A Clockwork Orange* , therefore, suggests that breastfeeding changes a child's psyche and provokes various behavioural and sexual deviations. The audience observes the young men spending their days brutally beating up innocent people, raping women, and having threesomes.

Whereas *A Clockwork Orange* focuses on the children's addiction to breastmilk, *Grace* showcases how the mother cannot stop breastfeeding the baby. This issue is raised in the film's subplot that narrates the story of the mother—Vivian Matheson—who loses her grownup son in a car accident. Her pregnant daughter-in-law, however, survives and eventually gives birth to a baby girl, who Vivian seems to view as a substitute for her son. In one of the scenes, the audience observes Vivian lying in bed with her husband. She starts touching her breasts, and eventually wakes up her husband to have sex with him. She intentionally unbuttons her bed gown, and the man starts to kiss her bosom. As he moves down, however, the woman forces him to return up and kiss her breast, which she now openly takes out for him. As the man sucks her breast, he tries to touch Vivian with his other hand, yet she aggressively stops him, and, from a sexual game, the act explicitly turns into a metaphorical breastfeeding. Later in the film, the viewer observes Vivian sitting in a room, which used to belong to her son when he was small, and taking her old milk pump out of the box. She is then shown in the bathroom with her breasts exposed and the milk pump fixed on her breast. Eventually, milk runs out of her breast. At this moment, the viewer realizes that Vivian played that sexual game with her husband intentionally because she wanted to be able to breastfeed her granddaughter, since, as she informed everyone in her family at the beginning of the film, "You can nurse past menopause. As long as the nipples get enough attention, it reactivates the hormones."

Vivian's desire to breastfeed the newborn is clearly perceived as a perversion. Desiring to nurse the baby, the woman views it not as her grandchild but rather as her own child. This idea is, however, provoked by her mental instability, which was arguably caused by her son's death. Vivian, thus, becomes possessive of the baby because it is her son's baby; she literally sees it as a part of her son. The newly emerged possessiveness reveals the tight bond between the mother and her son, which Vivian tries to restore after her son's death by exercising control over the baby. Indeed, the maternal dominance is noticeable already at the beginning of the film when the family is still expecting the baby: Vivian teaches her daughter-in-law what will be best for the soon-to-be-born baby; her irritation is evident when the pregnant woman expresses her disagreement. Vivian, therefore, embodies the stereotype of the possessive mother: she dominates her husband; she is jealous of her daughter-in-law (because she is the younger woman with whom Vivian has to share her son); but most importantly, she still controls her son's life. This relationship is a vivid example of one between "a dependant son" and "a mother who is caught in her own dependency trap," as described by Richard Bryant-Jefferies (vii). As soon as the mother is deprived of her son because of his death (the most psychologically difficult trial for any mother), she views his child as legitimately her child, too. Thus, keeping the baby with her and breastfeeding it is considered the only appropriate course of action. Being informed about Vivian's obsession, the audience, however, interprets the woman's desire to breastfeed the grandchild as an abnormality. Breastfeeding is, therefore, portrayed in *Grace* as some sort of female obsession rather than a natural practice.

The film's treatment of breastfeeding as an abnormal practice is also apparent when breastfeeding becomes synonymous with cannibalism. When the mother tries to suckle her baby, the audience observes how painful the process is for the young woman. Yet this happens not because she does not want to breastfeed the newborn girl or because of some medical issue. the baby does not need her mother's milk to survive—it needs human blood. Thus, sucking her mother's breast, she drinks blood instead of milk. On the one hand, substituting breastmilk with another liquid, *Grace* seems to undermine the vital role of the former. On the other hand, through this substitution, the film reinforces the tight bond between the mother and her infant, which is partially achieved through breastfeeding and is now overtly grounded in blood. Toward the end of the film, as the baby grows and begins to teethe, it starts eating her mother's breast, thus turning into a cannibal. Breastfeeding is, hence, displayed as a perversion because it literally turns the mother into food.

Both *A Clockwork Orange* and *Grace*, therefore, depict breastfeeding as an abnormal practice and claim that it can provoke psychological instability in both the mother and the breastfeeding child. Nevertheless, the films do not necessarily reject the positive aspects of breastfeeding; they rather use unnatural breastfeeding as an explanation for the characters' deviation. Indeed, neither cinematic example focuses on widely accepted portrayals of breastfeeding; instead, they display nursing of grownup men, a resurrected baby, and a psychologically unstable woman who considers it normal to breastfeed her grandchild. The films, therefore, impart the idea that there is such a notion as "abnormal breastfeeding" and warn about the possible ramifications.

VOYEURISM, PERVERSITY, AND REPULSION: UNDERSTANDING BREASTFEEDING SCENES IN *GROWN UPS* AND *GAME OF THRONES*

Unlike *A Clockwork Orange* and *Grace*, *Grown Ups* (2010) and *Game of Thrones* (2011-) focus on the visual side of breastfeeding, and claim that once the woman nurses her grownup son, breastfeeding turns into an act of perversion causing repulsion and disgust in the observer.

In *Grown Ups*, one of the heroines, Sally, continues breastfeeding her son who is already four years old. Thus, in one of the scenes, when the boy comes to her asking for "some milk," the woman happily reveals her breast to him. While the boy is nursed, the male friend of the woman, Kurt, turns away in disgust and eventually moves away, whereas Roxanne covers the eyes of her daughter. It is important that when Kurt asks how old the boy is, the boy's father, Eric, responds, "Forty-eight months," which shows although their son is already four, he is still treated like a baby. Breastmilk becomes the boy's caprice, and breastfeeding turns into the indulgence. Yet whereas the mother thinks that breastfeeding at four is right, the father—judging from his facial expressions—seems to be skeptical about it, but he does not articulate his opinion. Breastfeeding is later discussed among Eric and his male friends. One of them, Marcus, asks, "What's up with the boob-thing?" and then adds, "he's [the boy] gonna be rubbing the boob with his beard soon." Another man, Lenny, agrees: "He's gonna get a milk moustache on a real moustache. That won't look right." The men, therefore, do not consider breastfeeding of a four-year-old boy right or, for that matter, sexy in any way. More than that, they find the process absolutely unnatural, which hints at Sally being seen as an obsessed mother who does not allow her boy to grow into a normal man. Additionally, they underline the fact that observing Sally breastfeeding provokes repulsion and disgust in them; she is neither sexually attractive nor a good mother.

Later, the family is at a restaurant with friends. Eric orders food for everyone. When it is the turn of his four-year-old son, Eric realizes that the boy is being nursed. Yet the boy stops and asks for cookies, and Marcus comments that "cookies and MILF" are great. The explicit sexual reference to his wife's breasts makes Eric ask Sally to stop. When later in the film Sally uses a breast pump, Marcus hears the sounds and, lying on the sofa, states that they are "getting [him] horny." Interestingly, when some scenes later a drunken Marcus falls asleep in a closet—having "the sexiest dream about a little blond girl" (who turns out to be the dog that stayed with him in the closet)—and puts a milk pump on his chest, he only once again proves that he, indeed, considers milk pumping sexy. The scene when Sally uses a milk pump is perverse not only because she pumps her milk in front of her male friend (who becomes aroused) and Roxanne's daughter, but also because she does it to feed a bird that the girl found. Sally promises to continue feeding the bird later, when the weekend is over and everyone leaves, but her son intervenes: "Mommy that's my milk!" Sally responds that they "have to learn how to share, even with birds," to which the boy replies, "But he's going to drink you dry!" Later in the scene, when the woman gets too excited, she forgets to hold her milk pump and the milk sprays out of her breast onto her friend's face. Her son screams angrily, "You're wasting it!" which emphasizes his desire to control his mother's milk.

This obsessed motherhood is, however, most vividly raised in the fifth episode of the first season of *Game of Thrones*, titled "The Wolf and the Lion." It is worth mentioning that the series is filled with controversial scenes of sex, violence, and nudity, so the scene that portrays breastfeeding does not really stand out when viewed as part of the series. Yet taken out of the context, the scene is undoubtedly perverse in nature.

The scene depicts Lysa Tully who is visited by her sister Catelyn Stark and Catelyn's captive Tyrion Lannister. While talking to Catelyn, Lysa breastfeeds her son Robin Arryn, who seems to be around eleven years old. The boy greedily sucks his mother's breast, and when he stops (because the mother starts talking to him), Robin's mouth is completely covered in breastmilk. Moreover, the future lord is depicted as an imbecile; as his behaviour demonstrates, he is neurotic and psychologically unstable, and his mother indulges all of his whims. Listening to his mother and aunt talk, Robin sits calmly on his mother's lap, and sucks or leans on her breast. Yet when Catelyn's or Tyrion's words anger him, the boy jumps from his mother to display his displeasure. Robin's psychological instability is only intensified for the viewers when they learn he is the lord of the land. Despite his high status, he is overtly protected by his mother who still treats him like a baby. It is, however, apparent that Lysa is mentally unstable, too. Her psychological instability was caused by the murder of her husband—the man who loved her and their son. As Robin first speaks, he leans his head on his mother's fully exposed breast while keeping the skin-to-skin contact. Whereas in *Grown Ups* the boy always stands next to his mother while sucking her breast, in *Game of Thrones*, Robin sits on his mother's lap, which is an imitation of infant breastfeeding, where the mother holds her baby in her arms. Lysa's visitors are overtly shocked by what they see, and both Tyrion and Catelyn try not to stare. Nonetheless, both obviously realize that Lysa and her child are unstable.

Grown Ups and *Game of Thrones* suggest that it is unnatural and perverse to breastfeed boys who are no longer babies. Both examples illustrate this by accentuating the problem of gender difference between the mother and her child and hinting at mental instability of both. Such breastfeeding turns into a perverse spectacle that makes both the characters observing it, as well as the audience watching it, feel uncomfortable and disgusted.

CONCLUSION

The problem of perverse breastfeeding is evident in such cinematic and serial examples as *A Clockwork Orange*, *Grace*, *Grown Ups*, and *Game of Thrones*. Narrating the stories of mothers nursing their sons, the examined films and series overtly articulate a stance from gender and psychological perspectives: it is wrong for women to breastfeed older male children. It is significant, however, that the analyzed examples deal with such a significant issue through the genres of comedy (*Grown Ups*), horror (*Grace*), and fantasy (*A Clockwork Orange* and *Game of Thrones*), thus offering multifaceted commentary. Namely, they display breastfeeding as a comedic, horrific, or fantastic practice, and single out cases of perverse breastfeeding. Such breastfeeding practices, as the four examples suggest, unveil, first, the psychological instability of the mother, which is revealed through her obsession with being a truly good parent, and second, the immaturity, mental instability, and social deviation of the male child. More than that, as the examples suggest, late breastfeeding can also distort heterosexual male perception of women as solely potential sexual objects and hinder independence.

Cultural representations of late breastfeeding, therefore, display the process as an act of perversion rather than normality. The use of the same trope in the examined films and series reinforces the significance of the issue, and reveals a new perspective on breastfeeding. Indeed, breastfeeding has its pros and cons, and, hence, there are those who support and others who condemn it. It is crucial, however, that although breastfeeding is frequently represented as a natural and, importantly, positive practice—for it helps the baby grow healthy as well as facilitates the bond between the mother and the infant—the selected examples shrewdly examine a potentially dangerous side of breastfeeding, which results from the social pressure and cultural anxieties surrounding breastfeeding and women's breasts. These cinematic examples claim that normal breastfeeding should, first, involve only the mother and the infant—any deviation, as one can observe, for example, in *A Clockwork Orange* (the mother is absent) and *Grace* (the grandmother wants to nurse), is a perversion. Second, only infants should be breastfed. Breastfeeding older or grown children or men, as displayed in *Grown Ups*, *Game of Thrones*, and *A Clockwork Orange*, reveals the psychological deviation of both the mother and the child, and showcases the breastfeeding practice as a perversion. Although none of the examples seem supportive of breastfeeding—portraying it either as an act of cannibalism or as that of moral perversion—they censure this practice particularly strongly if it involves those participants who naturally do not belong to the process, and they condemn the role of society, which dictates specific rules to the mother and deprives her of the chance to decide for herself.

WORKS CITED

A Clockwork Orange. Directed by Stanley Kubrick, performances by Malcolm McDowell, Patrick Magee, Michael Bates, and Warren Clarke, Warner Brothers, 1971.

Bryant-Jefferies, Richard. *Relationship Counselling: Sons and Their Mothers—A Person-Centered Dialogue*. Radcliffe Publishing, 2004.

Grace. Directed by Paul Solet, performances by Jordan Ladd, Stephen Park, Gabrielle Rose, and Serge Houde, Anchor Bay Entertainment, 2009.

Grown Ups. Directed by Dennis Dugan, performances by Adam Sandler, Kevin James, Chris Rock, and David Spade, Columbia Pictures, 2010.

Ortner, Sherry B. *Making Gender: The Politics and Erotics of Culture*. Beacon Press, 1996.

Ruddick, Sara. *Maternal Thinking: Toward a Politics of Peace*. Beacon Press, 1995.

Sobchack, Vivian C. "Decor as Theme: *A Clockwork Orange*." *Literature/Film Quarterly*, vol. 9, no. 2, 1981, pp. 92-102.

"The Wolf and the Lion." *Game of Thrones*, season 1, episode 5, HBO, 2011.

Williams, Linda. "Of Kisses and Ellipses: The Long Adolescence of America Movies." *Critical Inquiry*, vol. 32, no. 2, 2006, pp. 288-340.

Young, Iris Marion. "Throwing Like a Girl: A Phenomenology of Feminine Body Comportment Motility and Spatiality." *Human Studies*, vol. 3, no. 2, 1980, pp. 137-56.

8.
"In This Whole Story, That's the Shocking Detail?"

Extended Breastfeeding in Emma Donoghue's *Room*

ANN MARIE A. SHORT

> "In reality, breastfeeding is both a 'simple and natural' process that flows from our human biological status as mammals, and a heavily *culturized* behavior that can be so modified by cultural perceptions away from a 'natural process' as to be almost unrecognizable" (Dettwyler, "Beauty and the Breast" 168)

Conversations about contemporary parenting—and more specifically, modern motherhood—have become as polarizing as they are ubiquitous. The so-called mommy wars have made their way into mainstream cultural consciousness in ways that many feminist mothers feel is unproductive, and such terms as "attached parenting," "immersion mothering," and "mommy martyrdom" have become lines in the sand, dividing good mothers from bad ones. So when Emma Donoghue's 2010 novel, *Room*, was published to wide popular and critical acclaim, including a Man Booker Prize nomination, it was not surprising that many of the readers who went online to review the novel responded explicitly to the novel's depiction of extended breastfeeding, a practice unusual even among breastfeeding mothers. Although Donoghue has noted in interviews that she had no intention of venturing into breastfeeding-related controversies when she imagined this particular facet of her five-year-old narrator's relationship with his mother, it was the reading public's discomfort with the idea of a school-aged child at his mother's breast that dominated many early online discussions of Donoghue's novel.

In this chapter, I examine how popular online book review forums such as *Amazon* and *Goodreads* reveal the reading public's anxieties about what many lay reviewers interpret as abnormal behaviour between mother and son in captivity. Without taking sides in the mommy wars, I argue that the novel, and the reading public's reaction to it, illustrates how estranged modern parenting has become from the type of mothering depicted in *Room*.[1] In fact, I suggest that the manner in which Ma parents Jack is made possible by the unnatural circumstances in which she is raising him—completely isolated from culturally constructed expectations regarding motherhood and childrearing. Indeed, as a work of fiction painfully invested in what Donoghue herself has called an "extraordinary act of motherhood," *Room* ultimately forces us to consider what we understand "natural" to mean with respect to parenting, and particularly with respect to motherhood, in the twenty-first century.

INTRODUCTION: DEPICTING THE UNUSUAL

Jack's perspective is circumscribed by a complete lack of knowledge about the world outside of "Room," his name for the eleven-square-foot garden shed in which he is imprisoned with his mother. For the newly five-year-old Jack, forced captivity is the only reality he has ever known, which also includes the intermittent breastfeeding that punctuates his days, which troubled so many of the novel's readers. Jack mentions breastfeeding, which he refers to as "having some," thirty-two times throughout the novel, and almost always describes it matter-of-factly: "I have some now, the right because the left hasn't much in it. When I was three I still had lots anytime, but since I was four I'm so busy doing stuff I only have some a few time in the day and the night. I wish I could talk and have some at the same time but I only have one mouth" (Donoghue 21).

Suckling throughout the day (and night) is presented as just another facet of Jack's daily routine in Room, alongside brushing his teeth, exercise, reading, and bath; in this context, his breastfeeding seems unremarkable. Yet the fact that I distinguish Ma's choice to nurse Jack as "extended" in the title of this chapter reflects current and prevailing cultural attitudes about breastfeeding: despite the capacity of most biologically sexed female bodies to lactate for years after the birth of a child, nursing past infancy is considered atypical in most Western societies. Indeed, in most industrialized cultures, nursing a child longer than twelve months is considered "extended" breastfeeding, even though the World Health Organization (WHO) recommends "up to two years of age or beyond" ("Breastfeeding").

In her article, "A Time to Wean: The Hominid Blueprint for the Natural Age of Weaning in Modern Human Populations," anthropologist Kathy Dettwyler argues that breastfeeding and weaning patterns are affected by cultural values and practices, and suggests that if the weaning process were based solely on physiological considerations, children would nurse much longer. Her findings, based in comparative primate life histories, indicate that natural weaning in humans should actually be between two and a half and seven years of age (Dettwyler "A Time to Wean" 39). In the U.S., however, the 2014 CDC "Breastfeeding Report Card" shows that only about one quarter of all babies are still breastfeeding at one year of age (the American Pediatric Association recommendation). Incidentally, research on women breastfeeding children past two years, as Jack does in Donoghue's novel, is far more difficult to find than research on infant breastfeeding, in part because of the social stigma associated with breastfeeding older toddlers and young children. This lack of data reaffirms the perception that breastfeeding past infancy is atypical, thereby discouraging women from admitting to nursing toddlers and young children, which, in turn, makes it more difficult to find credible information about extended breastfeeding practices in the U.S. and other industrialized countries.

For Dettwyler and other advocates of natural weaning, "natural" means that the decision to wean is made by the child, and without the consideration of cultural norms or expectations. However, she also notes that among humans, the "age of weaning is the *only* life history variable that is subject to direct and substantial cultural intervention, and the only life span segment for which shortening the duration or eliminating it entirely has come to be viewed as normal and desirable" (emphasis in original, qtd. in Hausman 132). These ideas help to contextualize my analysis of Ma's extended breastfeeding of Jack in the novel, since—imprisoned in a small soundproof garden shed by her abductor and rapist—societal norms and expectations are rendered meaningless by her circumstances. However, as soon as she and Jack escape, literally within hours of being free, Ma encounters shock and disgust over the fact that she still breastfeeds Jack. Initially, she defends that choice, snapping at the police officer who stares at her she breastfeeds, "I'm nursing my son, is that OK with you, lady?" (180), and informing her incredulous mother, "You don't know the first thing about it" (241). Yet by the end of the novel, a few months after their escape, Ma ends up weaning Jack in a manner that feels not just profoundly meaningful for her relationship with Jack, but also necessary for her reintegration into society.

Dettwyler's research also informs my analysis of the online responses readers have had to the breastfeeding in *Room* by articulating the ways in which cultural considerations shape attitudes about breastfeeding older children.[2] In May 2012, less than two years after *Room* was published, a *Time* magazine cover story featuring a mother nursing her three-and-a-half-year-old son precipitated a public debate that revealed just how removed these norms and expectations are from what Dettwyler's research suggests about the natural age of weaning. I mention this incident because the photograph of the little boy, standing on a wooden chair so that his mouth could reach his mother's breast, aroused shock and disgust expressed in rhetoric nearly identical to what reviewers on *Amazon* and *Goodreads* said about the depiction of Jack nursing in *Room*. To be fair, shocking is what *Time*'s editors seemed to be going for. The photographer himself said that he "liked the idea of having the kids standing up to underline the point that this was an uncommon situation" (Sun "Behind the Cover"). Placed on the chair, the boy is made to look taller, and therefore older; the mother is young, pretty, stylish, and with breast exposed, clearly sexualized. Consumers took to the cover story's comments section—one side raging over the mother's disgusting, unnatural, even abusive behaviour, and the other defensively arguing the moral superiority of breastfeeding mothers. Unfortunately, most of these emotionally charged conversations unproductively sidestep more relevant questions about how society—via breastfeeding education, lactation counseling, and changes to parental leave policy—may better facilitate all parenting choices. Indeed, these types of discussions consistently fail to acknowledge that most parenting choices, not to mention the beliefs and attitudes surrounding them, reflect patriarchal cultural norms shaped by a vast array of considerations outside of what is actually best for mothers and children.[3]

"SQUICKED OUT": LAY REVIEWERS RESPONSES TO THE DEPICTION OF BREASTFEEDING IN *ROOM*

A sample of reviews of *Room* on *Amazon* and *Good Reads* taken from July 2010 to February 2013 shows that early responses to the novel's depiction of extended breastfeeding articulated similar anxiety, disapproval, and often outright disgust as the responses to the *Time* cover.[4] Out of 129 reviews that address Jack's nursing, only 14 express satisfaction with Donoghue's choice, either because the reviewer felt strongly about the benefits of breastfeeding or because they felt that it worked as an artistic decision within the context of the plot. Twenty-eight reviews mention breastfeeding in a way that is neither explicitly positive nor overtly negative, and most of these neutral reviews are merely descriptive about the breastfeeding in the novel, noting that it happens. Nine of these neutral reviews, however, though not overtly negative, suggest that Ma's decision to nurse her five-year-old son was not adequately explained or justified in the novel. One neutral review says that there is "too much" of it; another asks, "Why is the author so obsessed with breastfeeding? I have nothing against it, but it doesn't need to be mentioned dozens of times ... to make a point." Yet another reviewer writes, "*Despite* a lot of page space dedicated to breastfeeding, I found it difficult to put down" (my emphasis). Reading these comments closely, therefore, shows that even about one-third of the neutral reviews are somewhat negative. By insisting the breastfeeding in the novel is superfluous and requires justification, these reviews suggest that Ma's breastfeeding of Jack is distracting at best and, therefore, at least somewhat off-putting.

In my analysis of "negative" marker words used in reviews expressing explicit dissatisfaction with the novel's portrayal of breastfeeding, a distinction emerges between reviewers that found it physically repellent and who found it to be sexually perverse. In the first group, I observed the prevalence of such words as gross, sickening, disgusting, distasteful, vulgar, revolting, offensive, ew, icky, queasy, cringe-worthy, and "squicked out." The reason these reviewers are so offended by descriptions of a breastfeeding five-year-old may, indeed, reflect their perception that the breastfeeding is sexual, which I discuss in more detail later in this section; however, this set of reactions more explicitly communicates the belief that breastfeeding is a bodily function—thus not to be seen or talked about (or depicted in a fictional novel)—than to a sexualized interpretation of Jack at Ma's breast.

In their study of negative psychosocial reactions to breastfeeding, Cox et al. suggest that these types of reactions reflect an existential aversion in humans to reminders of the "physical, animal nature of humanity" (111). This argument provides a useful framework for understanding the language I observed in this first group of negative reviews, as in, for example, "I grew weary of all the bodily functions—descriptions of poop, breast milk ... vomit, pee, blood etc." By associating breastmilk with other bodily excretions, this reader's reaction is representative of common arguments against the appropriateness of breastfeeding in public and the relatively common cultural imperative for nursing women to cover up or find a private space in which to nurse (although this, too, reflects anxiety about the exposure of the sexualized breast). It should not be surprising, then, that said "private space," when the nursing mother is outside the home, is usually a bathroom, the space to which other bodily functions are relegated. Although, in theory, breastfeeding may be accepted as beneficial, it is also true that "often people view it as indecent and disgusting; keeping it out of sight helps keep our animality, and ultimately our mortality, out of mind" (Cox et. al 111).[5]

The second grouping of negative marker words observed in the reviews suggests a sexual undertone to the nursing relationship between Ma and Jack. In addition to "unnatural," other related adjectives I noted were creepy, disturbing, weird, obsessive, abnormal, inappropriate, and twisted. In one particularly disheartening review, the reader comments on Jack's terminology for breastfeeding, asking, "Why then, would the ... child always refer to breastfeeding as ... 'having some'? Many readers were understandably creeped out by the constant breastfeeding ... I mean, don't we usually hear men say they are 'getting some' as a euphemism for sex?" This explicitly (hetero)sexualized interpretation of Jack's nursing represents the overall sentiment behind reviewers' reactions in this second group. Their language, with its suggestion of sexual deviance, is meant to arouse suspicion surrounding the mutual intentions and benefits surrounding the mother-son breastfeeding relationship depicted in the novel.

Similarly, readers also mention and take issue with the fact that when Jack actively requests to nurse, or "have some," he is articulating a desire for both breastmilk and the comfort he receives from nursing. One *Amazon* reviewer comments,

> I understand that being in "room" and having limited resources, breastfeeding was MAYBE a necessary thing (although, there were mentions of vegetables, broccoli, green beans, etc.), but the constant references to it were unnerving, especially Jack's *unnatural* cravings for it and his characterizations of it as "creamy." It was vulgar and revolting. Now, I know that Jack's attachment to "having some" was probably meant to be more of a comfort thing rather than a nourishment issue, but quite honestly, that made it worse for me. (my emphasis)

As with the reader who asserts, "If you're old enough to ask for it so plainly, you're too old to have it," this reviewer articulates a common reaction to extended breastfeeding. In addition to imposing an arbitrary rule on the complex factors informing a decision to wean, these comments also suggest that Jack's knowledge of the source of his milk and his ability to describe and express desire for it somehow marks the end of a previously sexually innocent breastfeeding experience. In *Mother's Milk: Breastfeeding Controversies in American Culture*, Bernice L. Hausman argues that "because most women do not publicly nurse toddler or older children, a routine complaint lodged against women who breastfeed for more than a year is that they are sexualizing these children; this view sees the mother's breasts as inherently sexual in an adult sort of way" (81).[6] Thus, a behaviour frequently touted as "natural" in discourses about infant feeding aimed at mothers becomes "unnatural" when the child reaches a certain age, particularly if the objective is comfort rather than nutrition.

These comments reflect complex anxieties surrounding sex, and maternal sexuality, in particular, which are projected onto breastfeeding, nursing mothers, and their breasts via cultural attitudes. Indeed, in "Beauty and the Breast," Kathy Dettwyler suggests that one of the "fundamental assumptions" about breasts that shapes cultural discourse about breastfeeding in the U.S. is the notion that "the primary purpose of women's breasts is for sex" (174). According to Dettwyler, women in industrialized Western societies would breastfeed more and for longer if breasts were as desexualized as they are in other many cultures around the world. Although the implications of this argument emphasizes the reproductive capacities of women's bodies and denies women the potential to experience sexuality as a function of their reproductive processes, it contextualizes the anxiety (expressed as disgust) palpable in the reviews I cited. The terms "natural" and "unnatural" are already culturally loaded, and readers' responses to *Room* show just how fluid and complicated these concepts are with respect to breastfeeding and maternal sexuality.

"STONE-AGE MOTHERING" IN *ROOM*: A FORCED ALTERNATIVE TO MODERN PARENTING

> "Now, figuring out how to raise him all on your own, without books or professionals or even relatives, that must have been terribly difficult."
>
> She shrugs. "I think what babies want is mostly to have their mothers right there." (Donoghue *Room* 262)

Breastfeeding five-year-old Jack, however, is not the only aspect of Ma's parenting in *Room* that falls outside the norms of mainstream parenting. Despite their most unnatural circumstances, her mothering in Room exemplifies behaviours characteristic of parenting styles known as "attachment parenting," or what

Hausman calls "Stone Age" or "evolutionary" parenting.[7] In fact, the Attachment Parenting International website calls this form of parenting "our biological imperative—the source of our most instinctual behaviors" ("API's Eight Principles of Parenting"). In addition to their breastfeeding relationship, Ma and Jack also co-sleep, interact almost constantly, develop routines around Jack's physical needs and natural inclinations, and foster a relationship built on mutual trust and respect because of their emotional attachment, all hallmarks of these parenting philosophies.[8] Moreover, both Jack and Ma indicate that they understand their relationship to be collaborative rather than hierarchical. Jack's contention that "maybe I'm a human but I'm a me-and-Ma as well" (308) is echoed in Ma's response when she asked about how she parented under the conditions available in Room: "I mean me and Jack ... We did it together" (262). In Room, Ma and Jack become extensions of one another, interdependent and efficient given their circumstances.

Hausman and other feminist motherhood studies scholars identify particular problems with the viability of this parenting style in contemporary culture, not the least of which have to do with the level of privilege it requires.[9] Moreover, in "The Impossibility of 'Natural Parenting' for Modern Mothers," Petra Bueskens argues that

> "immersion mothering" is synonymous, in the end, with social exile. Following the prescribed parenting practice creates for mothers an ontological and physical condition that cannot be readily accommodated in the structures of modern society. The result is either social exclusion or the exhaustion of trying to combine normative opposites (home and work, public and private, childcare and leisure). This is a contradiction at the heart of modern culture that cannot be ameliorated by spurious returns to nature or by appeals to an already invented tradition. (84)

Bueskens's use of the term "social exile" points to the psychological dangers accompanying this type of parenting, particularly for women, insinuating that it is neither desirable nor sustainable in modern life. Ironically, in *Room*, social exile is the cause rather than the effect of what Bueskens calls "intensive, romanticized caregiving carried out by biological mothers in the private sphere" (76). For Jack and Ma, Room's confinement and isolation facilitate Ma and Jack's physical and emotional intimacy—a point that is emphasized frequently in the second half of the novel as mother and son attempt to negotiate their relationship on the outside.

Frequently in the days after the escape, Ma denies Jack's requests to breastfeed, particularly when there are other people around, and he reacts with sadness, frustration, and confusion. He also must learn to compete for Ma's attention among so many new people, places, and things to do. Ma is only twenty-six, and in the seven years of her captivity, Facebook and iPods have become indispensable to her generation. Jack notices that when she puts "Dora the Explorer" on for him so that she can surf the Internet, or when she puts on her new ear buds she can listen to music he cannot hear, she is distracted from him (246-47). These moments mark an emotional separation new to them but not uncommon in modern parenthood.

In one of these particular separations, Jack's trip to the mall—with the uncle, aunt, and cousin he has only recently met—also serves as an opportunity for the novel to address such modern parenting issues as overstimulation, consumerism, and gender normativity in small children. Jack describes the mall as "extra bright and ginormous" full of shiny objects and brands marketed to children. Moreover, his hair is long and he has not yet been taught that Dora the Explorer isn't supposed to appeal to him, so when he begins to sport a pink Dora wheelie bag, he is mistaken for a girl and does not understand why. These instances serve to show that in his captivity, Jack has been shielded from the cultural norms that so many people internalize and accept. Through his perspective, these norms appear alien, subject to scrutiny and critique, and "unnatural" relative to his former existence.

Ma's negotiations outside Room reflect the tension between what seemed natural in her interactions with Jack in captivity and the imperative that she establish herself firmly as an individual separate from him now that they are free. This tension comes to a head when Ma must leave Jack in their hospital room for a televised interview and he clings to her, resulting in one of the most emotionally harrowing moments in the novel: "Get off me," Ma says, "You're not a baby. I said get off" (257). When Jack falls back and hits his head hard against a table, he cries from the shock of both the physical pain and the emotional rejection. This violently forced physical separation, the manifestation of Ma's inner conflict as she attempts to negotiate a new life outside of Room, marks the beginning of a new relationship with her son.

In the excruciating interview that immediately follows this incident in the novel, the reporter's line of questioning forces Ma to second guess everything about her parenting—from her decision to breastfeed Jack as long as she has to even her choice to raise him in captivity at all when she could have asked her captor to leave him on a hospital's doorstep. At first, Ma defends her decisions. Asked about breastfeeding a five-year-old, Ma scoffs, "In this whole story, that's the shocking detail?" (262). When the reporter asks her why she did not make the "ultimate sacrifice" and try to give Jack up so that he could have a normal life, Ma's initial response affirms the value she places on a strong bond between mother and child: she says, "I think what babies want is mostly to have their mothers right there" (262). However, the reporter's aggressive line of questioning ("You don't think he's been shaped—damaged—by his ordeal?") implies that Ma could not possibly have been enough for Jack and that her decisions in Room may have harmed Jack irreparably.

Yet despite the difficult adjustments Ma and Jack must make outside Room, the novel does not simply validate Bueskens's contention that "In the context of a globalizing, fragmenting society, women cannot meet the demands of 'immersion mothering' without breakdown pathologies (including depression, guilt, despair, and infanticide) because no one can comfortably—let alone happily—live outside the dominant values and social structure of the society they were born into" (84). My reading suggests that *Room* does not show that immersion mothering is in and of itself undesirable. Instead, in its depiction of this type of parenting under such extreme circumstances, it forces us to consider how and why modern life fails to accommodate parenting like Ma's productively for women who may choose it; in other words, why must immersion mothering require or cause "social exile"? If it is difficult for Ma and Jack to integrate their relationship in captivity into their new lives outside of Room, it is only in part due to the psychological consequences of having had to coexist as long as they did without physical or emotional boundaries. The more meaningful reason the parenting choices Ma makes inside of Room do not work outside, the novel suggests, is that modern social structures do not value or support all parenting choices equally.

Consider Jack's observation about parents and children at the end of the novel, once he has been integrated into society:

> Everywhere I'm looking at kids, adults mostly don't seem to like them, not even the parents do. They call the kids gorgeous and so cute, they make the kids do the thing all over again so they can take a photo, but they don't want to actually play with them, they'd rather drink coffee talking to other adults. Sometimes there's a small kid crying and the Ma of it doesn't even hear. (322)

What he observes in these families is the complete opposite of what he experienced with Ma in Room, where for better or worse, he was the centre of her universe. His thinly veiled critique of distracted, smart-phone wielding, latte-sipping parents suggests superficiality, and Donoghue caricatures these parents at the end of the novel to emphasize how easily children can become accessories.

There is nothing natural about Ma's kidnapping or the seven years of sexual assault and brutal imprisonment she endures at the hands of her captor. Neither did she have any choice over how or when she became a mother, or the conditions under which she is forced to parent. However, because of her horrifying situation, Ma is also isolated from all of the noise surrounding modern parenting, and her relationship with Jack is stripped of the expectations that define modern motherhood in particular. Therefore, in its depiction of Ma and Jack's relationship, *Room* shows that both "natural" and "unnatural" are cultural constructions. Ultimately Donoghue's novel gets to what is missing from too many contemporary parenting debates: an understanding of the multifaceted and overlapping negotiations parents make to ensure the safety and wellbeing of their children, even, or perhaps especially, under the direst circumstances.

ENDNOTES

[1]Though an imperfect term, I use "modern" throughout this chapter to describe contemporary parenting in the West, particularly in the U.S. in the age of technology, consumer capitalism, and discourses of "choice" in parenting.

[2] See Dettwyler "Beauty and the Breast," which I cite in my epigraph and in my analysis of readers' responses to what they understand to be sexualized breastfeeding in *Room*.

[3]As Adrienne Rich writes in *Of Woman Born*, motherhood has two meanings: it is at once a "relationship" that connects women "to [their] powers of reproduction and to [their] children; at the same time it is an "institution" that maintains male privilege, "ghettoiz[ing] and degrad[ing] female potentialities" (13).

[4]In the following paragraphs, I use the terms "readers" and "reviewers" interchangeably to refer to the writers of these reviews. When quoting these reviews, I retain original spelling and capitalization.

[5]For more on this, see Rebecca Lane's article, "Healthy Discretion? Breastfeeding and the Mutual Maintenance of Motherhood and Public Space," in which she connects breastfeeding advocacy and demands that nursing mothers breastfeed in private to patriarchal disciplining of women's bodies.

[6]In chapter two of her book, Hausman provides a comprehensive review of various feminist interpretations of maternal sexuality, from those who understand pregnancy, birth, and breastfeeding as an integral part of a woman's "sexual cycle." See also Kristen Norwood and Paaige K. Turner's "The Breast is (Always) for Sex: Breastfeeding Discourse in Response to May, 21 2012 *TIME Magazine* Cover" and Alison Bartlett's "Maternal Sexuality and Breastfeeding."

[7]In *Room*, Ma gives birth "under medieval conditions" (261) with no medical assistance, in the space where she lives during the seven years of captivity. Even this detail resonates with the calls for more natural ways to deliver babies (homebirths, midwife-assisted, etc.) prevalent in these parenting communities.

[8]Bill and Martha Sears and Attachment Parenting International are the two leading proponents of this style of parenting, and many of the tenets are also promoted by La Leche League International.
[9]See Katha Pollitt, Judith Warner, and Amy Tuteur for recent public feminist criticism of attachment parenting.

WORKS CITED

"AAP Reaffirms Breastfeeding Guidelines." *American Academy of Pediatrics*, 27 Feb. 2012, www.aap.org/en-us/about-the-aap/aap-press-room/pages/aap-reaffirms-breastfeeding-guidelines.aspx. Accessed 5 July 2016.

"About Us: API's Eight Principles of Parenting." *Attachment Parenting International*, 2017, attachmentparenting.org/principles/principles.php. Accessed 15 Apr. 2017.

"Attachment Parenting." *Ask Dr. Sears*, 2017,www.askdrsears.com/topics/parenting/attachment-parenting. Accessed 15 Apr. 2017.

Bartlett, Alison. "Maternal Sexuality and Breastfeeding." *Sex Education*, vol. 5, no.1, 1 Feb. 2005, pp. 67-77.

"Breastfeeding." *World Health Organization (WHO)*, 2016, www.who.int/topics/breastfeeding/en/. Accessed 5 July 2016.

"Breastfeeding Report Card." *Center for Disease Control (CDC)*, July 2014, www.cdc.gov/breastfeeding/pdf/2014breastfeedingreportcard.pdf. Accessed 5 July 2016.

Bueskens, Petra. "The Impossibility of 'Natural Parenting' for Modern Mothers." *Journal of the Association for Research on Mothering*, vol. 3, no. 1, 2001, pp. 75-86.

Cox, Cathy R., et al. "Mother's Milk: An Existential Perspective on Negative Reactions to Breast-Feeding." *Perspectives on Social Psychology Bulletin*, vol. 33, no.1, January 2007, pp. 110-122.

Dettwyler, Kathy. "A Time to Wean: The Hominid Blueprint for the Natural Age of Weaning in Modern Human Populations." *Breastfeeding: Biocultural Perspectives*, edited by Patricia Stuart Macadam et al., Gruyer, 1995, pp. 39-74.

Dettwyler, Kathy. "Beauty and the Breast." *Breastfeeding: Biocultural Perspectives*, edited by Patricia Stuart Macadam et al., 1995, pp. 167-215.

Donoghue, Emma. *Room*, Little, Brown, and Co., 2010.
Hausman, Bernice L. *Mother's Milk: Breastfeeding Controversies in American Culture*, Routledge, 2003.
Lane, Rebecca. "Healthy Discretion? Breastfeeding and the Mutual Maintenance of Motherhood band Public Space." *Gender, Place, and Culture*, vol. 21, no. 2, 2014, pp. 195-210.
Norwood, Kristen and Paaige K. Turner. "The Breast is (Always) for Sex: Breastfeeding
Discourse in Response to May 21, 2012 *TIME Magazine* Cover." *Qualitative Research Reports in Communication*, vol. 14, no. 1, 2013, pp. 79-86.
"Parenting." *La Leche League International*, 22 Mar. 2016, www.lalecheleague.org/nb/nbparenting.html. Accessed 15 Apr. 2017.
Pollitt, Katha. "Attachment Parenting: More Guilt for the Mother." *The Nation*, 4 June 2012, www.thenation.com/article/attachment-parenting-more-guilt-mother/. Accessed 15 Apr. 2017.
Rich, Adrienne. *Of Woman Born: Motherhood as Experience and Institution*, W.W. Norton and Co., Inc., 1976.
"Room: A Novel." *Amazon*, www.amazon.com/Room-Novel-Emma-Donoghue/dp/0316268356. Accessed 1 Mar. 2013.
"Room by Emma Donoghue—Reviews, Discussions, Bookclubs, Lists." *Goodreads,* http://www.goodreads.com/book/show/7937843-room. Accessed 1 Mar. 2013.
Sun, Feifei. "Behind the Cover: Are you Mom Enough?" *TIME*, 10 May 2012, www.time.com/3450144/behind-the-cover-are-you-mom-enough. Accessed May 2015.
TIME Magazine, TIME, Inc., 21 May 2012. Cover.
Tuteur, Amy. *Push Back: Guilt in the Age of Natural Parenting*. Harper Collins, 2016.
Ue, Tom. "An Extraordinary Act of Motherhood: A Conversation with Emma Donoghue."
Journal of Gender Studies, vol. 21, no.1, 2012, pp. 101-06.
Warner, Judith. *Perfect Madness: Motherhood in the Age of Anxiety*, Riverhead, 2005.

III.
The Politics of Breastfeeding and Lactation: The Implications for Identities

9. My Black Breast Friend

Breastfeeding and My Black Body

DIONNE IRVING

My father always swore that I would end up pregnant at sixteen. He would argue that with my mother's lax parenting style (a declaration I couldn't comprehend), and with my own lack of intelligence and grace (a declaration I'd come to believe), this was the fate that awaited me. Teenage motherhood was all I was suited for.

In the war of words lobbed back and forth during my parents' contentious divorce, my virginity, even at eight years old, was one of the rallying cries. It was a site where the battle began and often ended. My prepubescent body was a kind of trump card, a locus in the war they waged with each other. Even then, on a level that hadn't quite yet reached language, I knew that there was something in me that they—my parents—needed to tamp down for fear that someone else would take advantage of it.

"Even as a little girl," my mother says now, eyeing my postbaby body, "you always had a *shape*."

That shape needed management. It was to be contained and controlled. So less than a year later, I was outfitted with my first training bra. It was a pretty pink slip of fabric with lacey straps and triangle cups, made to hold my little bumps. They were hardly even breasts, just pockets of extra flesh positioned above my round little girl belly. The bra locked in the front with a clasp that clicked into a perfectly shaped rosebud.

And I hated it.

My mother told me that I was to wear it every single day underneath my regular undershirt, and she felt my back with the intensity of an overeager TSA agent before I left the house each morning for the fourth grade.

And I hated it.

The bra itched and felt tight. I missed the feeling of my bare skin against the soft fleece of my sweatshirt or the light cotton of t-shirts. Instead, there was a band of tightness across my chest, and every once in a while, the little rosebud would snap open and I would have to rush to the bathroom to click the little clasp back into place before anyone caught a glimpse of my breast.

And I hated it.

Somehow I knew what that bra meant. I knew it was insurance against my father's repeated claim that I was good for nothing but making babies. It was the first step in making sure that I wasn't just another pregnant black teenager. "*Yet*," he'd say. *Yet*. I'd started to believe that it was inevitable—that I didn't have a choice in the matter. *All* black girls got pregnant as teenagers, even if I didn't realize—exactly—how that worked.

* * *

2014 was the year I turned thirty-five and the year I first got pregnant. In a study released that year, the Center for Disease Control identified the median age for black, first-time mothers at 24.2 years. For white mothers, it was twenty-seven years. John Santelli, a professor of population and family health at Columbia University, explained that "Women are staying in school longer, they're going into the work force, they're waiting to get married, and they're waiting to have kids" (Sifferlin). I was one of those women, earning a bachelor's degree, a master's degree, and then a PhD. I got married and then divorced and then married again before I even considered having a child.

* * *

I haven't seen or spoken to my father in nearly seven years when I go to see him in a sterile room in an Atlanta hospital. A bulb embedded in the wall flutters and ticks. My father is suffering from colon cancer, but the prognosis is good. He won't die for another seven years.

I am startlingly thin, and I teeter into the hospital on the tallest pair of wedge heels I own and in the barest of summer dresses. I have gone down a cup size through my postdivorce weight loss. I am trying to make myself look like I did before I got married. My father's face lights up when he sees me. He doesn't know who I am. I was practically a teenager the last time I saw him.

"It's Dionne," I say.

His face falls a little.

"Oh. Hi, Dionne."

I am in the room no more than ten minutes when he asks, "So, do you have any children?" In some ways, I am surprised it takes him so long to get to that question.

I am thirty and newly divorced. Children are the last things on my mind.

"I have a cat," I say.

"Why don't you have a baby yet?" he asks.

"I am working on my PhD.," I say. "I don't have time for a baby."

"You're getting old," he says, his voice tinged with what he thinks is laughter. "You better hurry up."

I am thirty: single, in heaps of debt, recently divorced, in the midst of trying to finish my graduate degree. He doesn't care about any of that. In his mind, I'm good for one thing only. Always was.

***

When I become pregnant for the first time, I am in a new city. I have lived there less than a year, and I am starting my career. I am, this time, married happily. These are the pieces that will save me from being the girl my father has predicted I will be. I have a life, and a full one. The maternity leave from the small liberal arts college where I teach feels almost Parisian compared to the options available to my friends. I know women who have gone back to work six weeks after giving birth. I have friends who have gone to work hemorrhaging, with weeping C-section scars, with breastmilk wetting the front of their shirts when they cannot find a place to pump. Because I'm taking an entire semester of leave, I will have three months at home before the baby arrives, and after, I'll have six months before returning to work. Of course, this time will all come with only half my salary. However, I am lucky to have the financial support of my husband and family.

During the first weeks of my leave, I prepare by reading on the benefits of breastfeeding. And there are, of course, many. Not only does breastfeeding protect the baby against a host of illnesses, it also decreases rates of obesity in later life and lowers the risk of sudden infant death syndrome (SIDS). I am enthusiastic and convinced, and I'm excited to feed my son with and from my own body. For him, yes. Absolutely for him. But also for me. As an unexpressed counterargument to my father, my breasts are going to have their day; they are going to be the hero of this new narrative instead of villainous participant in the cautionary tale of teenage motherhood spun a hundred different ways by my father.

According to the Centers for Disease Control (CDC), black women are less likely to begin and to continue breastfeeding their children than any other group of mothers. And although the rate at which black mothers choose the bottle over the breast has declined in recent years, black mothers still have the lowest prevalence of breastfeeding initiation and duration among all groups of women. For complex reasons, infant mortality rates are highest among the children of black women. According to the CDC, "Although U.S. breastfeeding rates are increasing, rates remain relatively low among some groups of women, particularly those who are young, black, at or below the federal poverty level, and have less than a college education" ("Breastfeeding Initiation").

But this isn't me, I think. I did not get pregnant at sixteen. I have what constitutes several college educations. I live above the poverty level. The black women whom the CDC describes aren't like me. I recall a fragment of a yoga class years ago and tell myself I am an island and leave myself open to whatever the universe intends for me. I am hopeful that my baby will take the breast, but if I cannot breastfeed, I will simply give my baby formula. Everything will be fine.

This is the lie I tell myself. When I whisper "fine" in conversation or under my breath, when I repeat it in my head over and over again, a mantra bending the future to my will, I understand that—come hell or high water—I *will* breastfeed. And I *will* breastfeed because, if I am like those women in the CDC guidelines, then I am that girl my father said I was. I am a failure.

Absolutely nothing is fine about my birth experience. I cannot even hold my baby for the first few hours of his life, my arms still heavy and deadened from anesthesia.

Finally, my head still dense with the fog of medical sleep, I manage to cradle this new life. I undo my hospital gown in order to feed him for the first time, to reconcile my body to his. But his mouth is limp. He won't latch with his exquisite little duck mouth, the one we talked and laughed and smiled about during our childbirth classes. There is no connection between his being and mine. He doesn't suckle. I snap shut my sturdy black nursing bra after trying in vain to feed my son, after failing to do what may well be the most natural thing a mother can do. And then, click—the clasp against my clavicle—just like that, I'm brought back to the rosebud clasp on my training bra holding my tiny, budding breasts. The click of this bra seems to tell me the same thing: my breasts have failed me again. I've fallen short of even the most pathetic of parental aspirations. My father had misidentified how and even when I would fail, but he was right that I would.

***

In the article "Neutralizing the Maternal Breast," the authors point out the lacuna in current studies of black women breastfeeding: "Feminist scholars argue that hypersexualization of African American women's bodies in U.S. history and culture make breastfeeding in public particularly vulnerable for these women" (Owens et al. 2).

***

The summer before I turn fifteen, while vacationing in Key Largo with my father, sister, and four-year-old cousin, a man approaches me in the water as I splash at my little cousin, Nic.

"Are you here on vacation?"

"Yes," I answer. I raise my cousin in the air and dunk him into the warm water of the Atlantic.

The man is older, each of his arms covered in tattoos. In my head, he's cute in the way older guys are in part because they are older. He has the sun-bleached blonde hair and the good looks of the movie stars my girlfriends and I looked at in magazines. The kinds of men you have crushes on at fifteen. He is a man. Not a boy.

My bathing suit is old and pilling. It clings to my breasts and backside, the material thin in areas where the fabric is pulled too tight. He looks me up and down. He pauses at my breasts, already a full C cup, despite the fact that I weigh only 109 pounds. Seconds feel like minutes. Finally, he lowers his sunglasses and asks, "Is that your kid?"

"No. He's my cousin."

In the next few moments, he somehow manages to ask me to meet him at a local bar, to ask for my telephone number, and to offer me his. I do not know what to make of this man. What does he want? I remember a spate of kidnappings a summer or two earlier. I am still a kid. Abduction feels more real than romance.

"Have you ever dated a white guy before?"

Have I ever dated?

***

In the book *At the Breast: Ideologies of Breastfeeding and Motherhood in the Contemporary United States*, sociologist Linda Blum interrogates the lack of desire to breast feed on the part of black women: "Although most of the African-American mother gave multiple reasons for rejecting breastfeeding, nearly all touched on the public/private divide, the need for vigilance in keeping their suspect bodies private, and of how severely breastfeeding violates that privacy" (165).

On the Internet there are thousands of sites devoted to actress Halle Berry's breasts. Their shape, their size, the movies in which they have been featured bare and covered. There are interviews in which she discusses baring her breasts in certain films—a clip from *The Jimmy Kimmel Show* in which she defends her lopsided breasts as "natural" and "real," and an exchange with British interviewer Jonathan Ross where he becomes distracted mid-question and admits to losing focus because he was staring at Berry's breasts.

There is a rare instance in which Berry discusses her breasts in the context of feeding her two children. In a May 2014 appearance on *The Ellen DeGeneres Show*, in the midst of discussing her miracle geriatric pregnancy (she was forty-seven when her second child was born), Berry comments on the difference in the ways her children nursed. She pantomimes her daughter's dainty sucks and her son's intense nursing style. "He's sucking the life out of me!" she says to DeGeneres, who responds, "That was TMI in my opinion" (qtd. in Blickley).

Discussing how she uses her breasts to feed her child is too much information, yet marvelling at the size, shape, symmetry (or lack thereof), and firmness of Berry's breasts is de rigueur.

In an article recently posted on MTV News called "Black Women's Bodies Are More Than Your Fantasies," writer Kris Crews records a few all-too-familiar comments she's heard from men.

> "I've never been with a black girl before, but it's something that I'd definitely like to experience. I know black girls are really good in bed and do things that other girls won't."
>
> "I'd never date her, but I think it would be awesome to have sex with a black girl."
>
> "I don't really think black girls are all that pretty, but their bodies make up for it."

Of course, this sort of fetishizing of the black female body is nothing new. The image of the Jezebel has long been constructed as hypersexual and knowingly, intentionally provocative, which either causes or is caused by the formation of black body as sexualized object, a trope that's haunted the white imagination from the very beginning. One famous example comes from the early 1800s, when Saartjie "Sara" Baartman, a black South African woman, was presented as "The Hottentot Venus" in freak shows throughout Europe. Baartman's living body was displayed as a spectacular object—one that elicited revulsion because of its "abnormal" proportions and supposedly overdeveloped sex organs. Her physicality became the genesis for scientific theories that sought to demonstrate the connection between black bodies and those of beasts, and to differentiate between so-called normal European women and abnormal African women. The black female body was "scientifically" fixed as the locus of exotic difference teeming with rampant sexuality. Even after her early death at the age of twenty-six, Baartman was not permitted any rest. Her body—and most specifically her brain, skeleton, and sexual organs—remained on display in a Paris museum until 1974 (Parkinson).

A search of the Getty Image database for images for black women breastfeeding does turn up a few images of Westernized black women feeding their children as well as some of white women breastfeeding their children. Most of the images, however, feature some variety of tribal women, headscarves, and beads. These women wear colourful cloth skirts, or carry baskets atop their heads. Many are topless, but the images lack anything that even slightly smacks of the sexual. These women's breasts are long and pendulous. Asexual. Unlike Halle Berry's perfectly round and perky breast, these are utilitarian. The African women featured in these pictures cannot be both mothers *and* sexual beings. Their fundamental purpose is clear and essentializing, and it reveals an uncomfortable either/or binary: a black woman is perceived as a hypersexual(ized) American woman or she is an African earth mother. There is no other category, no space, no room to be both.

* * *

I made sure that I kept my own breasts covered as soon as I realized their terrifying power. Turtlenecks, sweaters, loose fitting shirts. No matter what men and boys said, I was not flattered or pleased by their attentions, their grabs, and pokes. Their snaps and touches on the sly. That pretty pink bra was the first one I hid—and I worked to hide each subsequent bra as I moved rapidly through an alphabet of cup sizes.

"You dress like a professional nun," my friend told me in college.

I hadn't even realized it.

"You have a great body," she said. "Show it off."

I was tentative and a bit ashamed at first, but I took her advice and experimented with accenting my breasts. Growing more adept, I bought blouses with V-necks, tight t-shirts from Gap Kids that showed off my big breasts and small waist. I was, after all, an undergraduate. On a Friday night, we drank syrupy wine coolers and skunked malt liquor, working toward the kind of buzz that left a sticky film on our tongues. My white girlfriend and I went into her bedroom to change into our club uniform: dark jeans, rhinestone-encrusted tops. We rubbed glitter infused body lotion onto our hands, on our arms, chests, and midriffs. Body glitter was *so in*. As we tried to make ourselves sparkle—giggling at our own ridiculousness—her boyfriend sat out in the living room watching music videos on MTV. He was an odious person; we both knew it even then. Even so, we were surprised to hear him call out, unprompted, from the living room. He wanted his girlfriend to check the colour of my nipples. He wanted to know about black nipples. Is it true, he wondered, that they're dark instead of pink? *Abnormal. Normal.* Is it true that they are bigger than hers? *Abnormal.* Are they bigger than the size of a quarter, like hers? *Normal.* And finally he yelled to ask me outright if he could get a look at those "big titties."

This is what the female black body represents, a shadowed force of desire. Sex. A thing. Flesh. Object. But what's most difficult is that these projections are what my female and black body represented to *him*—and to so many others—but it's not at all what my female and black body represents to *me*. I think of all of these experiences, pulling them apart like the fibres of a rope and looking at each one in turn, seeing how, when braided, they become strong, capable of holding enormous weight. In my first blush of motherhood, my great desire is to recast my breasts, to create a new context to eclipse the old. With the birth of my son, I want to remake them. He will be a male for whom my breasts—my body—will not be a sexual or sexualized object. For him, my breasts will be devoid of anything other than their simultaneously mundane and miraculous function. For him, they will be life.

***

At my baby shower held three months before I gave birth, a white friend gave me something called "My Breast Friend"—a contraption meant to fit around my waist, a foam pillow designed to make breast-feeding easier, more comfortable. This fluffy pillow ring was going to be what got me through the trials and tribulations of breastfeeding. No village, no partner. A piece of foam.

No one at the shower asked me if I planned on breastfeeding because the expectation was that I would. Of course I would. I work at a college in a small city, and guests at the baby shower were mostly professors and their spouses. These are the kinds of people who buy organic food and ride their bicycles to work—people who can recite the benefits of breastfeeding in their sleep. The question isn't *would* I breastfeed, but for how long. My friends tell me about the La Leche League Meetings in our town. They tell me that breastfeeding is hard work but the very best thing that I can do. They tell me about how they breastfed for a year, eighteen months, two years even. They tell me about how their children refused to take bottles. I looked at My Breast Friend lying there among the stuffed toys, onesies, teething remedies, and receiving blankets. I'd never felt lonelier in my life.

* * *

On the day I give birth, back from the OR and in the hospital room where another bulb flutters and ticks, my son refuses to latch. The trauma surrounding his birth has left him lethargic. His head and body are floppy. His mouth is limp and won't grip the nipple, which I push into his mouth. Again. Then again. He doesn't suck, doesn't latch. He just lets it lie there.

In come the lactation consultant and a gaggle of nurses, with various contraptions, bottles—a series of confusions. My breasts feel empty. Where is my milk?

"We are going to have to give him formula," says one of the nurses. "He must eat." I feel panic surging through my body. This is what I hear: you cannot care for your baby.

"I want to breastfeed," I tell the nurse. "I don't want him to get nipple confusion."

She looks at me pityingly, as though there have been countless other women with the same demand. She leaves the room and comes back with a plastic spoon. "You can feed him off this," she says.

"Still not eating?" the lactation consultant says when she comes back later in the day. I have not yet stood up, or used the bathroom. My legs are cocooned within giant blood pressure cuffs to maintain circulation after my emergency C-section.

"Where is my milk?" I ask.

The lactation consultant shrugs and takes my baby out of my hands. "If he doesn't start eating soon, they will have to put him in the NICU."

I have lost so much blood and I am on so many drugs that I am having trouble focusing, having trouble talking. This all feels like it's taking place underwater. Like this is happening to someone else.

The nurse feeds my son Similac off the plastic spoon, which he finally starts to sip. Later I hand-express colostrum onto the same plastic spoon that my husband holds to my nipple, and I cry softly. And I think, *maybe I waited too long*. I click the strap closed to restrain the breasts I had tried to contain for years and which now seem to have a mind of their own. They sense *need*—my son's need—and begin to expand. They leak, they flow, and they ache. And still, my baby won't latch.

* * *

Slaves were expected to wean their babies when they were between eight and twelve months old. Slaveholders enforced this practice by gradually limiting the amount of time that slave mothers were allowed to feed their infants. By the time infants were walking, breastfeeding during the day was prohibited. Slaves caught breastfeeding exposed themselves to potential punishments as bad as can be imagined. One slave, Peggy Perry—devastated that she was unable to adequately nurse her baby in the fifteen minutes she was allotted by the overseer—prayed to God "that the infant would soon die and end her misery as well as his" (Schwartz 225). Such a prayer must've been common.

There is a growing body of scientific study showing we can inherit fear from our ancestors (Kase). It can create biases, and it falls under the category of what psychotherapist Carl Jung has defined as the collective unconscious and what other scientists describe as genetic memory (Treffert). A 2013 study at Emory University School of Medicine shows that a trauma could affect DNA and alter the brains and behaviours of subsequent generations (Gallagher). We are only 150 years removed from the nearly 250-year institution of slavery in America. If this science is true, is it feasible that black mothers who prayed for the death of their infants might have hardwired into their own descendants a hesitation in relation to their own children, children who, as recently as 150 years ago, were not only liable to be removed from their mother's breast, but to be beaten, raped, or wrenched away from their family at any time?

In *At the Breast*, several black mothers consider the attachment that breastfeeding creates between them and their child. In their discussion with the author, they are ambivalent about the desire for that kind of closeness. Andrea Bronson, a young black mother, describes the process this way: "When they breastfeed, they get attached. I don't want that hassle, especially with me going back to work. I want my babies to be attached, but not that attached" (164). According to Bronson, the benefits of breastfeeding don't outweigh her concerns. She explains, "The doctors said breast milk was the best, but I told them I didn't want to. They tried to talk to me into it, but they couldn't. They gave me a videotape and papers, but I didn't want to breastfeed!" (161). It is difficult to imagine, with the lingering spectre of a child being whisked away, that a mother would listen to any authority figure who encouraged attachment.

In her 1996 speech to the Democratic Convention, Hilary Clinton spoke about the importance of family and community. She mentioned parents who worked the second shift, who can't afford childcare, and she highlighted the importance of community in raising families:

> For Bill and me, there has been no experience more challenging, more rewarding and more humbling than raising our daughter. And we have learned that to raise a happy, healthy, and hopeful child, it takes a family. It takes teachers. It takes clergy. It takes business people. It takes community leaders. It takes those who protect our health and safety. It takes all of us. Yes, it takes a village. ("Clinton Speaks")

Taken, perhaps, from a Swahili proverb, Clinton's notion of the necessity of "a village" is often a part of the narrative of childbearing and raising (Goldberg). It is the idea that a community will support childrearing. In the same speech, Clinton says that we are each a part of the same family—the American family. But what, really, does that family look like for each of us?

The annual CDC report card for breastfeeding is posted each year on its website. Starting in 2013, the site features an image on its cover of a black woman breastfeeding her child. Next to her, an older woman cradles the baby's head. Both women have light complexions, and the baby's got a head full of curly hair. The baby whose skin is even lighter than the two women reaches up for her mother's partially covered breast. In 2014, the CDC features a trio of dark-skinned black women on the cover. This time, two older women bookend a younger black woman who peers down at her baby. The women on each side of her cradle the baby's head and feet. The message is clear. It takes a village. But this village doesn't often enough include male partners.

In the DNC speech, Clinton also talks about how her husband was by her side when she left the hospital, and she uses this discussion to laud her husband for the Family and Medical Leave Act. The act requires employers to provide job-protected, unpaid leave for medical or family reasons. Clinton connects the additional provisions in the law to a surrogate village. She points out that, often, there are no grandparents, insurance, or additional incomes for many parents.

When my husband and I come home from the hospital, my mother and stepfather—so unlike my biological father—are there, waiting for us. No less than two hours later, my milk comes in. And like a kind of miracle, the baby latches almost immediately. I weep with relief. He is eating. He is eating! My joy barely lasts a week before I—chilled, feverish, and exhausted—realize that something isn't right. I am still recovering from the birth, but I know something is wrong. The doctor diagnoses me with mastitis. A bacterium from my son's mouth has infected my breasts. "Keep breastfeeding if you can," my gynecologist says. "But it's okay if you have to stop."

The mastitis causes me to feel like hot, crushed glass is coming through my nipples. My breasts feel like they are being ripped apart and then devoured by my son's hungry mouth and incessant need. I cry each time I breastfeed, which is upward of twelve times a day. I try not to scream, to scare the boy. I kick my coffee table so hard I am worried that I break a toe. My in-laws come to stay with us, but after two weeks, they are gone. Everyone is gone. The house feels empty. I am without a village. When my husband leaves in the morning, being alone with my son's naked need terrifies me.

He still won't latch well and he screams and screams and screams. He will not lie on the beautifully moulded My Breast Friend. And we both cry. I nurse lying in bed on my side for hours. I watch *Mad Men* on an iPad propped behind my head, and scenes of Betty Draper's bleak suburban existence bring me to tears. Eventually, my son falls asleep, and I worry that I am starving him. When my husband comes home, he pops the baby's mouth open and guides him to the nipple. It is hard for my son to keep hold. The nipple falls from his mouth, and he can't seem to find it again. He is hungry all the time. He is angry all the time.

It's okay to use formula if you need to. My friends who are mothers write and text to tell me this. My paediatrician, my gynecologist, and my own mother all tell me the same thing. Logically, I know that they are right. But in my head, I keep going over the idea that if I can't feed my child, what else am I good for?

During his first paediatrician's visit, my son is underweight. He is hungry. The paediatrician suggests waking him up every two hours to feed him, day or night. My husband sets alarms and like zombies, we wake up, and then we wake up the baby. Once awake, he screams and resists. Or he screams, and then my husband forces him onto my breast.

I work harder at breastfeeding. I feel like if I work harder and harder at it, I will get better. He will get better. So, I drink gallons of water. I make lactation cookies to up my supply. I offer him my breasts every two hours. I have never been more tired in my life.

At home, the hours are endless. When I can finally drive again, we go to Target nearly every day. We make slow circles around the store, and when he wakes up, I take him into the changing room to feed him. In the full-length mirrors inside the accessible dressing rooms, I look at myself. I am unrecognizable. My body seems distended and my face is puffy. Where is my village?

The mastitis returns, this time more painful than the last. The doctor prescribes a more intense round of antibiotics, and I start to wonder if instead of my body giving life, my baby's biology is rejecting mine. Is his genetic memory pulling him away from my breast? Have I imparted some psychic DNA strand in him that means he can't form an attachment to me? Outside of my body, his mouth has rejected my breasts on a cellular level.

"You need support," friends write to tell me electronically. "Find some other moms."

La Leche League was founded in 1956 when breastfeeding rates across the United States had dropped to 20 percent. At the meeting held in a park on a warm spring day, the gathered women were uniformly white. They all seemed to casually embody a kind of earth mother vibe—flowy skirts, practical wash-and-wear bobbed hair, and trail sandals. I felt overdressed in a pair of pre-pregnancy jeans and a maternity sweater. Although I cradled my son, they looked at me suspiciously as I approached the group of mothers with infants.

"Is this the La Leche group?" I asked timidly.

Their faces changed suddenly, the suspicion gone.

"Yes," they said. "Welcome."

"Look at you, wearing earrings," one of the mothers, said. "Aren't you *fancy*."

Was I fancy? I regretted immediately my choice to put on earrings. It seemed like years since I had connected with other adult woman, and I had wanted to look nice. Earrings were as far as I had energy to go. These were all stay-at-home mothers; most were from the area or had lived there long enough to develop a network of friends with children of similar ages.

I barely spoke. But my son cooed in the sunshine, content for the first time in over a month. He smiled at the gentle breeze ticking his face, and I took a moment to experience it with him, to take his little hand and to reflect on how nice it felt to be outdoors.

When he started to get fussy, I left. I said goodbye, but no one responded. Perhaps I spoke too quietly. Perhaps I did not fit into whatever it was they had going. I never went back.

Instead, I join three groups on Facebook: Mocha Milk Mommies, the Breastfeeding Support Group for Black Moms, and the Indiana Black Breastfeeding Coalition. All of the members of these groups have made a commitment to breastfeed. Their stories, unfortunately, are the same: grandmothers and aunts who advise expectant or new mothers not to breastfeed; women whose partners tell them they are "gross" or unsexy because they breastfeed; rude comments from people in public spaces; frustration at the lack of places to feed or pump. There are women who despair because their jobs only allow fifteen minutes to pump during the workday, and the women must do it in the bathroom or cars. There are stories of women's milk drying up as soon as they return to work. One woman posts, "This and other communities like it helped me realize that what I'm doing is normal. I'm not singled out for wanting to do what's best for my baby." Members echo this sentiment, over and over. But the effects of class run like a river through these posts. Many of these new black mothers are struggling with work, with relationships, with *everything*. As Blum highlights in *At the Breast*, breastfeeding among black women is on the rise. But the obstacles they face are consistent.

Many of these women live in major metro areas—Atlanta, D.C., L.A. These women, the ones who are stay-at-home mothers, meet for play dates and coffee. They offer networks of support services in their areas. They share names of good preschools, birthing coaches, and breast pumps. They are insured. They help each other; support each other, lean on each other. They are a village.

> "My family has been very supportive of breastfeeding. However, I've been encouraged not to be the 'boob out in public' mom. This forum has been a good resource because I can connect with other moms who struggle with breastfeeding especially for us that pump with no latching. It's good to know we're not alone, almost two months strong—my minimum goal is six months but I'd be blessed to make it to a year."

> "Man this wasn't easy but when you have a village and a great support system anything is possible."

> "From the moment N. was born, I have been supported, loved and encouraged by a community of women that weren't initially a part of my village. These ladies were at the hospital, have made a meal train link for anyone to sign up and cook my family meals, given me breast pumping bras, activities for my children."

And other women—the ones who post at midnight or 3:00 a.m.,

after they are home from work, who stayed up to pump milk at night or to commiserate in the safe space of the Internet—talk about their struggles with low pay, lack of maternity leave, poor employers or spouses:

> "My oldest two sweeties are ten and six years old now and I was never able to successfully breastfeed them past two or three months mainly because I didn't have support at home, no one around me knew about breastfeeding so I had no one to go to for advice. So I quickly got on WIC and got formula. Having this group has helped me to not only learn more about nursing but also to learn more about TRULY bonding with my baby in general. It has been a huge blessing and I have now added anyone and everyone of color that I know to the group as soon as I know they are pregnant."

> "I had no support family-wise or otherwise. [Breastfeeding] was looked at as unnecessary and at the age he is now, nine months, it's seen as crazy. They think he's too 'big.' It's been suggested even by my mother that I 'give that boy a bottle' so he will sleep and so I can sleep through the night."

> "I Googled some lactation consultants but they are really expensive, one of them said the initial consultation price is $180.00, which is wayyyy out of my budget, as I am not being paid for my maternity leave."

In many ways, these concerns are typical, of course. But in others, they are not. What do these women need? What are we getting from this group? I see in it the "village" thread that runs through the posts of women of a certain class, a network of friends, parents, and caregivers. It is the desire to afford things like doulas, childcare, and lactation consultants and a willingness to commiserate with those who can't. It is the women who have lengthy maternity leaves, and those who worry that their bosses will fire them despite the Family Medical Leave Act.

I click on photos of all these different women breastfeeding their babies. Mothers in these groups post images of black babies at black breasts sucking enthusiastically. They look confidently, directly into the camera, proud, their breasts exposed, the heft of a fat, well-fed baby arm splayed across them. I look at these women, and I feel tears welling from deep and from far back. I see women marking their six-month, one-year, two-year breastfeeding milestones, and I catch my breath. If all these women can do it, can't I? I find the community heartening in all ways. I look down at my son nursing on the bed beside me, angled at my breasts, larger than they have ever been, performing the task they were built for. And for the first time I feel something else. Pride. In myself. For doing this.

I search desperately for women who live close to the small city where I do, but they are in Indianapolis, or Fort Wayne, places where there are communities for them, networks of other women who are close by and with whom they can commiserate. I feel deep gratitude for this virtual community, and I still feel so utterly alone—the Internet's blessing and curse.

Around the end of the second month, my son turns a corner. He begins to latch on his own. He reaches for my breasts independently. He takes the skin on the underside of my breast and curls it around his fist as if to intensify our closeness. He gazes up at me, studying my face, barely blinking as if considering this woman who is his mother. And I feel so acutely aware of the paradox of motherhood—that if I do the best I can for him, someday he will grow up and move away from me. He may someday think it "weird" that I breastfed him so long. He probably won't want to talk about it and won't remember these moments we had together, figuring out the beginnings of our relationship. He won't know that in these moments, I was leaving behind the echoes of my father.

Around the fourth month, my mother begins pressuring me to give my son cereal, and in the seventh, she asks, "Hasn't this gone on long enough?"

"How long did you breastfeed, Mum?"

"Six months," she says. "After that, it got weird."

She makes a funny face but I don't push her on it. Despite her education, she did not have the support I do. She had no family, no community, and no supportive partner. She was in a country that was not her own, and there was no Internet to buoy her. But I am not ready to stop yet. I enjoy our quiet time, uninterrupted, early in the morning or late in the evening, when I see his face relax and his body loosens as he nuzzles toward my breast. When we look at each other, I am struck by the sheer wonder that my body has grown and is feeding another human being. This most mundane of miracles.

In truth, My Breast Friend ended up being electronic, not a tube of foam. It was my electronic village. It was the friends from all over the country who texted and emailed and wrote, and who answered my questions at 3: 00 a.m. or 3:00 p.m. My village was also the networks of other women of colour grappling with their bodies and with the politics attendant to feeding your child as a black mother—all of this—who made this community feel like a safe space, an embrace. But my journey, the one that transported my breasts from the level of the pornographic to realm of the political, concludes with my making a statement that is, finally, almost completely for my own benefit. And though my ideas about breastfeeding have not changed, the way I look at my own breasts has.

WORKS CITED

"A Brief History of La Leche League International." *LaLeche League International*, www.llli.org/llliihistory.html. Accessed 22 Feb. 2016.

"Black Mother Breastfeeding Pictures and Images." *Getty Images*, www.gettyimages.com/photos/black-mother-breastfeeding?excludenudity=true&mediatype=photography&phrase=black%2bmother 2bbreastfeeding&sort=mostpopular. Accessed 22 Feb. 2016.

Blickley, Leigh. "Halle Berry Overwhelms Ellen DeGeneres With Breastfeeding Reenactments." *The Huffington Post*, 20 May 2014, www.huffingtonpost.com/2014/05/20/halle-berryellen-breastfeeding_n_5357978.html. Accessed 22 Feb. 2018.

Blum, Linda M. *At the Breast: Ideologies of Breastfeeding and Motherhood in the Contemporary United States*. Beacon Press, 1999.

"Breastfeeding Initiation and Duration at 4 Weeks." Centers for Disease Control. PRAMS, the Pregnancy Risk Assessment Monitoring System, 2011, www.cdc.gov/prams/pdf/snapshot-report/breastfeeding.pdf. Accessed 22 Feb. 2018.

"Breastfeeding Report Cards." Centers for Disease Control and Prevention, Centers for Disease Control and Prevention, 22 Feb. 2018, www.cdc.gov/breastfeeding/data/reportcard.htm. Accessed 22 Feb. 2018.

Crews, Kris. "Black Women's Bodies Are More Than Your Fantasies." *MTV News*, 25 Aug. 2016, www.mtv.com/news/2923514/black-womens-bodies-are-more than-your-fantasies/. Accessed 22 Feb. 2018.

"First Lady Hillary Rodham Clinton Speaks at the Democratic National Convention." *PBS,* www.pbs.org/newshour/bb/politics-july-dec96-hillary-clinton/. Accessed 22 Feb. 2018.

Gallagher, James. "'Memories' Pass between Generations." *BBC News*, 1 Dec. 2013, www.bbc.com/news/health-25156510. Accessed 22 Feb. 2018.

Goldberg, Joel. "It Takes A Village To Determine The Origins Of An African Proverb." *NPR*, 30 July 2016, www.npr.org/sections/goatsandsoda/2016/07/30/487925796/it-takes-a-village to-determine-the-origins-of-an-african-proverb. Accessed 22 Feb. 2018.

Kase, Aaron. "Science Is Proving Some Memories Are Passed Down From Our Ancestors."*Resetme*, 20 Feb. 2015, www.reset.me/story/science-proving-memories-passedancestors/. Accessed 22 Feb. 2018.

Owens, Nicole, et al. "Neutralizing the Maternal Breast Accounts of Public Breastfeeding byAfrican American Mothers." *Journal of Family Issues*, 2016, pp. 1-21, www.journals.sagepub.com/doi/pdf/10.1177/0192513X16650229. Accessed 22 Feb. 2018.

Parkinson, Justin. "The Significance of Sarah Baartman." *BBC News*, 7 Jan. 2016, www.bbc.com/news/magazine-35240987. Accessed 22 Feb. 2018.

Schwartz, Marie Jenkins. *Birthing a Slave: Motherhood and Medicine in the Antebellum South*. Harvard University Press, 2006.

Sifferlin, Alexandra. "The Average Age of First-Time Moms Is Higher Than Ever." *Time Magazine*, 14 Jan. 2016, www.time.

com/4181151/first-time-moms-average-age/. Accessed 22 Feb. 2018.

Treffert, Darold. "Genetic Memory: How We Know Things We Never Learned." *Scientific American* Blog Network, 28 Jan. 2015, www.blogs.scientificamerican.com/guestblog/genetic-memory-how-we-know-things-we-never-learned1/. Accessed 22 Feb. 2018.

10.
Breastfeeding in the Military

A Feminist Communicology Analysis

PATTY SOTIRIN

As of 2014, women comprised 15.1 percent of active-duty military personnel (Department of Defense iii). Of these women, 90.8 percent are of childbearing age (less than forty-one years old); in 2010, approximately 17,000 of these women gave birth while on active-duty status (Rychnovsky 38). Thus, lactation and breastfeeding are increasingly present in the military workplace and assert maternal bodies, relations, identities, and cultural associations within the dominant masculinist military culture. This chapter considers military mothers' breastfeeding as overlapping communicative relations, including (1) everyday interactions; (2) identity performances; (3) military culture; and (4) representational politics. By considering a complex of communicative relations, the chapter constructs a more multifaceted understanding of the gendered dynamics of breastfeeding by military mothers. A feminist communicology framework offers a multidimensional approach that engages the complexities of breastfeeding in the military and reveals dynamics of struggle and change.

FEMINIST COMMUNICOLOGY: A THEORETICAL FRAMEWORK

Karen Ashcraft and Denns Mumby's feminist communicology addresses conflicting *in situ* meanings and practices, the negotiation of cultural identities, and dynamics of change and resistance in work and popular cultures. Thus, feminist communicology facilitates a multidimensional inquiry into the cultural implications of breastfeeding in the military.

Feminist communicology takes gender as a cultural construction rather than a biological pregiven: "a complex, ongoing, and contradictory accomplishment" that involves embodied action "in an intricate field of discursive and nondiscursive relations of power, accommodation, and resistance" (Ashcraft and Mumby 115). Hence, gender identity is enacted at the juncture of micro and macro social forces. Personal desires, capacities, energies, and material circumstances are situated and shaped within sociocultural-historical enablements and constraint. Furthermore, a dialectic of power and resistance riddles identity and meaning: gender identities, interactions, and discourses are resources and products of intricate struggles that create and contest, accept and resist, significances and possibilities. The focus is, thus, on a dynamic conception of hegemony (consensual social order) played out in everyday, interactional, institutional, and cultural routines and contestations. Analyses pay particular attention to the play of power and resistance in ironies, ambiguities, and contradictions. The critical goals are to analyze how dynamics of marginalization and privilege are enacted in everyday interactions and entrenched in institutional structures (129) and to unsettle and even transform prevailing dynamics so that alternative, more equitable possibilities for identity and action may be realized.

Looking across dimensions of lived experience offers a rich appreciation for the complexities of everyday struggle, from mundane interactions to cultural and representational politics. A communicology framework thus explores how women engage with prevailing practices and assumptions that marginalize the breastfeeding active duty mother even as official policies promote integrating and accommodating these mothers. For example, in day-to-day interactions, the effort to pump breastmilk or find ways to breastfeed an infant can encounter stigmatizing perceptions and practices. The following section explores the strategies active duty mothers use to counter such stigmas.

EVERYDAY (GENDERED) INTERACTION: INTEGRATING BREASTFEEDING

In 2015, the Army was the last U.S. military service to issue a general directive requiring private rooms and adequate time to express breastmilk during the workday. Army Directive 2015-43 "Revised Breastfeeding and Lactation Support Policy" states that soldiers (not women) lactate and breastfeed; commanders are directed to designate a private space (not a restroom) and ensure adequate time to breastfeed or express milk. Yet, integrating breastfeeding into the schedules and expectations of military worklife is fraught with practical difficulties—when, where, how often, how long, what to do with the milk, and how to manage temporary duty travel assignments and longer-term deployments (Rychnovsky; Sleutel; Stevens and Janke). Furthermore, despite military efforts to neutralize gender differentiations, service members continue to enact gendered communicative behaviours, perceptions, and styles, often reinstating gender-based discriminations and privileges.

To understand the lived difficulties and strategies of active-duty mothers and breastfeeding, I turn to women's stories about their active-duty breastfeeding experiences collected by Robyn Roche-Paull for her insightful and useful book and website, *Breastfeeding in Combat Boots: A Survival Guide to Successful Breastfeeding While Serving in the Military*. Roche-Paull addresses a broad range of concerns for military women returning to active duty across a variety of assignments, including deployment, field exercises, and various workplace environments (shipboard, air flights, hazardous duty, and so on). Although the intent of her book is to provide a comprehensive guide for breastfeeding military mothers, the anecdotes Roche-Paull collected from active-duty women about their experiences and their creative strategies are insightful and poignant, and I draw on those comments to give voice to breastfeeding experiences.

In the chapters devoted to active-duty breastfeeding, Roche-Paull provides advice and resources for women who want to express milk both by hand and with breast pumps throughout the workday. Yet pumping milk clearly interrupts military work schedules and inserts maternal activities into the workday. Furthermore, because breastfeeding epitomizes nonmilitary responsibilities and biological necessities, such interruptions may stigmatize individual servicewomen. Although accommodating lactation is military policy, mothers who pump in military workplaces face stigmatizing perceptions such as slacking, lack of career commitment, unprofessionalism, and selfishness. Given their awareness of stigmas, it is little wonder that returning to active duty is the chief reason many military mothers choose to formula-feed their infants (Roche-Paull 45). Stigma strategies are, thus, central to breastfeeding women for managing day-to-day interactions in the military workplace. Although Roche-Paull does not address stigma, I read many of the anecdotes in her book as perceptions of and strategies countering stigmas.

Stigma is an identity discrediting perception that may be based on physical, social, or moral differences from the norm in a given time, place, and population (Goffman). Rebecca Meisenbach's stigma communication theory assumes that stigmas are materially and discursively constructed through both public and workplace perceptions of the stigma as well as specific perceptions of the stigmatized individual. Two categories of defensive responses to stigma acknowledge the negative perception of breastfeeding at work; they either accept that it applies to the individual's own situation or seek to avoid the negative ramifications of the stigma. Two categories of strategies accept that the stigma applies to the individual's situation but seek to change the general understanding of breastfeeding at work. Finally, two strategy categories seek to challenge both the general perception and its application to the individual's case. Many of the mothers' comments about breastfeeding experiences included in *Breastfeeding in Combat Boots* can be categorized into one or another of the six stigma response categories—illustrating the everyday interactions that make active-duty breastfeeding so personally, socially, and professionally difficult. The following analysis excerpts their comments to demonstrate stigma strategies used by active-duty breastfeeding mothers.

Defensive stigma strategies accept both the workplace perceptions and their applications to one's own case. Many anecdotes in Roche-Paull's book are about the negative comments and humiliating situations women had to endure while pumping milk during the workday. For example, an Air Force Staff Sargent recalls, "I had to pump in the galley with a blanket over. . . . That sucked, crew dogs are not nice when it comes to comments, but you just have to crew dog up and tell them to keep their comments to themselves"

(Roche-Paull 197). Another defensive strategy is to subtly disparage mothers who use formula; a Navy Petty Officer says, "I got lots of grief for not pulling my weight because I had to break once every two hours to keep my supply up. It didn't help that all but one of them fed their babies formula" (241). This strategy creates an "us versus them" orientation that divides those who pump from those who do not, despite their obvious shared interests and struggles to mother well in the context of military demands.

A second category of stigma response is "passing" or acknowledging the stigma of breastfeeding in uniform but deflecting its negative implications. Whereas some mothers went to extraordinary lengths to send pumped milk home while on travel or deployment, others hid their pumping and engaged in "pump and dump," as this Army Major explains: "When I went to the field for four days, I took my pump. I had planned to send the milk back to the OB floor via a daily runner, but conditions in the field were too dirty. So I just pumped and dumped.... I pumped in the tent that I shared with about twenty other people, both male and female, and used my rain parka to keep covered" (201).

A third category of stigma response seeks to change perceptions of the stigma itself, even as the woman may acknowledge her own culpability. Two such strategies are evading responsibility and reducing the offensiveness of the stigmatized behaviour. For example, a Navy Petty Officer seems to evade responsibility by charging her chain of command with being supportive "by the book" but failing to address her coworkers' negative comments; the implication is that coworkers' stigmatizing perceptions might change with more proactive support from the command: "LPOs [leading petty officers] would be right there when comments either about breastfeeding moms or me in particular were made.... I wish the upper chain of command at any level would have been mature enough to say something positive instead of turning their heads" (242). A refocusing strategy attempts to reduce the stigma of breastfeeding in uniform by equating it with other personal habits that require accommodation, evident in this Army Major's argument: "They were surprised to hear my suggestion of considering pumping as the same as a smoke break. So many Soldiers smoke and since smoking is prohibited inside, they must take a break to go outside … it is no less than what would be required for a pumping mom to go to the bathroom and pump" (241). Equating breastfeeding with smoking as two personal needs that require appropriate time and space throughout the workday normalizes breastfeeding accommodations.

The fourth category of stigma strategies attempts to both challenge public perceptions and deny that the stigma applies to the woman's individual case. A Senior Airman mother advises deflecting perceptions of pumping as slacking: "If you can get a [pumping] schedule that works for you and your job, that would be best, so that way no one can accuse you of 'trying to get out of work'" (194). One Air Force servicewoman recounts pumping milk for her infants in the squadron rest area which was "dubbed the 'crew breast area' by my squadron mates" (187). As a stigma strategy, her account provides evidence for challenging the stigma as well as its application to her own situation. She says, "I was never shy about pumping, and I think that put my squadron at ease about it. People would sit there and talk to me while I was pumping" (187). As she explains to Roche-Paull, not only was her own squadron comfortable with pumping, but she relied on other crews who were flying home to bring her expressed milk back to her son. *Breastfeeding in Combat Boots* includes many such testimonies that provide evidence countering the stigmas of breastfeeding in uniform.

The newly adopted policies about accommodating breastfeeding support integrating this activity; yet stigma still haunts everyday interactions given that breastfeeding emphasizes biological and private sphere differences between women and men in service. At the same time, responses challenging dominant stigmatizing perceptions are emerging. However, it must be noted that the tenacity of stigmatizing perceptions about active-duty breastfeeding is not due to embodied difficulties and social interactions alone. Rather, stigmatizing perceptions and available responses draw on cultural-historical discourses about working mothers and warrior heroes.

IDENTITY PERFORMANCE: BREASTFEEDING LIKE A SOLDIER

Breastfeeding in uniform is not only embedded in workplace

interactions but is just as importantly an identity performance that actualizes contrary discourses of the professional soldier and the moral imperative to breastfeed as an enactment of the good mother (Holmer-Nadesan and Sotirin; Marshall et al.; Murphy; Shaw). As Roche-Paull ruefully observes, "Sometimes, bringing something as feminine as breasts into the warrior culture of the military can cause uncomfortable feelings and possible problems amongst your co-workers" (237). The heteronormative masculinity of military service has long put women in uniform at a disadvantage (Pawelczyk). Women in uniform may be said to "pass" by mimicking the performance of requisite masculinity at the centre of military culture. For example, women's military uniforms are styled on existing men's uniforms with subtle adjustments to accommodate but deemphasize breasts, waists, buttocks, and size. There is a uniform designed for pregnant soldiers to accommodate their changing shape.

Yet women are not men, and the distinction remains a critical one in military culture. Military socialization enacts a strict bifurcation between masculine and feminine attributes and capacities, often including ritual objectification of women and emasculating taunts about "engirlment." Thus mimicry is requisite so that women soldiers can "pass" not as pseudo-men but in their performance of a masculine standard or a "militarized femininity" requiring both the capabilities of a male soldier and the vulnerability of a civilian woman (Sjoberg 93; qtd. in Mathers 136). Hence, women in uniform face what Laura Prividera and John Howard III call a "female soldier paradox"—negotiating conflicting injunctions to enact embodied signs of masculinity and femininity simultaneously.

This paradoxical injunction to be and not be both masculine and feminine is further complicated for breastfeeding service women who, after all, are working mothers. Working mothers in general face contrary disciplinary discourses of "good worker" and "good mother" (Buzzanell and Liu), which are especially troublesome for pregnant and breastfeeding working mothers (Payne and Nicholls; Turner and Norwood). This is even more the case for breastfeeding during active duty. The good-worker discourse complements contemporary expectations about professionalism and careerism, which requires dedication to the profession, long hours, personal sacrifices for the good of the organization, and self-discipline to maintain habits of mind and lifestyle (Turner and Norwood). Conversely, the good-mother discourse requires prioritizing maternal duty above everything else including self and work (Hays). Thus, working military mothers must negotiate a complex of paradoxical discourses—the good soldier, the good worker, and the good mother—that are all the more implacable for those who wish to breastfeed in uniform. As one military mother succinctly puts it in *Breastfeeding in Combat Boots*: "I … felt pulled between my responsibilities to the Air Force and my responsibilities to my child" (Roche-Paull 238).

These paradoxical discursive injunctions are often played out on the body of the mother. Some military mothers recall leaking breasts, engorged breasts, and being caught in the act of pumping—all moments when good worker and good soldier identities seem "tainted" by the workplace unruliness of female bodies (Nadesan and Trethewey). Similarly, a frequent response to popular photographs of women breastfeeding in uniform is the question of whether such an act violated regulations because the women were "out of uniform." Exposed breasts reveal bodies that cannot be contained by uniforms designed to mask female difference. The female body simply does not perform the disciplined military body in the same way that a male body does.

The recent military directives supporting breastfeeding across the services provide discursive resources for negotiating the paradoxes of good mother, worker, and soldier. Yet, there remains another chilling paradox that spoils the good-mother identity of military mothers: good mothers nurture life, whereas good soldiers must be ready to take life. The good soldier must prioritize killing over nurturing and loyalty to comrades over children and family. Thus, breastfeeding soldiers are caught in an intractable paradox of life giving and life taking.

Yet paradoxes are points of instability. The paradoxes besetting the breastfeeding military mother have been the subject of public deliberations over the role of women soldiers more generally. Such discussions evidence a shift in public acceptance of rights protecting marginalized identities as well as technological and political shifts in the conduct of war that portend changes in the gendered culture of military organizations.

ORGANIZATIONAL CULTURE: THE GENDERED MILITARY CULTURE

It perhaps goes without saying that the various military organizations—Army, Navy, Air Force, Marines—are historically and structurally gendered organizations premised on male bodies, masculine attributes, men's work-life patterns, and patriarchal values (Acker, "Hierarchies," "Inequality"; Carreiras). Across the services, the substructure of worklife continues to enforce militarism, masculinity, and intensive worklives. Yet there are shifts in the construction of military service that have begun to temper the hypermasculinity of the warrior ideal. In their analysis of LGBTQ military service, Anna Young and Pauline Kaurin point to a critical articulation of contexts leading to the elimination of the "Don't Ask Don't Tell" policy, including shifts in political culture and public values toward greater acceptance of diverse identities (sexual, racial/ethnic, disabilities); a shift in international engagement toward diplomacy and technological warfare rather than ground combat; and an expansive enforcement of civil and legal rights in liberal political culture. In such shifting cultural, political, and historical contexts, the gendered hegemony of military culture has begun to admit multiple images of the warrior: "Warriors may still be fit and strong and brave but they are also culturally sensitive, smart, and compassionate" (Young and Kaurin 427).

Notably, some researchers maintain that breastfeeding military mothers reframe strength, determination, resilience, and protectiveness by problem solving and overcoming the physical and cultural obstacles to breastfeeding, thus enacting the army's model of soldier resilience and readiness (Parcell; MacGuire). This construction of the breastfeeding military mother redefines military strength and resilience, and contributes to the tempering of the warrior hero image. Concurrently, the number of "dual military" marriages has increased—in 2014, 55.3 percent of military personnel were married, and 11.7 percent were in dual military marriages (Department of Defense). These statistics suggest that more military men are dual-career partners bringing the conflicts between work and home into the immediate purview of military command. Both a caring masculinity and the need to change patterns and expectations to accommodate birth, lactation, and motherhood and/or fatherhood may contribute to shifts in organizational structure and culture.

At the same time, the gendered culture of military organizations affects a well-established consensual order in which even the recent image of sensitive masculinity is absorbed into dichotomies between masculinity and femininity, men and women. Thus, women continue to "carry a burden of proof" to legitimize their capacities and status as soldiers (McFarlane). In military culture, values of obedience, conformity, and standardization discipline working bodies, protocols, missions, and visions. Such a disciplinary regime aims at sameness through a logic of equivalence—treat male and female soldiers the same, different but equal. As Ashcraft points out, pursuing equality through organizational standardization assumes a foundational sameness. Difference is, thus, disciplined through conformity and obedience to a one-size-fits-all standardization.

Such a logic entails a critical impasse for women and other marginalized groups most readily apparent at the level of the body. Embodied difference is disciplined through standardization—for example, uniforms that mask sexual differences. In such a culture, full-blown system transformation to eliminate discriminatory bias and marginalization is deterred by focusing on disciplining individuals and introducing piecemeal reforms like breast-pumping policies. The assumption is "tackle individual bias and you will eventually correct the system distortions it creates" (Ashcraft 128). Thus, military coworkers and commanders are instructed to avoid bias while breastfeeding mothers are responsible for fitting in to military schedules, patterns, and workplace spaces. Assimilating difference through a logic of equivalence and standardization reforms rather than transforms the extant culture.

Breastfeeding in uniform is accommodated in the military workplace by disciplining lactating bodies to pumping schedules and social sanctions; in this way, the differences that such bodies offer is assimilated into a hegemonic cultural order. Even though a variety of programs and regulations now address mothering as a soldier, the visibility of breastfeeding support does not necessarily indicate that the invisible patterns and relations governing military conduct have been dramatically altered. Nonetheless, the warrior hero myth historically critical to military organization and war culture is undergoing change (Young and Kaurin)—in part thanks to the visible emergence of alternative identities, such as breastfeeding military mothers, and concurrent shifts in political culture.

THE GENDERED MILITARY: BREASTFEEDING IN UNIFORM AS SUBVERSIVE

Rather than a frontal assault on the gendered culture of military organizations, the subversiveness of breastfeeding in uniform may have more impact as a subversive cultural act (McFarlane). Public perceptions of breastfeeding in uniform reveal ambivalences over expectations for military conduct and bodies and over sanctions on breastfeeding as a public versus a private act. For example, in 2012, a photograph of two Air Force mothers breastfeeding, one mother with a twin on each breast, went viral and elicited a plethora of public comments (Sitt). Some hailed the image as a sign of support for military mothers and the military's accommodation of breastfeeding; others found the image to be a positive sign of change based in women's integration into the services. But negative comments focused on whether breastfeeding in uniform violated regulations, military decorum, and professionalism. Some comments speculated on whether the women in the photograph were promoting a lactivist "cause" while in uniform, casting the photograph as lactivist activism like nurse-ins and public breast-feeding advocacy (Boyer; Carpenter; Cassidy). (The photo was commissioned by Mom2Mom, a breastfeeding support group.) The conflicting reactions point to the photograph as a site of cultural contestation and contradiction.

Megan McFarlane argues that there is more at stake in the popular response than celebrating or disciplining military mothers: comments tapped an ideological chain of associations between U.S. national identity, U.S. global military dominance, and a gendered image of military service. Representing military personnel as breastfeeding mothers troubles the links between U.S. nationalism and militarism because such representations reframe national strength and readiness, betray patriotism for maternalism, and emasculate the military's image in the country and globally. At the same time, the increased visibility of women in uniform across all services and in most military assignments, including combat roles, has altered prevailing perceptions of gender roles. Breastfeeding in uniform can be seen as a testament to women's public sphere access and achievements.

Yet McFarlane points out that the visible breasts of a mother feeding twins confound the functional desexualization of nursing breasts with the highly sexualized breasts that are fetishized in male military indoctrination, socialization, and bonding rituals (Thompson). The photograph constructs a "discordant" perception of women in the military by blurring the boundaries between motherhood and sexuality as well as by confounding the roles of mother and combat soldier (signified by their camouflage uniforms), and by denying the uniformity required of military bodies. The photograph thus "antagonizes U.S. military culture" by showing women embracing their embodied difference, which complicates the depiction of patriotism, national identity, and gendered militarism (McFarlane 205). Ultimately, this photograph and others like it have the potential to subvert dominant categories and perceptions that underwrite hegemonic acceptance of the conflation of military might, U.S. global dominance, and gendered order. However, as the following section argues, this subversive potential is undermined by the representational politics of these photographs because they deflect possibilities for reflective public discussion.

REPRESENTATIONAL POLITICS: MILITARY BREASTFEEDING AS A "MISFITTING" SPECTACLE

The photographs of breastfeeding in uniform are visual arguments that invite particular ways of understanding what is at issue and why it matters. Photographer Tara Ruby's portrait of ten mother-soldiers in camouflage uniforms breastfeeding their infants went viral in 2015 (Bologna; Mosbergen). Ruby argued that her portrait makes a case for normalizing military breastfeeding. Yet the public responses to such images suggest that they circulated as what Stephen Best and Douglas Kellner identify as "interactive spectacles"—mediated and momentary amusements that spur collective response but deflect reflective deliberation and democratic action. I turn to Rosemarie Garland-Thomson's conceptualizations of disability representations to show how Ruby's photograph and others like it cast these breastfeeding mothers in an exotic rhetorical perspective that, rather than normalizing breastfeeding in uniform as intended, distances the viewer and draws attention to these figures as out of the ordinary.

In an insightful essay on the visual rhetorics of disability, Garland-Thompson argues that popular photographs of disabled bodies persuade viewers to see and understand disability in particular ways ("Seeing"). Rather than an unvarnished image of disability, such photographs "manipulate the viewer" to adopt a particular view of the photographic subject and "appropriate the disabled body" in the service of constructing such a viewpoint (339-40). One of the visual tropes she identifies is a "rhetoric of the exotic" in which the photographed figure is set at a distance from the viewer and cast as "sensationalized, eroticized, or entertaining in their difference" (343). Although lactation is certainly not a disability, the trope of the exotic marks the photographs of breastfeeding in uniform. In Ruby's portrait, exposed breasts and awkwardly held nursing infants set against camouflage uniforms and in an outdoors setting do not convey an image of normality. Instead, the viewer is positioned to stare rather than look away—a form of looking that takes the subject as a public spectacle in contrast to looking away which would be more typical if the image posed breastfeeding as a private act. In this way, cultural ambivalence over public breastfeeding is put on display, and the photograph sets up an exotic spectacle rather than an invitation to normalize breastfeeding at work.

Furthermore, the photograph poses breastfeeding as an interruption of work by showing these women in uniform but not working. The stigmas attending time and space accommodations for breastfeeding and/or pumping were discussed earlier; the photograph's ostensible purpose is to counter such stigmas, but instead they are implicitly present. Thus, the portrait of breastfeeding women in uniform ironically estranges the viewer, and invites admiration, ambivalence, or a sense of spectacle for an out-of-the-ordinary practice. In this way, the image unsettles its assurances that there is a place for breastfeeding (even in the military). As was evident in the anecdotes Roche-Paull included in *Breastfeeding in Combat Boots*, breastfeeding is hard to fit into a military workplace. A lactating body, a breast pump, uncomfortable spaces and inconvenient times for pumping—these are materialities that do not fit and resist material and policy accommodations.

Garland-Thomson develops the concept of "misfitting" as a feminist materialist understanding of embodied particularities and material environments. Rather than discursive constructions, she holds that identities are dynamically embodied: "Every body is in perpetual transformation not only in itself but also in its location within a constantly shifting environment" (600). Fitting is when the body that has been anticipated in the conceptualization, design, and construction of a material world navigates that world, the "uniform, standard, majority bodies" of such a material environment (595). This is an apt description of military regimens disciplining bodies and workplace environments fitted to standard male shapes, sizes, comportments, and sensory capacities. In contrast, lactating bodies resist such generic environments: "A misfit occurs when the world fails flesh in the environment one encounters" (600). For Garland-Thomson, such failures can produce new sensibilities about material experience along with strategies for navigating human, built, and natural environments in ways that do not deny but embrace relational and locational dependencies and vulnerabilities.

Ruby's portrait conveys "misfitting" not just in the discordance of uniforms, babies, and breasts but in the discomfort of the positions and relations among the twenty bodies—ten mothers and ten babies—in the frame. It is the discomfort itself that calls attention to the difficulties of integrating breastfeeding bodies into militarized environments. The image unsettles its assurances that there is a place for breastfeeding even in the military. In this sense, the military breastfeeding mothers as "misfits" offer a troublesome intrusion into military environments. That they do not "fit" is politically potent; rather than being assimilated into prevailing material arrangements, these "misfitting" bodies challenge the logic of sameness and equality and policies of fitting bodies to environments. Beyond the military organizations per se, these breastfeeding "misfitting" bodies mark a location from which to critique the gendered polarities, intensive labour, and discursive-material environments that configure contemporary work worlds.

CONCLUSION

The focus in this chapter has been on struggles over the meanings, identities, possibilities, and value of breastfeeding by active-duty servicewomen. Breastfeeding in uniform provokes contradictions and antagonisms that have significance for U.S. military culture, worklife arrangements, and the politics of gender. The chapter explores the challenges of breastfeeding through strategic interactions, discursive identity contradictions, the logics of organizational accommodation, and the subversive potential of breastfeeding images whether as confronting dominant understandings or as insisting on the "misfitting" relation of bodies and arrangements. Across these dimensions, a feminist communicology approach identifies multiple points for rearticulating prevailing constructions that marginalize breastfeeding military mothers. Breastfeeding is a critical site of struggle and possibility in military life carried out through the multifaceted dynamics of gendered communicative relations.

WORKS CITED

Acker, Joan. "Hierarchies, Jobs, Bodies: A Theory of Gendered Organizations." *Gender & Society*, vol. 4, no. 2, 1990, pp. 139-58.

Acker, Joan. "Inequality Regimes: Gender, Class, and Race in Organizations." *Gender & Society*, vol. 20, no. 4, 2006, pp. 441-64. *Sagepub.com*, doi: 10.1177/0891243206289499.

Ashcraft, Karen Lee. "Feminist Theory." *The Sage Handbook of Organizational Communication: Advances in Theory, Research, and Methods*, Third Ed., edited by Linda L. Putnam and Dennis K. Mumby, Sage, 2014, pp. 127-150.

Ashcraft, Karen, and Dennis K. Mumby. *Reworking Gender: A Feminist Communicology of Organization*. Sage Publications, 2003.

Best, Steven, and Douglas Kellner. "Debord and the Postmodern

Turn: New Stages of the Spectacle." *Illuminations: The Critical Theory Project*, pages.gseis.ucla.edu/faculty/kellner/Illumina%20 Folder/kell17.htm. Accessed 1 Oct. 2016.

Bologna, Caroline. "Working Moms Breastfeed in Uniform in Stunning Photos." *Huffington Post*, 21 Apr. 2016, www.huffingtonpost.com. Accessed 25 June 2016.

Boyer, Kate. "'The Way to Break the Taboo Is to Do the Taboo Thing': Breastfeeding in Public and Citizen-activism in the UK." *Health & Place*, vol. 17, no. 2, 2011, pp. 430-37. Elsevier, doi: 10.1016/j.healthplace.2010.06.013.

Buzzanell, Patrice M., and Meina Liu. "Struggling with Maternity Leave Policies and Practices: A Poststructuralist Feminist Analysis of Gendered Organizing." *Journal of Applied Communication Research*, vol. 33, no. 1, 2005, pp. 1-25. *Taylor & Francis Online*, doi: 10.1080/0090988042000318495.

Carpenter, Faedra Chatard. "'(L)Activists and Lattes': Breastfeeding Advocacy as Domestic Performance." *Women & Performance: A Journal of Feminist Theory*, vol. 16, no. 3, 2006, pp. 347-67. *Taylor & Francis Online*, doi: 10.1080/07407700600955354.

Carreiras, Helena. *Gender and the Military: Women in the Armed Forces of Western Democracies*. Routledge, 2006.

Cassidy, Tanya M. "Making 'Milky Matches': Globalization, Maternal Trust and 'Lactivist' Online Networking." *Journal of the Motherhood Initiative for Research and Community Involvement*, vol. 3, no. 1, 2012, pp. 226-40.

Department of Defense. *2014 Demographics: Profile of the Military Community*. Washington DC: Office of the Deputy Assistant Secretary of Defense, 2014.

Garland-Thomson, Rosemarie. "Misfits: A Feminist-materialist Disability Concept." *Hypatia*, vol. 26, no. 3, 2011, pp. 591-609. *Wiley Online Library*, doi: 10.1111/j.1527-2001.2011.01206.x.

Garland-Thomson, Rosemarie. "Seeing the Disabled: Visual Rhetorics of Disability in Popular Photography." *The New Disability History: American Perspectives*, edited by Paul K. Longmore and Lauri Umansky, New York University Press, 2001, pp. 335-374.

Goffman, Erving. *Stigma: Notes on the Management of Spoiled Identity*. Simon and Schuster, 2009.

Marshall, Joyce L., et al. "Being a 'Good Mother': Managing

Breastfeeding and Merging Identities." *Social Science & Medicine*, vol. 65, no. 10, 2007, pp. 2147-159. *Elsevier*, doi: 10.1016/j.socscimed.2007.06.015.

McFarlane, Megan D. "Breastfeeding as Subversive: Mothers, Mammaries and the Military." *International Feminist Journal of Politics*, vol. 17, no. 2, 2015, pp. 191-208. *Taylor & Francis Online*, doi: 10.1080/14616742.2013.849967.

Mathers, Jennifer G. "Women and State Military Forces." *Women & Wars*, edited by Carol Cohn, Polity Press, 2013, pp. 124-45.

Meisenbach, Rebecca J. "Stigma Management Communication: A Theory and Agenda for Applied Research on How Individuals Manage Moments of Stigmatized Identity." *Journal of Applied Communication Research*, vol. 38, no. 3, 2010, pp. 268-92. Taylor & Francis Online, doi: 10.1080/00909882.2010.490841.

Mosbergen, Dominique. "Stunning Photo Shows Soldiers Breastfeeding in Full Uniform." *Huffington Post*, 15 Sept. 2015, www.huffingtonpost.com. Accessed 25 June 2016.

Murphy, E. "Risk, Responsibility, and Rhetoric in Infant Feeding." *Journal of Contemporary Ethnography*, vol. 29, no. 3, 2000, pp. 291-325. *Sagepub.com*, doi: 10.1177/089124100129023927.

Holmer-Nadesan, Majia, and Patty Sotirin. "The Romance and Science of 'Breast Is Best': Discursive Contradictions and Contexts of Breastfeeding Choices." *Text and Performance Quarterly*, vol. 18, no. 3, 1998, pp. 217-32.

Maguire, Kathryn C. "Military Family Communication: A Review and Synthesis of the Research Related to Wartime Deployment." *A Communication Perspective on the Military*, edited by Erin Sahlstein Parcell and Lynne M. Webb, Peter Lang, pp. 19-38.

Parcell, Erin Sahlstein. "Research at the Intersections of the Military and Communication: A Preview and Review." *A Communication Perspective on the Military,* edited by Erin Sahlstein Parcell and Lynne M. Webb, Peter Lang, pp. 1-18.

Pawelczyk, Joanne. "Constructing American Female War Veterans' Military Identity in the Context of Interviews." *Women & Language*, vol. 37, no. 1, 2014, pp. 87-112.

Payne, Deborah, and David A. Nicholls. "Managing Breastfeeding and Work: A Foucauldian Secondary Analysis." *Journal of Advanced Nursing*, vol. 66, 2010, pp. 1810-818. *Wiley Online*

Library, doi: 10.1111/j.1365-2648.2009.05156.x.

Prividera, Laura C. and John W. Howard III. "Paradoxical Injunctions and Double Binds: A Critical Examination of Discourse on Female Soldiers." *Women & Language*, vol. 35, no. 2, 2012, pp. 53-73.

Roche-Paull, Robyn. *Breastfeeding in Combat Boots: A Survival Guide to Breastfeeding Successfully While Serving in the Military.* Hale Publishing, 2016.

Rychnovsky, Jacqueline D. "Postpartum Fatigue in the Active-duty Military Woman." *Journal of Obstetric, Gynecologic, & Neonatal Nursing*, vol. 36, no. 1, 2007, pp. 38-46. *Wiley Online Library*, doi: 10.1111/j.1552-6909.2006.00112.x.

Shaw, Rhonda. "Performing Breastfeeding: Embodiment, Ethics and the Maternal Subject." *Feminist Review*, vol. 78, no. 1, 2004, pp. 99-116.

Sitt, Pamela. "Military Mom 'Proud' of Breastfeeding, Despite Criticism." *Today*, 30 May 2012. www.today.com. Accessed 1 Oct. 2016.

Sleutel, Martha Rider. "Breastfeeding During Military Deployment." *Nursing for Women's Health*, vol. 16, no. 1, 2012, pp. 20-25. *Wiley Online Library*, doi: 0.1111/j.1751-486X.2012.01696.x

Stevens, Kevin V., and Jill Janke. "Breastfeeding Experiences of Active Duty Military Women." *Military Medicine*, vol. 168, no. 5, 2003, p. 380.

Thompson, Marie. "Military Sexual Trauma: Bridging the Chasm Between Trauma and Support." *Women & Language*, vol. 37, no. 1, 2014, pp. 131-38.

Turner, Paaige K. and Kristen Norwood. "Bounded Motherhood: Embodying a Good Working Mother Identity." *Management Communication Quarterly*, vol. 27, no. 3, 2013, pp. 396-424. *Sagepub.com*, doi: 10.1177/0893318913491461.

Young, Anna M. and Pauline Kaurin. "The Myth of the Warrior: Rhetorics of Masculinity and Don't Ask Don't Tell." *A Communication Perspective on the Military*, edited by Erin Sahlstein Parcell and Lynne M. Webb, Peter Lang, pp. 411-30.

11. Legal Representations of Breastfeeding

On Angela Ames and Sex Discrimination

DANA LLOYD[1]

In an introductory chapter to his book *Fear and Trembling*, the Danish philosopher Søren Kierkegaard imagines alternative scenarios to that of the sacrifice of Isaac in the book of Genesis. In each of these portraits, Abraham, the father who is about to murder his son, is compared with a figure of a mother weaning her child (9-14). Without digressing into the details of this original and intriguing introduction, I want to point out that Kierkegaard, albeit a childless man, saw something that is usually invisible to nineteenth-century philosophers: philosophers tend to assign meaning to our mortality rather than our natality, to the fact of our death as opposed to the fact that we are all, as Adrienne Rich has reminded us, "of woman born." Kierkegaard, on the other hand, focuses on weaning as an event in a mother's life—and in a child's life—that is not only rich with meaning but also with terror. The moment of individuation is compared with that of the most (in)famous sacrifice in Western culture. And if weaning is given such status, it means that Kierkegaard recognizes the significance of breastfeeding both to the mother and to the child. The uniqueness of this introduction to a book in philosophy reveals that breastfeeding is something that philosophers (as opposed to psychoanalysis theorists, for example) usually do not see or do not want to see or to think about. As Sarah LaChance Adams and Caroline R. Lundquist note,

> conception, pregnancy, childbirth, the child's first word, the first steps, and so on ... are the experiences that women

> are usually more involved in than men. Yet, since women have largely been excluded from the practice of academic philosophy, their experiences have rarely found just representation in the canon. As a result, philosophy has a long history of ignoring, misunderstanding, reappropriating, and denigrating pregnancy, childbirth, and mothering. (1)

Joshua Shaw adds that: "There is a tradition ... of philosophers philosophizing about fatherhood. Yet they seem to be oddly unwilling to philosophize about motherhood.... Virtually all philosophers who have taken motherhood as a topic worthy of sustained and serious inquiry have been women philosophers" (139). Not only is breastfeeding regarded as meaningless in the history of philosophy, it is also too messy, too emotional, too bodily, and too private to write about analytically. Breastfeeding as a private and domestic practice has to do both with its equation with so-called good motherhood and with the sexualization of the female breast (Smith 375; Braudo 223).[2] As we will see in this chapter, not only philosophy but also law tends to ignore pregnancy, childbirth, and breastfeeding (Christrup 263). The absence of nursing mothers from law and from philosophy—two authoritative realms of knowledge to which we often turn to determine what is right—is related to a more general cultural approach that restricts motherhood to the private sphere. As such, the absence of breastfeeding mothers from philosophy and from the law can begin to explain the case of Angela Ames v. Nationwide Mutual Insurance.[3]

In 2012, Angela Ames lost her job at Nationwide Insurance Company because she was a breastfeeding mother. She filed a sex-discrimination suit that was rejected because "men can lactate under some circumstances" (Sherwin). Not only does this rationale sound absurd and outrageous ("silly," as described by Amanda Marcotte in *Slate*), it also seems, at first glance, to contradict the rationale of previous cases (e.g., Martinez v. N.B.C., Inc., a breastfeeding-related sex-discrimination suit, was rejected because men cannot breastfeed).[4] But a closer look exposes the underlying notion common to all those cases—one that understands pregnancy, childbirth, and breastfeeding scientifically, as mere biological functions. In this chapter, I argue that this scientific notion blinds the courts from seeing the deep gender inequality that their decisions promote.[5] What will happen if we give up the biomedical definition of pregnancy, childbirth, and breastfeeding? A focus on pregnancy, childbirth, and breastfeeding as socially constructed will reveal, I argue, norms of good motherhood and of the ideal worker as well as the regime of domesticity of which these norms are a part. This regime, together with the scientific approach to pregnancy, childbirth and breastfeeding, not only domesticates (privatizes) motherhood but individualizes it—making each case seem as a unique case of a bad employee who happens to be a mother who chose to "go home and be with [her] babies."[6] For social change to become possible, norms of good motherhood and of ideal workers must be exposed and addressed together.[7]

This collection of essays is about cultural representations of breastfeeding, and this chapter focuses on legal representations. A few words of explanation about the relation between law and culture are, therefore, necessary. Law and culture maintain a close and dynamic relationship. Cultural representations of breastfeeding both construct the legal meaning given to breastfeeding and reflect legal ideologies about gender equality and the position of the nursing mother in the workplace. In Renée Ann Cramer's words, we can see "law and culture as mutually constitutive, as mutually self-reinforcing, and as mutually regulatory" (20). In other words, the way courts understand motherhood is detached neither from motherhood's representation in popular culture nor from the lack of representation of motherhood in the history of philosophy; court decisions about nursing mothers also reinforce notions about women's equality already common in our society. Pregnancy, breastfeeding, and motherhood are socially constructed and culturally situated; they are not merely natural phenomena. Law is understood as culture, Greg Johnson argues, "not only in the sense of being contained by culture, but in the more particular sense of doing the work of culture: making and marking the distinctive boundaries of human sociality, meaning, and power" (282-83).[8] Therefore, the decision in Angela Ames's case is not only a legal document but also cultural one.

Part one of this chapter will retell Angela's story and recount the decisions of the courts that heard it. Part two will locate the case in the context of previous case law and relevant legislation, showing that even though the decision in Ames seems unique, it is actually in line with other cases of sex-discrimination based on pregnancy and breastfeeding. The Conclusion will propose to abandon the biomedical understanding of pregnancy and breastfeeding and to expose the social norms that are at the background of gender inequality, specifically in the context of motherhood. It will finally raise the question what may happen to the popular imagination when the social construction of pregnancy and breastfeeding is revealed, and social policies are tailored to address it.

ON ANGELA AMES

Here is Angela's story as it is told in the decision of the Iowa District Court.[9] Angela Ames was hired as a loss-mitigation specialist at Nationwide Mutual Insurance in October 2008. She gave birth to her first child in May 2009, and discovered that she was pregnant again in October 2009. Having suffered pregnancy complications, Angela was ordered on bedrest in April 2010. She encountered hostile reactions from the head of her department, Karla Neel (who rolled her eyes and said that she had never had to go on bedrest when she had been pregnant) and from her immediate supervisor, Brian Brinks (who remarked to others in the office: "Oh, yeah, I'm teasing her about only taking a week's worth of maternity leave. We're too busy for her to take off that much work" [Ames v. Nationwide Mutual Insurance, 765]).

Angela gave birth to her second child prematurely in May 2010. Nationwide, thereafter, informed Angela that her Family Medical Leave Act (FMLA) maternity leave would expire on 2 August 2010. In June, Neel called Angela to inform her that there had been a mistake in calculating her maternity leave and that it would expire three weeks earlier than she had been told previously (Ames v. Nationwide Mutual Insurance, 766). Neel also told Angela that she could take additional unpaid leave until August, but that doing so would "cause red flags," that she "[did not] want there to be any problems like that," and that she "[did not] want there to be any issues down the road" (766). Neel finally offered to extend Angela's maternity leave an additional week. Angela had, therefore, two months to recover from childbirth before returning to work. During her maternity leave, Angela was told that she would be able to use a lactation room to express milk after her return to work.

Angela returned to work in July, as agreed, when her son was two months old and, according to the court, was breastfeeding every three hours (Ames v. Nationwide Mutual Insurance 766).[10] By the time Angela arrived at work that first morning, more than three hours had passed since her son had last nursed. Angela asked Neel to use a lactation room. Neel replied that it was not her responsibility to provide her with one. Angela then turned to the company nurse, who informed her of Nationwide's lactation policy, which required the completion of paperwork that took three days to be processed. When Angela told the nurse that she needed to express milk immediately, the nurse suggested that Angela use a wellness room, but the wellness room was occupied, and Angela's breastmilk would be exposed to germs there. While waiting for the wellness room, Angela met with Brinks to discuss her work. Brinks told Angela that none of her work had been completed while she had been on maternity leave, that she had two weeks to complete that work, that she would have to work overtime to accomplish this, and that if she failed to catch up, she would be disciplined. After that meeting, Angela returned to Neel's office to see if she could help her to find a place to pump milk, and Neel refused again. Angela was visibly upset and in tears, and so Neel handed her a piece of paper and a pen and told her, "You know, I think it's best that you go home to be with your babies." Neel dictated to Angela what to write on the piece of paper to effectuate her resignation (Ames v. Nationwide Mutual Insurance 766).

Angela sued Nationwide, alleging sex and pregnancy discrimination. Her complaint asserted that the unavailability of a lactation room, "her urgent need to express milk," and Nationwide's "unrealistic and unreasonable expectations about her work production" (5) forced her to resign from her position. The Iowa District Court ruled that there was no constructive discharge (33), and that even if there was, it would not have counted as sex discrimination (38, 41). And here is its reasoning:

> Ames has not presented sufficient evidence that lactation is a medical condition related to pregnancy ... lactation can be induced by stimulating the body to produce milk even though the person has not experienced a recent birth or pregnancy ... Additionally, the Court takes judicial notice of the fact that adoptive mothers can also breast-feed their adoptive babies ... Furthermore, it is a scientific fact that even men have milk ducts and the hormones responsible for milk production. (12, n. 28)

The court of appeals upheld this ruling,[11] and the U.S. Supreme Court refused to hear the case,[12] effectively affirming that there was no sex-discrimination in Angela's case because breastfeeding is not the exclusive practice of a mother who recently gave birth to a baby. In doing so, writes Laura Iris Mattes, "the court is concluding that no reasonable juror could find that these circumstances reflect pregnancy discrimination as prohibited under the PDA.[13] This deeply undermines the purpose of the PDA, shifts attention away from the employer's poor behavior, and places unreasonable burdens on the employee" (381).

Although a reading of this case as radically subverting the heteronormative order by refusing to treat breastfeeding as an exclusively feminine practice is possible, I doubt that a court who uses such reasoning to deny a woman her right to breastfeed is likely to protect the right of a transman to do so (Matambanadzo).

This ruling reveals something about the court's conception of equality as well as its conception of parenthood. Equality, as understood in this case, is formal. If both men and women can produce milk, and they are both subject to the same policy with regards to accessing the lactation room—then there is no sex-discrimination in Angela's case. Traditionally, women were excluded from the workforce based on stereotypical notions of essential womanhood; women are different from men, and they naturally belong in the private sphere. The case of Angela Ames shows us that the same exclusion can be easily achieved using the rhetoric of sameness. This rhetoric treats women as identical to men in terms of their position in the workplace, and ignores the reality of inequality that affects women's participation in the paid-work market.

Because equality is conceived of formalistically,[14] it becomes an individual right. Women's precarious position is not considered at all when thinking of discrimination. Here are some numbers. Women comprise almost half of the workforce in the United States and two-thirds of the low-wage workforce, according to a 2014 report by the National Women's Law Center.[15] In 2015, according to the Bureau of Labor Statistics, around two-thirds of mothers with children under six worked.[16] According to a report by the Pew Research Center, in 40 percent of households with children, women are now the sole or primary breadwinners.[17] Since women are now having children at a much later age than they used to a few decades ago, they now have babies right in the middle of their peak earning periods, and their earnings are crucial to the economic stability of their families (Traister 14). And motherhood takes an economic and practical toll on their careers. On average, whereas men's earnings increase by 6 percent after having children, a woman's earnings decrease by 7 percent for every child she has (Matambanadzo 200). The difficulty with conceptualizing the problem in terms of inequality is that it individualizes it and allows the courts to treat each of the cases brought before them as private cases of bad workers or overly dedicated mothers, whose dismissal by an unsatisfied employer is justified.

The court does not understand parenthood as a right that deserves its protection, especially not active parenthood. Motherhood (or so-called good motherhood) is still understood as something that is done in private, and it has no room in the public sphere. It is not that the court understands good motherhood as anything other than active motherhood. Neel's words—"you should go home and be with your babies"—are quoted several times in the court's decision.[18] Good motherhood equals active motherhood, but it belongs in the private sphere, not in the workplace. Indeed, as long as a woman can successfully be an ideal worker and an ideal mother at the same time, everything is okay. Once her performance as an ideal worker conflicts with her ability to be an ideal mother, she is sent home.

Angela is represented as a unique woman, who chose motherhood over good performance at work, and whose case does not raise any doubts about the employer's policy. Angela's case is privatized and individualized. It also neutralizes her motherhood, turning it into "parenthood." As Noya Rimalt notes, "In an age of neutral parental equality, when the right to motherhood has officially become the right to parenthood, an explicit discussion of especially-devoted motherhood practices ... presents activists who strive to promote women's position in the workforce with a significant ideological difficulty" (624-45).[19] Given all this, is equality the best potential route to take in cases related to mothers' paid work? Could there be an alternative conceptual route? Can we talk about the right to parenthood in this context? And if there is such a thing as a right to parenthood, is it possessed by both mothers and fathers? Can good mothers take part in the realm of paid work? Although these questions are largely outside the scope of this chapter, I believe that examining them through the lens of breastfeeding has a unique potential to reveal their complexity because breastfeeding exists in an in-between space, between the biological (pregnancy) and cultural (childrearing)—a space that allows norms of good motherhood to enter the scene and play an essential role. Angela's case may seem unique, but what can we discover if we read it against the background of relevant case law and legislation? The next section is dedicated to this background.

ON SEX DISCRIMINATION

Henry Wiatt Christrup writes that "Every year more than one million women are forced to choose between breastfeeding their children and keeping their jobs" (263). This rhetoric of choice repeats itself in the literature on breastfeeding and work. Thus, for example, a 2011 article in the *American Journal of Public Health* suggests that "improving the ability of mothers to breastfeed or to express and store milk in the workplace would likely contribute to higher U.S. breastfeeding rates" (Murtagh and Moulton 217). The rhetoric of choice goes hand in hand with a focus on the benefits of breastfeeding, and although I share the belief in the many advantages of breastfeeding, I find this focus as problematic as the rhetoric of choice it accompanies. Instead of counting the ways in which breastfeeding benefits mothers and children alike, then, I would like to shift our attention to the norms of good motherhood at play here; if social change is what we are interested in, it is social explanations that we need to seek and critique.[20]

Breastfeeding one's child is often equated with good motherhood, and not only by those whose explicit agenda is to domesticate women. Take, for example, a chapter in an edited collection with a clear feminist agenda, in which the authors declare that "Part of being a good mother is breastfeeding one's infant, or at least attempting in good faith to do so" (Overall and Bernard 49). Although the authors undoubtedly mean well—calling not for social interference with maternal practices but for "finding ways to provide support for women's role as breastfeeders" (50)—their equation of good motherhood with breastfeeding demonstrates the way in which the norm of the good mother is enforced. Clair O'Hagan critiques the rhetoric of choice and the privatization of the issue of pregnancy and breastfeeding discrimination as closely related:

> The inequalities women experience are constructed as private troubles, and their privileges are constructed as the outcome of their freely made choices, which is why women appear to accept a situation which is patently unfair.... Women experience powerless responsibility, and because they are seduced by the illusion of choice, they do not see the operation of power, but accept their inequalities as personal troubles. (180)

Not surprisingly, the rhetoric of choice in the literature is repeated in the case law. Let us begin the (brief) exploration of the case law and legislation that are at the background of the Ames decision with the case of General Electric Co. v. Gilbert[21] and its notorious interpretation of Title VII of the Civil Rights Act of 1964 as excluding pregnancy discrimination from the category of sex discrimination.[22] Title VII counts as protected classes race, colour, religion, sex, and national origin. A sex-discrimination claim under Title VII can be made within different legal frameworks, including disparate treatment and disparate impact.[23] The respondents in General Electric Co. v. Gilbert filed a disparate impact claim, concerning the company's disability plan, which covered all temporary conditions except pregnancy-related disabilities. According to the court, the policy did not discriminate against women because its pregnancy exclusion "was not in itself discrimination based on sex" (135). The reasoning the court provided was that the two relevant classes are "pregnant women and non-pregnant persons. While the first group is exclusively female, the second includes members of both sexes" (135). In order to prove sex discrimination, claimants have to show that a group comprised only of women is disadvantaged in comparison with a group comprised only of men. Justices Brennan, Marshall and Stevens dissented, noting that "Surely it offends common sense to suggest ... that a classification revolving around pregnancy is not, at the minimum, strongly 'sex related'" (149). The classifications "pregnant women" and "non-pregnant persons" strongly suggest that pregnancy is a matter of choice and that a woman who is also a good worker can choose not to become pregnant; it portrays as legitimate the choice of a career over family life.

Two years later, in 1978, Congress passed the Pregnancy Discrimination Act (PDA) in response to the Gilbert decision.[24] The PDA amends Title VII of the Civil Rights Act by defining sex discrimination to include pregnancy, childbirth, and related medical conditions:

> The terms "because of sex" or "on the basis of sex" include, but are not limited to, because of or on the basis of pregnancy, childbirth, or related medical conditions; and women affected by pregnancy, childbirth, or related medical conditions shall be treated the same for all employment-related purposes, including receipt of benefits under fringe benefit programs, as other persons not so affected but similar in their ability or inability to work.

Although the purpose of this legislation was "to guarantee women the basic right to participate fully and equally in the workforce, without denying them the fundamental right to full participation in family life,"[25] one of its major limitations "emerges from the fact that it does not explicitly define pregnancy or provide guidance for determining the scope of related medical conditions that the Act addresses" (Matambanadzo 189). Therefore, the courts can apply Gilbert's reasoning to breastfeeding discrimination claims.

The Gilbert decision created the absurd situation in which "while only women could become pregnant, no discrimination was established because there were nonpregnant women in the second group" (Hansen 901). But in the dissent (which was embraced by Congress), the two classes compared are not pregnant women versus everyone else, but, instead, "*those who face a risk of pregnancy* (women) versus *those who do not* (men)" (Hansen 901, emphasis in original). If we accept this as the logic of the PDA then breastfeeding should be recognized as protected by Title VII. And although the terminology of "risk" has obvious negative connotations, it at least abandons the rhetoric of choice. Nevertheless, the courts have used sex-plus analysis to create two categories: breastfeeding employees versus all other employees, which embraces the rhetoric of choice once again.[26]

In Martinez v. N.B.C., Inc., the plaintiff alleged that her employer failed to accommodate her need to express breastmilk following her pregnancy. The court cited the Gilbert case approvingly, holding that there was no sex-plus discrimination "*for the quite simple reason that men are physiologically incapable of pumping breast milk*, so plaintiff cannot show that she was treated less favorably than similarly situated men" (309-10, emphasis in original). Similarly, in Derungs v. Wal-Mart Stores, Inc.,[27] plaintiffs filed a claim of sex discrimination after they were not allowed to breastfeed their children in the defendant's stores. The court held that "for there to be impermissible sex discrimination, there must be one gender that is treated differently than another. Feeding infants is not something that only one parent can accomplish, and even the feeding of breast milk may be done by either parent from a bottle" (437). The court concluded that "the Plaintiffs cannot establish such 'sex-plus' ... discrimination, absent evidence that Wal-Mart treated a corresponding sub-class (i.e., men who breast-feed) better by allowing them to engage in breastfeeding activity in its stores" (437). This reasoning may not be as absurd as the Ames reasoning (that not only women but also men can lactate), but it reinforces the rhetoric of choice that we find in other cases, according to which women can (and must) choose between breastfeeding their children and participating in public life.

CONCLUSION

At a first glance, the Ames decision—breastfeeding is not the exclusive practice of women who recently gave birth—seems to contradict the logic of the cases surveyed above, which rejects sex-discrimination claims because men cannot breastfeed. Nevertheless, I argue that Ames ultimately follows the same notion that justifies discrimination scientifically. The scientific fact cited may be that men cannot become pregnant and cannot breastfeed or that men can, indeed, breastfeed. Whatever the supporting evidence, the outcome is always the same: breastfeeding discrimination is not sex discrimination. Saru M. Matambanadzo terms this reliance on scientific approaches "biomedical essentialism," which she defines as "an ideological perspective that reduces the process of pregnancy to its biological and physiological facets, obscuring the important ways in which society and culture shape the meaning of pregnancy and structure our experience of it" (190). The biomedical approach to pregnancy is extended to breastfeeding because both legal decisions and feminist legal scholarship present an understanding of breastfeeding as an extension of pregnancy.[28] Understanding breastfeeding as merely an extension of pregnancy, a biological fact, conceals the centrality of breastfeeding—as a phenomenon separate than that of pregnancy—to the common definition of good motherhood as a form of motherhood that is incompatible with being a good worker.

What may we see if we look beyond this biomedical essentialism, and beyond the scientific justification for discrimination? There is an unbridgeable gap between the realities of mothers' lives—such as that of Angela—and the legal discourse in which the ideal of equal parenting frames the discussion of women's rights (Rimalt 625). In our social reality, sex discrimination overlaps with discrimination on the basis of parenthood. Although the courts have adopted a view of equal parenting, society still sees mothers as mainly responsible for childrearing, and women are disproportionally affected by discrimination on the basis of parenthood in the workplace (625). Even though it is generally positive that the law can now imagine active fathers (who cannot only bottle-feed but even breastfeed their babies!), this notion is still being used to exclude women from the workforce rather than to allow for their inclusion, as the Ames decision demonstrates.[29]

The rhetoric of gender neutrality is tightly related to the rhetoric of choice that dominates court decisions. As Daphna Hacker and Michal Frankel argue, the ideology of "choice" between paid work and caring for one's child is itself a part of the apparatus that reproduces and legitimates gender inequality in the workplace as well as in the domestic sphere. In fact, this is not a matter of free choice but of subjection to social norms of the ideal mother and the ideal worker (281). If we are to challenge these norms, we need to challenge both at the same time because they are defined in opposition to each other: "Anything that constructs or favors men as Breadwinners also constructs or favors women as Mothers ... The only way out of this cycle is change in the nature of waged labor, that is, change in both discriminatory practices *and* the norm of the Ideal Worker ... men and women must become *both* workers and parents at the same time" (Slaughter 74, emphasis in original).[30]

For change to be possible, breastfeeding mothers—real breast-feeding mothers—must be present in the public sphere and represented culturally. As long as breastfeeding mothers only appear in professional debates—the debates of nurses and doctors who want to guide young mothers or of courts that have to decide cases related to breastfeeding—our lives will remain limited to the private sphere, where we ought to be if we want to be good mothers. A "thick description" of the social and cultural aspects of motherhood and breastfeeding transcending the biomedical model is not available to lawmakers and judges who have to make decisions with regards to breastfeeding mothers' lives.[31] Indeed, the cultural representations of motherhood in general are limited. Although some "accounts idealize the mother's relationship to her child, emphasizing love, connection, and fecundity" using metaphors of motherhood and ignoring its reality, "those who resist the poetic impulse tend to consider pregnancy, childbirth and mothering as obstacles to women's participation in public life and to their financial independence" (Adams 4). As we saw at the opening of this chapter, nursing mothers are generally absent in the history of philosophy; given the way that the law looks at nursing mothers, I would suggest we understand this absence as reflective of a generalized attitude about nursing mothers that firmly relegates them to the private sphere. With such a limited understanding of motherhood and of breastfeeding, it is impossible to expect courts to decide cases such as Angela's differently. If we want change to become possible, a "thick description"—drawing on interdisciplinary scholarship and on other cultural materials—of the phenomenon of breastfeeding must be available to the judges who make decisions about nursing mothers' lives and work and about women's equality more generally. Rebecca Asher writes that "In so many ways modern society is intent on overcoming biological constraints, from assisted conception to athletic prowess. Yet giving birth and breastfeeding permanently define a woman's life, and differentiate it from a man's, in a way that is drearily unimaginative and restrictive" (5). Only diverse representation of nursing mothers—and of parenthood in general—in the public sphere, in popular culture, in philosophy, and in the legal realm, I believe, will enable the broadening of our social imagination to include images of women and men that are more than good mothers or good workers.

ENDNOTES

[1]A previous version of this chapter was presented in the annual conference of NWSA in Milwaukee in 2015. I am grateful for the comments and encouragement of the organizers, participants and audience in the panel in which it was presented. I also wish to thank the anonymous reviewer for her helpful comments.

[2]Although in this chapter I focus on the equation of breastfeeding with so-called good motherhood and not on the sexualization of the breast, I think the two are inseparable.

[3]Ames v. Nationwide Mutual Insurance Co., 760 F.3d 763, 766 (8th Cir. 2014), cert. denied, 135 S. Ct. 947 (2015).

[4]Martinez v. NBC, Inc., 49 F. Supp. 2d 305 (S.D.N.Y. 1999).

[5]As Paige Hall Smith notes, "although there are biological differences between men and women, these differences are not responsible for the arrangement of social institutions that construct gender inequalities. Instead, culturally elaborated distinctions between

men and women can form the basis of a socially constructed distribution of power that values masculinity over femininity" (376).
[6]Ames v. Nationwide Mutual Insurance Company, 760 F.3d, 763, at 766.
[7]According to Patricia Boling, this privatization is a uniquely American issue, and it has prevented American women from uniting across class and racial divides to demand state sponsored quality childcare (172-73).
[8]See also Rosen.
[9]Ames v. Nationwide Mutual Insurance, No. 4:11-cv-00359 RP-RAW (S.D. Iowa, Oct. 16, 2012).
[10]I believe that the absence of nursing mothers from popular culture and from intellectual discourse, as well as the 'scientific' approach to breastfeeding allows the courts to determine that at the age of two months, infants nurse every three hours. Every mother knows that this is not the case, and I find this remark particularly outrageous.
[11]Ames v. Nationwide Mutual Insurance, 760 F.3d 763, 766 (8th Cir. 2014).
[12] Certiorari denied, 135 S. Ct. 947 (2015).
[13]Pregnancy Discrimination Act (1978).
[14]U.S. courts understand equality as Aristotle did: treating like cases alike and different cases differently. This notion has been critiqued extensively by feminist scholars. See, for example, McKinnon 33 and Williams 205.
[15]National Women's Law Center.
[16]See United States Government.
[17]See Wang, Wendy, et al.
[18]The ACLU amicus brief talks about this norm in terms of "the illegal sex stereotype that women would prioritize child care responsibilities over paid employment" (7) and about Neel's statement as completely embodying this stereotype (8).
[19]Lisa Hansen writes that:

> Ironically, American feminists have unwittingly contributed to the difficulties working mothers face because, unlike European feminists, who sought to lessen the dual burdens of home and work, the American feminist movement focused on a notion of parity and equality between women and men. Rather than acknowledging women's sex-specific

> differences, and advocating for recognition and accommodation of these traits, including support for working mothers in the workplace, American feminists have shied away from making these demands out of fear that the fight for women's equality will be diluted (Hansen 892).

Paige Hall Smith adds that "Because the bodily and biological differences between men and women are not the true source of social gender inequities, the social and feminist decisions to ignore real differences in biological abilities or needs does not necessarily lead to gender equality" (376).

[20]If the balance between nurturing one's child and participating in the workforce is a matter of choice, then we can define a "good" mother as she who chooses to "go home and be with [her] children" and a "good" worker as he who chooses otherwise.

[21]General Electric Co. v. Gilbert, 429 U.S. 125 (1976).

[22]For a more extensive survey of the case law and the legislation that preceded the Ames decision, see Kasdan 317-32, and Hansen 897-905.

[23]Disparate treatment means that an employee was subject to an adverse employment action because she belongs to a protected group. A claim of disparate impact is established by demonstrating that an employer had a specific employment practice that, though facially neutral, had a disproportionate effect upon a protected class. Disparate impact, unlike disparate treatment, does not require proof of intentional discrimination by an employer.

[24]See Newport News Shipbuilding & Dry Dock Co. v. EEOC, 462 U.S. 669 (1983).

[25]California Federal Savings & Loan Ass'n v. Guerra, 479 U.S. 272, (1987), at 289.

[26]The sex-plus theory involves a comparison between two similarly situated groups of men and women who share an additional characteristic. Sex-plus discrimination occurs when an employer subjects a person to discrimination based on the person's sex, plus the additional factor (Hansen 901-2).

[27]Derungs v. Wal-Mart Stores, 374 F.3d 428 (2004).

[28]This equation is also related to the language of the PDA, which extends the protection of Title VII to "pregnancy, childbirth, or related medical conditions," although the courts have tended to

reject breastfeeding as a medical condition related to pregnancy and childbirth (Hansen 903).

[29]Rebecca Asher argues that "Society chooses to base the entire parenting structure on this one biological fact. We magnify the differences between men and women instead of recognising that their commonalities are greater and acknowledging that both parents can play a part in the day-to-day care of their children as well as in the wider world" (5).

[30]See also: ACLU Amicus Brief 6-7; Braudo 232; O'Hagan 195; and Abrams, who calls women with children to "challenge the notion of a natural or pre-ordained line dividing work and family" (1223).

[31]This argument follows that of Matambanadzo's in the context of pregnancy.

WORKS CITED

Case Law

Supreme Court

California Federal Savings & Loan Ass'n v. Guerra, 479 U.S. 272, (1987).

General Electric Co. v. Gilbert, 429 U.S. 125 (1976).

Newport News Shipbuilding & Dry Dock Co. v. EEOC, 462 U.S. 669 (1983).

Circuit Courts

Ames v. Nationwide Mutual Insurance Co., 760 F.3d 763, 766 (8th Cir. 2014).

District Courts

Ames v. Nationwide Mutual Insurance, No. 4:11-cv-00359 RP-RAW (S.D. Iowa, Oct. 16, 2012).

Derungs v. Wal-Mart Stores, 374 F.3d 428 (2004).

Martinez v. NBC, Inc., 49 F. Supp. 2d 305 (S.D.N.Y. 1999).

Other Legal Documents

American Civil Liberties Union Foundation, Brief of *Amici Curiae*,

No. 12-3780, Ames v. Nationwide Mutual Insurance Co., 760 F.3d 763, 766 (8th Cir. 2014).

Articles and Books

Abrams, Kathryn. "Gender Discrimination and the Transformation of Workplace Norms." *Vanderbilt Law Review*, vol. 42, no. 4, 1989, pp. 1183-1248.

Adams, Sarah LaChance. *Mad Mothers, Bad Mothers, and What a "Good" Mother Would Do: The Ethics of Ambivalence*. Columbia University Press, 2014.

Adams, Sarah LaChance, and Caroline R. Lundquist, editors. *Coming to Life: Philosophies of Pregnancy, Childbirth, and Mothering*. Fordham University Press, 2013.

Asher, Rebecca. *Shattered: Modern Motherhood and the Illusion of Equality*. Random House, 2011.

Boling, Patricia. *The Politics of Work–Family Policies*. Cambridge University Press, 2015.

Braudo, Yael. "Looking Medusa in the Eye: Breastfeeding and the Public Sphere." (Hebrew) *Labor, Society and Law*, vol. 12, 2010, pp. 219-59.

Christup, Henry Wyatt. "Litigating a Breastfeeding and Employment Case in the New Millennium." *Yale Journal of Law and Feminism*, vol. 12, no. 2, 2000, pp. 263-86.

Cramer, Renée Ann. *Pregnant with the Stars: Watching and Wanting the Celebrity Baby Bump*. Stanford University Press, 2016.

Hacker, Daphna, and Michal Frankel. "Active Parenthood and Employment Equal Opportunities: The Need to Change the Characteristics of the Labor Force" (Hebrew). *Labor, Society and Law*, vol. 11, 2005, pp. 275-303.

Hansen, Lisa. "A Comprehensive Framework for Accommodating Nursing Mothers in the Workplace." *Rutgers Law Review*, vol. 59, no. 4, 2007, pp. 885-916.

Johnson, Greg. "Courting Culture: Unexpected Relationships between Religion and Law in Contemporary Hawai'i." *After Secular law*, edited by Winnifred Fallers Sullivan et al., Stanford University Press, 2011, pp. 282-301.

Kasdan, Diana. "Note, Reclaiming Title VII and the PDA: Prohibiting Workplace Discrimination Against Breastfeeding Women." *New York University Law Review*, vol. 76, 2001, pp. 309-43.

Kierkegaard, Søren. *Fear and Trembling and Repetition*. Translated by Howard V. Hong and Edna H. Hong, Princeton University Press, 1983.

Matambanadzo, Saru M. "Reconstructing Pregnancy." *Southern Methodist University Law Review*, vol. 69, no. 1, 2016, pp. 187-264.

Marcotte, Amanda. "Breast-Feeding Mom Loses Discrimination Case Because Men Can Lactate Too." *Slate*, 4 Feb. 2015, www.slate.com/blogs/xx_factor/2015/02/04/angela_ames_sex_discrimination_case_breast_feeding_mom_loses_because_men.html. Accessed 23 Feb. 2018.

Mattes, Laura Iris. "Ames v. Nationwide Mutual Insurance Company: Breastfeeding Battlegrounds and the Fight against Pregnancy Discrimination." *Berkeley Journal of Employment and Labor Law*, vol. 36, no. 2, 2015, pp. 377-85.

McKinnon, Catharine. *Feminism Unmodified: Discourses on Life and Law*. Harvard University Press, 1988.

Murtagh, Lindsey and Anthony D. Moulton. "Working Mothers, Breastfeeding, and the Law." *American Journal of Public Health* vol. 101, no. 2, 2011, pp. 217-23.

National Women's Law Center. *Underpaid and Overloaded: Women in Low-Wage Jobs*. 2014, nwlc.org/sites/default/files/pdfs/final_nwlc_lowwagereport2014.pdf. Accessed 23 Feb. 2018.

O'Hagan, Clare. *Complex Inequality and "Working Mothers."* Cork University Press, 2015.

Overall, Christine, and Tabitha Bernard, "Into the Mouths of Babes: The Moral Responsibility to Breastfeed." *Philosophical Inquiries into Pregnancy, Childbirth, and Mothering*, edited by Sheila Lintott and Maureen Sander-Staudt, Routledge, 2012, pp. 49-63.

Rich, Adrienne. *Of Woman Born: Motherhood as Experience and Institution*. Norton, 1976.

Rimalt, Noya. "Good Mother, Bad Mother, Irrelevant Mother: Parenthood in Law between the Ideal of Equality and the Reality of Motherhood" (Hebrew). *The Hebrew University Law Review*, vol. 39, 2010, pp. 573-632.

Rosen, Lawrence. *Law as Culture*. Princeton University Press, 2006.

Shaw, Joshua. "Why Don't Philosophers Tell Their Mothers' Stories? Philosophy, Motherhood, and Imaginative Resistance." *Philosophical Inquiries into Pregnancy, Childbirth, and Mothering*, edited by Sheila Lintott and Maureen Sander-Staudt, Routledge, 2012, pp. 138-50.

Sherwin, Galen. "Firing a Mom Because She's Breastfeeding is Sex Discrimination." *ACLU*, 2 Feb. 2015, www.aclu.org/blog/speakeasy/firing-mom-because-shes-breastfeeding-sex-discrimination?redirect=blog/womens-rights/firing-mom-because-shes-breastfeeding-sex-discrimination. Accessed 22 Feb. 2018.

Slaughter, Marty M. "The Legal Construction of 'Mother'." *Mothers in Law: Feminist Theory and the Legal Regulation of Motherhood*, edited by Martha Albertson Fineman and Isabel Karpin, Columbia University Press, 1995, pp. 73-100.

Smith, Paige Hall. "Breastfeeding and Gender Inequality." *Journal of Women, Politics and Policy*, vol. 34, no. 4, 2013, pp. 371-83.

Traister, Rebecca. "Labor Pains." *New Republic*, vol. 246, no. 1, 2015, pp. 12-17.

United States. "Employment Characteristics of Families Summary." Bureau of Labor Statistics, www.bls.gov/news.release/famee.nr0.htm. Accessed 23 Feb. 2018.Wang, Wendy, et al. "Breadwinner Moms." Pew Research Centre, 29 May 2013, www.pewsocialtrends.org/2013/05/29/breadwinner-moms/. Accessed 23 Feb. 2018.

Williams, Joan. *Unbending Gender: Why Family and Work Conflict and What to Do About It*. Oxford University Press, 2001.

12.
The Politics of Mothers' Milk in Modern India

SUCHARITA SARKAR

> "Like mother's love, there is no substitute for mother's milk." (Anand et al., *Breastfeeding and Complementary Feeding: A Guide for Parents*)

> "Then there's the breastfeeding, which is (f)actually beast-feeding ... and no, you never get used to it." (Anawnimiss, "So, Worth It?")

In traditional Hindu Ayurvedic medical practice, breastmilk is eulogized for its life-giving powers. The valorization of breastfeeding and the ideal maternal breast becomes politically implicated in the context of the simultaneous glorification of motherhood and subjugation of mothers in Indian patriarchal systems. In the dominant narratives of contemporary culture, good mothers and milk continue to be glorified as the site and resource that (re)produce the nation. Expectedly, the official state position on breastfeeding—evidenced in the advocacy literature of the Department of Women and Child Development, in various governmental legislations, and in such recent government initiatives as MAA—Mother's Absolute Affection—is to "protect, promote and support" breastfeeding. These discourses have also shaped the agenda and the literature of such voluntary national networks as the Breastfeeding Promotion Network of India (BPNI), which has been working since 1991 toward "putting child nutrition at the forefront of social change" (BPNI, "Information Sheet-2").

The strategic overlapping of breastfeeding with good motherhood results in the stigmatization of mothers who cannot or will not breastfeed and also in the marginalization of mothers' lived experiences of the stresses and pains of (non)breastfeeding. These experiences are documented in mothers' self-writing where they articulate their satisfactions, frustrations, and exhaustions, and also when they negotiate their choices with the cultural expectations and policing of breastfeeding. A close reading of these maternal narratives reveals how these mothers internalize, reassert, resist, reject, and interrupt the dominant expectations of good lactating motherhood. In this chapter, I investigate traditional Ayurvedic breastfeeding discourse and the allied public discourse, and compare it with personal maternal discourse by analyzing selected posts from contemporary blogs in which Indian mothers write about their breastfeeding experiences. I argue that this comparison helps to unpack the complicated politics of mothers' milk in modern India, particularly in relation to social constructions of motherhood and the effects on mothers' identities.

THE HINDU AYURVEDIC DISCOURSE ON THE NECTAR OF LIFE

> "May four oceans, full of milk, constantly abide in both your breasts, you blessed one, for the increase of the strength of the child!" (*Sushruta Samhita* III.10; qtd. in Laroia and Sharma 95)

In Ayurveda, the foundational text *Atharva Veda* metaphorizes lactating breasts as pitchers full of divine nectar granting humans strength and longevity (Laroia and Sharma 94). This significant metaphor objectifies the maternal body and also indicates that the Ayurvedic discourse of *Kaumaara bhrityam* (study of mother and child welfare) has always been not only child centred, but focused on the mother only as the producer and conduit of milk. Such ancient Ayurvedic texts as *Charaka Samhita*, *Sushruta Samhita*, and *Kashyapa Samhita* have extensive sections on the merits of "ideal" breast ("*stana sampat*"), the characteristics of "pure" breastmilk, and the possible abnormalities and loss of breastmilk ("*stanyanasha*") (Masram and Singh 23-24). Foucauldian analysis suggests that an intrusive inspection and surveillance of maternal bodies would be necessary for such diagnoses. The concern for infant health and breastmilk purity is often inimical to maternal agency. The practices of discarding the colostrum, of giving the baby prelacteal feeds, and of initiating breastfeeding on the third or fourth day are recommended in the *Sushruta Samhita* and have become popular and persistent traditions mothers are coerced to follow (Laroia and Sharma 96; Masram and Singh 24). Such scripturally sanctioned rituals control the mother-child dyad. The rituals include a forty-day period of rest and confinement for a new mother, usually in her natal home, where she can exclusively nurse the child while female elders monitor her breastfeeding performance and feed her galactogogues to increase breastmilk supply (Laroia and Sharma 97). Such a natal familial network is undoubtedly a source of support for new mothers, and the focus on maternal nutrition a necessary intervention. However, such constant scrutiny and dietary supervision also marginalize and silence the mother's autonomy and opinions.

Under such tightly controlled and institutionalized motherhood, it is unsurprising that most Ayurvedic texts stigmatize mothers whose breastmilk is "vitiated": the *Sushruta Samhita* states that "excessive anger, grief, and lack of maternal love result in suppression of lactation," contraindicates certain kinds of mothers with "abnormalities" from breastfeeding, and prescribes elaborate "treatments" for such "abnormalities" (Masram and Singh 25-27). Such public and medicalized scrutiny of breastmilk "abnormalities" allows for stricter disciplining of the maternal body and exacerbates the feelings of inadequacy in mothers. It also contributes to the cultural shaming of those mothers who do not adequately respond to the prescribed treatments, and are regarded as failed mothers. Thus, the glorification of mother's milk as "the sap of the immortal life divine" is paradoxically embedded in a culture where maternal choice is delegitimized and the maternal body is objectified, regulated, and exploited (Laroia and Sharma 95). The privileging of breastmilk in Hindu medico-religious and cultural discourse—as in the Western medical model of breastfeeding advocacy—positions and disempowers mothers as "disembodied providers of milk who must be educated and scrutinized" (Wall 594).

THE STATE DISCOURSE OF NATURE'S GIFT AND NATIONAL RESOURCE

> "Breastfeeding is nature's way of nurturing the child, creating a strong bond between the mother and the child." (*National Guidelines on Infant and Young Child Feeding* 7)

The official breastfeeding discourse of the Indian government—which is also echoed by state-supported, voluntary organizations such as BPNI—has been shaped by the Ayurvedic valorization of breastmilk, but recasts the breastfeeding narrative in a more modern, maternalist vocabulary that is, in many ways, more sensitized to mothers' needs and experiences. The National Guidelines on Infant and Young Child Feeding states that its goals are to promote exclusive breastfeeding practices for the first six months after birth, followed by the introduction of complementary foods in addition to continued breastfeeding for two years; it also claims that these goals are "consistent with the Indian traditions of prolonged breastfeeding" as well as with the "Global Strategy on Infant and Young Child Feeding" (8). Successive legislations passed by the government have been consistent with these goals. The recent proposed amendment of the 1961 Maternity Benefit Act—to increase paid maternity leave (to women working in public and private sector organizations) to twenty-six weeks—addresses the anomaly between the goal of exclusive breastfeeding for six months and the earlier state policy of only twelve weeks of maternity leave, which often forced working mothers to opt out of exclusive breastfeeding before the recommended six months. However, since these proposed benefits will exclude mothers working in the unorganized sectors, the reach and impact of such legislation will be very limited (Rao). The state breastfeeding narrative's attempts to modernize old Ayurvedic practices are often confusing and not easily accepted by many Indian families. (I say families instead of mothers because childcare decisions are rarely taken autonomously by Indian mothers.) For instance, despite the various state narratives providing information about the "value of colostrum," deeply entrenched ancient Ayurveda-authorized practices, such as prelacteal feeding and discarding of colostrum, continue to persist, although studies indicate a gradual decrease (National Guidelines 11). Yet the valuing of traditional knowledge sources along with a readiness to adapt to modern medical findings indicates a progressiveness and flexibility of approach in the state discourse that gives hope to mothers' rights activists. They have for long been advocating for public policies that would educate mothers as well as address the social factors and other constraints—such as emotional stress and the burden of domestic or paid work—that underlie breastfeeding. There are vast numbers of Indian mothers, including those in underprivileged positions, who engage in paid or unpaid work in organized and unorganized sectors. According to feminist activists, the state must take this into account and consider breastfeeding as "a multi-faceted social issue which needs to be addressed by the family, society, employers and government, in order to create appropriate support structures for the mother-child dyad," rather than as an exclusive and freely chosen maternal decision (Narayanan 31).

This flexibility to changing social conditions is evidenced in the BPNI narrative, which engages supportively with the problems faced by working mothers who wish to continue breastfeeding. Their guidelines specify the conditions under which working mothers can continue with the "optimum practices" of breastfeeding: it is possible if these mothers are "fully supported by the family and the community" and if there are "adequate maternity leave," breaks for feeding or expressing, and "nearby childcare facilities" ("Information Sheet-1," 4). Such guidelines address the complexly intertwined structures and arrangements that enable breastfeeding, and they also distribute the responsibility of continuing breastfeeding from the mother alone to the wider context of family, community, and the employing organizations in which she works. There has also been a gradual change in the state-approved discourse in breastfeeding toward a less gendered, more inclusive approach. The BPNI parental guidebook has a section on "A father's role in successful breastfeeding," in which the father is instructed not only to make his wife "feel good about herself by *praising her job* as a mother," but also to "spend *some time* with your baby" to enable the mother to rest and "not *feel embarrassed* if she is feeding baby outside home" (Anand et al. 41; my emphasis). Although the extent of the father's participation appears to be limited instead of equal, and although the patriarchal strategy of glorification of motherhood persists, even such small steps—the father supporting the mother to rest at home and to breastfeed outside home—are significant in the context of conventional mothering roles and responsibilities in India, and could positively impact the mother-blaming perceptions that currently prevail.

However, there are several aspects of the state discourse that need to be critiqued and contested. When listing the advantages of breastfeeding, the BPNI parental guidebook not only lists the benefits to the child and the mother, it also details the "benefits the society enjoys"— which includes lowering of "health-care costs" by reducing infant illness and mortality, reducing the "strain on the family budget," and "reducing absenteeism from work as exclusively breastfed children are less prone to diseases"—thus proving to be "less costly" for the family, the employer, and the nation (Anand et al. 4). The breastfeeding mother is, thus, constructed as an ideal neoliberal state subject: as a "good mother" as she also a "responsible citizen" (Simon-Kumar 146). She reproduces to create future human resources for the nation; produces the most low-risk, low-cost food for the budding neoliberal workforce; and is herself a model, never-absent labourer in this workforce. The government of India introduced neoliberalism when it implemented the New Economic Policy in 1991; it is not a coincidence that subsequent studies treated breastmilk as a "major national resource," and attempted to quantify the "tremendous economic value of mother's milk to the nation" (Gupta and Rohde 1391). Yet if the mother is unable to balance her productive and reproductive labours, or if she fails in her reproductive duties of breastfeeding, she is castigated and stigmatized. Arun Gupta and Jon Rohde write: "Those who opt for the difficult and *undesirable method* of bottle-feeding in order to seek work outside the home, may be gaining small fiscal benefit at considerable health and nutritional risk to the infant" (391, my emphasis). Refracted through the prism of macroeconomics, the bottle-feeding, working mother is projected as an irresponsible parent who deliberately ignores the risks to the nation's future citizens for trivial and selfish financial gains. Indian feminists have also critiqued such studies for "ignoring social realities"—such as the fact that most working women in India are poor and work out of necessity rather than choice (Swaminathan 2099).

The parental guidebook of the BPNI, though using a more mother-friendly vocabulary, also ignores certain physical realities, such as the inescapable reality of maternal fatigue and exhaustion. It advises working mothers to breastfeed "early in the morning," "frequently after you come back in the evening," as well as "as many times as possible" during the night if they want to "successfully" combine work and breastfeeding (Anand et al. 29-30). The BPNI narrative, in its zeal to promote breastfeeding, also often exaggerates the risks attached to breastmilk substitutes: their parental guidebook warns that "Even a single bottle a day can harm your child" before listing details of the "dangers of artificial feeding" for both babies and mothers (Anand et al. 5). One of the primary areas of BPNI's activism is the proper implementation of the 1992 Infant Milk Substitutes, Feeding Bottles, and Infant Foods (Regulation of Production, Supply, and Distribution) Act (IMS Act) and its subsequent amendment in 2003, which regulates the marketing and promotion of commercial breastmilk substitutes. Maternal rights activists have objected to the limitations of such legislation. Restricting artificial feeding "without providing for positive social support measures may be damaging to children, besides being unfair and unjust to women" (Swaminathan 2100). The state and BPNI discourse excludes and demonizes the bottle-feeding mother while it ostensibly supports (and also polices) the breastfeeding mother. The *BPNI Information Sheet-2* quotes and endorses the government's claim that "inappropriate feeding practices lead to infant malnutrition, morbidity and mortality in our children. Promotion of infant milk substitutes and related products like feeding bottles and teats do constitute a health hazard." This claim omits the data on healthy bottle-fed babies and marginalizes the root causes of mortality of bottle-fed babies: poverty and lack of education. Poor and uneducated mothers often feed their children overdiluted milk from unsterilized bottles. In her study of lactation consultants in the United States, Miranda Waggoner cites current research to examine how "risk discourse in contemporary public health tends to exploit notions of blame and guilt to perpetuate social control over health behaviors" and how such "regulatory advice" can potentially make mothers "feel guilty about their infant feeding choices while ignoring the realities of women's lives" (155). By implying that all artificial feeding is inappropriate and hazardous, the state and BPNI narratives similarly exacerbate the guilt and shame many bottle-feeding mothers already feel.

This guilt, shame, and sense of inadequacy are often felt by mothers who are unable—for a variety of reasons—to breastfeed, especially when breastfeeding is regarded as a natural function of the maternal body. This breastfeeding discourse "overlaps" with "cultural constructions of nature" (Wall 596). Stating that breastmilk is nature's perfect food, and therefore pure and good, and that women can breastfeed naturally exclude those mothers who cannot breastfeed from the constructed category of "natural." The state discourse valorizes breastmilk as nature's gift to nurture the child and considers it essential for mother-child bonding (*National Guidelines* 7). The recent government initiative to promote breastfeeding is called MAA, an acronym for Mother's Absolute Affection (Singla). These associations of breastfeeding with loving and natural motherhood covertly project mothers who cannot breastfeed as "artificial," unloving, unnatural, and, therefore, monstrous. The tagline of the MAA campaign states "*Stanpaan vikalp nahi, sankalp hai*" ("Breastfeeding is not an option, but a commitment") (Singla). The framing of the breastfeeding narrative in terms of responsibility rather than of choice overdetermines maternal consent to breastfeed, legitimizes public scrutiny of maternal bodies, and, again, places a burden of guilt on those mothers who cannot honour this commitment. What Glenda Wall writes about Canadian public discourse of breastfeeding is applicable in the Indian context, too: "the emphasis is on maternal responsibility while taking for granted a cultural model of natural, intensive, self-sacrificing and isolated motherhood" (605). Thus, despite the valuable support and education of breastfeeding mothers that is provided by the state discourse, there is a need for more inclusiveness of mothers' heterogeneous experiences and positions, and less judgment of maternal bodies and decisions.

THE MOTHERS' DISCOURSE OF BREASTFEEDING AGENCY

> "And for all mothers and to-be-mothers: If you want to breastfeed—It is fine!
>
> If you do not want to breastfeed—It is fine!
>
> If you want to but can't (any medical condition)—It is still fine!"
>
> (Mutteringsofmemyself, "Breastfeeding—Why it was NOT an Option for Me")

A more inclusive, diverse, and multitudinous breastfeeding discourse emerges in the self-writings of mothers, especially online, in mom blogs and social networks. Many of the blogposts prioritize the mother's experience and perspective over the prescriptive advice and informational support that they share, thus privileging the "maternalist" over the "medical" models of breastfeeding discourse suggested by Linda Blum. Blogger Preethi, for instance, interweaves advice—about mixed feeding, lactation consultants, galactogogues—with encouragement ("Hang in there! It gets better") as she narrates her personal breastfeeding story, which had a "rocky start" when she "gave her [child] formula but kept up the nursing." It eventually becomes a "great journey," as she is able to "exclusively breastfeed" after her struggles (Preethi). Blogger Namrata, mother to twin boys, also contests the official discourse and asserts that "formula is not evil," even though "breastfeeding came very naturally" to her: "Breastfeeding doesn't have to be all or nothing. Give your babies as much breast milk as you can and if you have to supplement with formula, do not feel guilty" (Sadhvani). Through both experience and empathy, mothers reject the breastmilk-formula binary and decide to use either or both according to their own convictions and convenience, not according to medical convention.

Jacqueline Wolf notes that "Women should indeed be free to choose between formula and human milk, but women also have the right to be fully informed when they make that decision"

("What Feminists" 414). This kind of noncoercive information support is more possible in a mother-to-mother situation (for instance, when a blogger shares such information with her mother readers) than in a more intimidating expert-to-mother situation. Such community blogs as *Indian Moms Connect* have attempted to "build a resource for new moms who may be struggling with breastfeeding" through posts providing links and discussions that would help to "get the right idea about breastfeeding, the issues related to it, alternatives which are possible, what can go wrong, and how exactly can we overcome the issues" (Team IMC). The bloggers reject "those blissful images of women breastfeeding" that produce "mommy guilt," contend that "we should set expectations about how difficult breastfeeding can be, so we know what to prepare for," and suggest that mothers should "start off with formula if nothing works" because they do not think "there is anything wrong with it" (Team IMC).

Sometimes, the mom bloggers open up more choices for mothers. The BPNI guidebook for parents does not mention breast pumps; instead, it focuses on teaching mothers "how to hand express" their milk (Anand et al. 31). Though reaching a much narrower and more affluent readership than the BPNI literature, mom blogs provide information on breast pumps and how they can help to "increase milk supply" as well as to cope with the "guilt-trip of low breast milk supply" (Kejal). The blogs are a space for alternatives like "a rapidly emerging section—Pumping Moms," who "pumps out her breast milk to feed the baby through a bottle": such "pumping moms" choose to do so because of multiple reasons like working away from home, or having "sore nipples," or needing "some freedom for [her]self" (Nancy). Articulating such a radical desire (for time for oneself) destabilizes the culturally imposed ideal of devoted, self-sacrificing motherhood.

In the Ayurvedic and the state-approved discourse, the breastfeeding mother is expected to spend all her time and energy in controlling her body, diet, and environment to protect her child from multiple risks. This conforms to the culturally determined, normative stereotype of "total motherhood" critiqued by Joan Wolf (*Is Breast Best?*). There are mom bloggers who internalize the prescriptive association of motherhood with breastfeeding and who advise mothers to police their bodies in order to live up to the standards of "total motherhood." In her post on "Breastfeeding Guide for Indian Moms" (which includes links to "complete Indian meal plan" for lactating mothers and daily schedules for working mothers who breastfeed), blogger Mansi writes, "The best part of being a new mother for me was definitely breastfeeding.... It made me feel wanted. It made me understand what is nurturing" (Zaveri). Yet in spite of her adherence to the norms of total motherhood, blogger Mansi shares her blogspace with guest blogger Rati Girish, who writes a defiant post titled "I Chose to Formula Feed my Children, Are You Going to Mom Shame Me Forever?" She explains that she was "convinced that they would benefit a lot more from a happy, caring mom than they would from forced breastfeeding," and provides links to join the movement to "End Mom shaming right now." Mansi inserts a disclaimer at the end of this post, "Mother's milk is best for baby but we also do not endorse mom shaming" (Girish). Although blogger Anu Prabin ends her post on a self-congratulatory "I pat myself on the back for not giving up on breastfeeding" and feels happy and proud, she also begins her post on breastfeeding by disclosing her own problems: "In this post I pour my heart out on the unpleasant experiences about breastfeeding that I went through as a mother" (Prabin, "Unpleasant"). Most bloggers subvert the dominant homogenized concept of the perfect breastfeeding mother by deploying their blogging agency and blogspace to narrate their own problems and to support other mothers who may have similar or different problems and make similar or different choices.

As has been noted, the charge of insufficient milk stigmatizes mothers as inadequate when compared to the ideal of the bountiful, giving, nurturing, good mother. Many of the mom bloggers articulate an anxiety about their breastfeeding capabilities, and a persistent fear about not being able to perform good motherhood. Suffering from "engorged leaky breast, sore nipples, restless days, sleepless nights, a gagging and choking baby," blogger Anu Prabin writes: "I felt I was doing something wrong. I felt defeated, helpless, frustrated" (Prabin, "Unpleasant"). This anxiety is embedded in an awareness of being the object of constant public scrutiny. Blogger Shaivi writes, "The new mom is often judged on parameters set by relatives and neighbours—'She couldn't get a simple latch right?', 'We never had issues with breastmilk supply'" (Sharma). Another mom blogger, who shifted to soya milk because she had a retracted nipple and her child was lactose-intolerant, recollects feeling confused by the familial and expert policing before she took her "tortured" decision to shift: "My mother upset! She felt some evil eye had been cast on her grandson. My mother-in-law wary! She was sure it was something wrong with me and my diet.... My grandmother-in-law aghast! She felt I was unwilling to give my son what was best for him! ... My husband's family doctor convinced! I should stop breastfeeding!" (Mutteringsofmemyself).

These posts reveal how women in patriarchal families are often complicit in blaming and shaming mothers who cannot match the ideal standards of breastfeeding. This shaming extends to mothers breastfeeding in public, especially in urban spaces, where mothers are expected to breastfeed discreetly, if at all. Blogger Prerna recollects how she was constantly "reminded by older women – my mother-in-law included – to cover up while feeding, even if I was alone in the room" so that the baby would "get used to feeding under a blanket." Conservative mom bloggers also advise mothers to practise before a mirror, to "use a cover-up," to "turn away to latch," to ensure "the least skin exposure while nursing," and to try and be "least visible to strangers": this puts the onus of behaving responsibly on the mothers themselves (Prabin, "9 Sure Shot"). The diversity of maternal narratives in the blogosphere, however, enables other mothers to share their own traumatic stories of nursing in public, and empowers them to challenge those who sexualize and criminalize such acts. Blogger Prerna shares her distressing experience of breastfeeding her "forty-day-old baby sitting on a commode in Delhi airport"; and how her "social life came to a standstill" because even when she breastfed her baby under a shawl in a restaurant, "waiters gawked, people in the restaurants stared and men gaped" (Prerna). In a post that had been widely reblogged, blogger Anawnimiss narrates how she nursed her baby "in full public view in a Starbucks outlet" and posted a photograph of this as her Facebook profile picture: she counters those who advise her that "feeding in public can make some men uncomfortable" by arguing that her "photo's staying" because there is a "need to normalize breastfeeding so people get used to women nursing in public" (Anawnimiss, "Fuck Sensitivity"). The circulation of such posts help mothers to enact their mothering in radically empowering ways, and also raise consciousness about the need for changing public perceptions of breastfeeding.

THE POLITICS OF THE GIVEN AND THE HIDDEN IN INDIAN BREASTFEEDING DISCOURSE

> "But then motherhood is all about bending rules to suit oneself, isn't it? To each, her own." (Iyer)

The politics of breastfeeding in India encompasses and imbricates both state policies and public perceptions, and impacts how mothers feed their children, how they judge themselves, and how they are judged by others. Contradicting the traditional perception that breastfeeding is an easy and natural act and a given attribute of motherhood, mom bloggers insist on revealing the difficulties that mothers experience. Blogger Kejal confirms, "Till date I have come across only 2 mothers who have NOT had an issue with breastfeeding." The maternal counter-discourse, thus, exposes the hidden problems and subverts the given agenda of the public breastfeeding discourse. Samira Kawash writes, "The evidence for the advantages of breast-feeding for both maternal and infant health is, by now, unequivocal" (992). The unequivocal championing of "breast is best" is the given aim of the public discourse and state policies. What is hidden is the cost—in terms of time, effort, and bodily discomfort—that mothers have to bear. Most mom bloggers also acknowledge, document, and circulate the advantages and satisfactions of breastfeeding. What they expose and insert into the Indian breastfeeding discourse is the lived experience and the maternal cost of breastfeeding. Blogger Mansi says, "Breastfeeding is natural and normal but that does not mean it comes easily. Every mother has a different story and different struggle" (Mittal). The blogosphere prioritizes maternal experience and maternal choice, and enables the sharing of mothers' individual stories and struggles, which are often omitted or hidden in the official discourse. As Lalita Iyer contends in the quote at the beginning of this section, mothering should entail the freedom of mothers to decide what works for them. Although the official breastfeeding discourse in India is gradually shifting toward a more mother-friendly approach, it is the mothers' self-written counter-discourse that interrupts, contests, and sometimes co-opts the official narrative to provide a more nuanced, comprehensive, and individualized perspective on the politics of mothers' milk in India. In doing so, it encourages and empowers mothers to engage with breastfeeding in agentic rather than coerced ways. Even if such online maternal counter-discourse is too limited (as blogs are written and read by a minuscule section of mothers who are urban, educated, middle/upper-class, and digitally connected) to impact state policies, I would still conclude that such emerging discourse is necessary to change, albeit in small ways, the mother-blaming and mother-shaming that dominate perceptions of breastfeeding in India.

WORKS CITED

Anand, R.K., et al. *Breastfeeding and Complementary Feeding: A Guide for Parents*. BPNI, 2005.

Anawnimiss. "Fuck Sensitivity." *Anawnimiss*, 11 Apr. 2016, anawnimiss.wordpress.com/2016/04/11/fuck-sensitivity. Accessed 23 Feb. 2018.

Anawnimiss. "So, Worth It?" *Anawnimiss*, 6 Feb. 2016, anawnimiss.wordpress.com/2016/02/06/so-worth-it. Accessed 23 Feb. 2018.

BPNI. "Information Sheet-1: Guidelines for breastfeeding and complementary feeding." Breastfeeding Promotion Network of India, 2001.

BPNI. "Information Sheet-2: Protecting Mothers and Children; A Law to Protect, Promote and Support Breastfeeding." Breastfeeding Promotion Network of India, 2003.

Blum, Linda M. *At the Breast: Ideologies of Breastfeeding in the Contemporary United States*. Beacon, 1999.

Gupta, Arun, and Jon E. Rohde. "Economic Value of Breast-Feeding in India." *Economic and Political Weekly*, vol. 28, no. 26, 1993, pp. 1390-1393, *JSTOR*, www.jstor.org/stable/4399902. Accessed 23 Feb. 2018.

Girish, Rati. "I Chose to Formula Feed my Children, Are You Going to Mom Shame Me Forever?" *KidsStopPress*, 22 June 2016, www.kidsstoppress.com/2016/06/whats-wrong-with-formula-feeding-asks-a-puzzled-indian-mom. Accessed 23 Feb. 2018.

Government of India, Ministry of Human Resource Development. *National Guidelines on Infant and Young Child Feeding*. 2004.

Iyer, Lalita. "Why I Went the Extended Breastfeeding Way." *Mommy Go Lightly*, 20 Sept. 2011, mommygolightly.com/2011/09/20/an-ode-to-my-girls. Accessed 23 Feb. 2018.

Kawash, Samira. "New Directions in Motherhood Studies." *Signs*, vol. 36, no. 4, 2011, pp. 969-1003, *JSTOR*, www.jstor.org/stable/10.1086/658637. Accessed 23 Feb. 2018.

Kejal. "The Guilt-trip of Low Breast Milk Supply." *Being Momma*, beingmomma.com/the-guilt-trip-of-low-breast-milk-supply. Accessed 23 Feb. 2018.

Laroia, Nirupama and Deeksha Sharma. "The Religious and Cultural Bases for Breastfeeding Practices among the Hindus." *Breastfeeding Medicine*, vol. 1, no. 2, 2006, pp. 94-98, doi.org/10.1089/bfm.2006.1.94.

Masram, Pravin, and B.M. Singh. "Review on Ayurvedic and Modern Concept of Human Breast Milk and Breast Feeding." *Pharmagene,* vol. 2, no. 2, 2014, pp. 23-29, www.genesisjournals.org/vol2issu2.php. Accessed 23 Feb. 2018.

Mittal, Mansi. "Breastfeeding: My Journey and Debunking Myths." *Parentous*, 6 Aug. 2016, www.parentous.com/2016/08/06/breastfeeding-myths-debunked-breastfeeding-week. Accessed 23 Feb. 2018.

Mutteringsofmemyself (Shyama). "Breastfeeding—Why It Was NOT an Option for Me." *Indian Moms Connect*, 6 July 2013, www.indianmomsconnect.com/2013/07/06/breastfeeding-why-it-was-not-an-option-for-me. Accessed 23 Feb. 2018.

Nancy. "Pumping MOMs." *The Thinking Hat*, 4 Aug. 2014, thethinkinhat.com/2014/08/04/pumping-moms. Accessed 23 Feb. 2018.

Narayanan, Rama. *At What Cost? Women's Multiple Roles and the Management of Breastfeeding*. M.S. Swaminathan Research Foundation, Jan. 1997.

Prabin, Anu. "Unpleasant Experiences about Breastfeeding no

Mom would ever Reveal." *Bumpsnbaby*, 29 Oct. 2014, www.bumpsnbaby.com/unpleasant-experiences-breastfeeding. Accessed 23 Feb. 2018.

Prabin, Anu. "9 Sure Shot Strategies for Confident Breastfeeding in Public." *Bumpsnbaby*, 2 Jan. 2015, www.bumpsnbaby.com/confident-breastfeeding-public. Accessed 23 Feb. 2018.

Preethi. "Rocky Start to a Great Journey." *Indian Moms Connect*, 5 Dec. 2011, www.indianmomsconnect.com/2011/12/05/rocky-start-to-a-great-journey. Accessed 23 Feb. 2018.

Prerna. "Why We Need World Breastfeeding Week." *Indian Moms Connect*, 7 Aug. 2015, www.indianmomsconnect.com/2015/08/07/why-we-need-world-breastfeeding-week. Accessed 23 Feb. 2018.

Rao, Menaka. "Maternity Leave Increases to 26 Weeks—But Only for a Small Section of Indian Women." *Scroll.in*, 13 Aug. 2016, www.scroll.in/article/813888/maternity-leave-increases-to-26-weeks-but-only-for-a-small-section-of-indian-women. Accessed 23 Feb. 2018.

Sadhvani, Namrata. "My Breastfeeding Story." *Indian Moms Connect*, 6 Aug. 2015, www.indianmomsconnect.com/2015/08/06/my-breastfeeding-story. Accessed 23 Feb. 2018.

Sharma, Shaivi. "I Am Just a Mom, Not God." *Parentous*, 9 Aug. 2016, www.parentous.com/2016/08/09/dealing-with-childbirth-new-mom-advice-shaivi. Accessed 23 Feb. 2018.

Simon-Kumar, Rachel. "'Productive' Reproducers: The Political Identity of Mothering in Contemporary India." *Journal of the Association for Research on Mothering*, vol. 11, no. 2, 2009, pp. 143-152.

Singla, Neha. "Actress Madhuri Dixit Launches MAA, Mother's Absolute Affection, an Indian Campaign to Promote Breastfeeding." *MediaIndia.eu*, 12 Aug. 2016, mediaindia.eu/social-vibes/actress-madhuri-dixit-launches-maa-mothers-absolute-affection. Accessed 23 Feb. 2018.

Swaminathan, Mina. "Breast-Feeding and Working Mothers." *Economic and Political Weekly*, vol. 28, no. 39, 1993, pp. 2099-2100, *JSTOR*, www.jstor.org/stable/4400206. Accessed 23 Feb. 2018.

Team IMC. "Conversations—Breastfeeding Troubles." *Indian*

Moms Connect, 19 Apr. 2012, www.indianmomsconnect.com/2012/04/19/conversations-breastfeeding-troubles. Accessed 23 Feb. 2018.

Waggoner, Miranda A. "Monitoring Milk and Motherhood: Lactation Consultants and the Dilemmas of Breastfeeding Advocacy." *International Journal of Sociology of the Family*, vol. 37, no. 1, 2011, pp. 153-171, *JSTOR*, www.jstor.org/stable/23029791. Accessed 23 Feb. 2018.

Wall, Glenda. "Moral Constructions of Motherhood in Breastfeeding Discourse." *Gender and Society*, vol. 15, no. 4, 2001, pp. 592-610, *JSTOR*, www.jstor.org/stable/3081924. Accessed 23 Feb. 2018.

Wolf, Jacqueline H. "What Feminists Can Do for Breastfeeding and What Breastfeeding Can Do for Feminists." *Signs*, vol. 31, no. 2, 2006, pp. 397–424, *JSTOR*, www.jstor.org/stable/10.1086/497279. Accessed 23 Feb. 2018.

Wolf, Joan B. *Is Breast Best? Taking on the Breastfeeding Experts and the New High Stakes in Motherhood*. New York U.P, 2010.

Zaveri, Mansi. "Breastfeeding Guide for Indian Moms". *KidsStopPress*, 5 Aug. 2016, www.kidsstoppress.com/2016/08/breastfeeding-guide-for-indian-moms. Accessed 23 Feb. 2018.

IV.
The Challenges of Feminist Breastfeeding and Lactation Discourse

13.
"We Chose the Hardest Road"

Examining Self-Representations of the Exclusive Pumper

LEE ANN GLOWZENSKI

Many women who breastfeed rely on a pump to express milk from time to time, but very few women call themselves "exclusive pumpers." Borrowing the notion of exclusivity from its usual pairing with "exclusive breastfeeding," exclusive pumpers do not nurse directly; instead, they feed their children mechanically expressed breast milk, sometimes in combination with formula but more often as the sole source of nutrition until solid foods are introduced. Unlike women who only pump when physically separated from their breastfed children, the exclusive pumper may initially attempt direct breastfeeding, but her breast pump eventually becomes the means by which all milk is transferred from herself to her child. Although exclusive pumpers certainly exist, breastfeeding research rarely addresses their realities and experiences. When pumping mothers do appear in studies of breastfeeding, they are most often working women who must balance the demands of feeding at home with pumping at the job site. Otherwise, in academic research, mainstream journalism, and popular culture alike, pumps are considered as tools that support direct breastfeeding but not as the nursing mother's sole means of producing breastmilk.

This chapter shifts the focus of the pumping discussion from women who pump in combination with nursing to the exclusive pumpers—women who, as a result of choice or circumstance, perform the labour of breastfeeding via pumping and bottle-feeding.[1] I begin with a brief survey of existing studies of pumping. Just as in mainstream culture, where pumps are depicted as a (usually humorous) part of the return to so-called normal work and home life, academic research presents a similarly limited image of the pump as a means of regaining autonomy after childbirth. This notion of pumping as an ultimately self-serving act partly accounts for the invisibility of exclusive pumpers in representations of breastfeeding life. Precisely because breastfeeding is an act of solely maternal labour (Stearns, "Work" 76), pumping—traditionally constructed as a means by which a woman regains time "for herself"—conflicts with popular notions of breastfeeding as self-sacrifice. Additionally, breast pumps exhibit a strong relationship with errant bodies: if not pumping for a positive reason (paid or unpaid time away from the child), a woman usually pumps to compensate for a negative aspect of her own or her child's body. Exclusive pumpers, thus, often choose not to self-identify for fear of revealing the nonstandard aspects of the body. And finally, women who pump inadvertently technologize the work of breastfeeding by turning a supposedly spontaneous, natural act into one necessarily mediated by science. Hardly the liberating experience of technology that would at least allow for infants to be reared by, if not "born to both sexes equally" (Firestone 11), exclusive pumpers more often experience the dystopian than utopian possibilities of the convergence of body and machine. Accordingly, the exclusive pumper assumes these negative associations as well, lacking as she does any possible "redemption" through direct breastfeeding.

In the second part of this chapter, I turn to exclusive pumpers (EPers)[2] themselves to examine real-life experiences on the pump. As with members of any contemporary subculture, EPers may never meet other women who share their struggles, but they find each other online. Searching for information on how to pump comfortably, maintain supply in absence of nursing, and navigate the parenting world as women who breastfeed indirectly, EPers form communities such as BabyCenter's "The Exclusive Pumpers!" and Reddit's /bbpumpers. Significantly, these women actively challenge negative representations of pumping by subverting the normal association of the pump with work, play, and autonomy. If some women "frame pumping and providing breast milk as being a good effort, but never the best effort" (Stearns, "Breast Pump" 20), EPers assert that the labour of exclusive pumping performed alongside the usual duties of parenthood, in fact, requires more effort than nursing—and for less reward. Together, exclusive pumpers work to reframe discussions about their work and reimagine previously negative representations of their bodies and their relationships with their families. Online communities for EPers, thus, function as vital spaces for women who perform a unique and underrepresented act of maternal labour.

PUMPING AS WE KNOW IT: STUDIES ON THE WORK AND PLAY OF PUMPING MOMS

Because breast pumps are not usually considered a woman's sole means of breastmilk production, it is useful to first place them in the context of assisted reproductive technologies (ART)—processes such as in vitro fertilization and ovulation induction that are, for some women, the sole means of reproduction. Examined in this light, breast pumps represent either a step toward the liberation of the female body or a slip into further control of that body by an overwhelmingly male-dominated field of science. In *The Dialectic of Sex*, Shulamith Firestone argues advances in "artificial reproduction" ensure that "the dependence of the child on the mother (and vice versa) would give way to a greatly shortened dependence on a small group of others" (11). Although breast pumps do not completely shift the responsibility for infant feeding away from mothers alone, they do alter the relationship between maternal and infant bodies by allowing mothers to provide nourishment while pursuing separate work or leisure activities. As I will explore later in this chapter, exclusive pumpers take issue with this perception of the breast pump as tool of autonomy because they do not experience the pump in this way, but it is worth noting here that breast pumps can and do free some mothers from the significant labour of exclusive breastfeeding. Despite these liberatory possibilities, however, breast pumps more commonly come to represent the negative aspects of technological advances in maternal and infant care. Writing on ART as a male-dominated and patriarchal science, Robyn Rowland claims that "the process of reproductive technology is distancing women from our bodies, from our own procreative processes, and from birth" (8). Breast pumps can be seen as sharing in this same legacy. First, they do not merely enable but, in fact, require physical distance between mother and child so that the mother might retrieve her milk. Holding an infant while pumping is possible but so difficult as to be impractical, especially as the infant grows in size and gains the ability to grasp the pump's cups, bottles, tubes, and dials. Second, this physical distance can result in a psychological distance between the mother and her own body as she comes to rely exclusively on the pump to perform the labour of milk transfer. Placing pumps in the context of feminist writings on ART, thus, contributes to our understanding of the positive and negative impacts of this form of technology on a mother's relationships with her body, child, and community. However, just as in the case of ART, for some women, there is no choice but the pump and the pump alone.

Moving from general considerations of technology to pumps specifically, existing pumping research generally focuses on breastfeeding women who work outside the home and pump to maintain their milk supply. According to Cindy Stearns's survey on the use of breast pumps, women report that they pump "to accommodate paid employment outside the home"; "to enable short time periods away from their child for leisure activities and/or errands"; "to continue producing breast milk when the physical act of breastfeeding directly to a child was not possible (e.g., poor latch, maternal use of short-term medication, engorgement, maternal surgery, infant illness, etc.)"; and "to enable ... vacations" ("Breast Pump" 17). Paid employment and leisure activities—work and play—account for most pump use. Although the quick mention of difficult breastfeeding could be a nod to women who pump exclusively rather than supplementally, the difficulties listed apply more to nursing women; a woman coping with poor latch is more likely to EP, but women using short-term medication or facing surgeries/illness are likely to otherwise nurse. As evidenced by Stearns's list, breast pumps continue to grow in popularity because they meet a variety of needs. According to Kate Boyer, "Expressing breast milk has become a normative aspect of maternal practice in the U.S., with over 77 percent of American mothers reporting having used breast pumps at least once" (270). Yet although pumping is a common activity, as well as one that seemingly should be supported in the workplace,[3] Stearns has found that "women who worked outside the home had the most to say about pumping and much of their discourse was complaint. They were unhappy with the lack of privacy in pumping ... the difficulty in being able to relax and produce milk quickly, the ... sound of the pump, and the physical exhaustion" ("Breast Pump" 17). An examination of online narratives of pumping at work supports Stearns's findings. Women report their struggles to find clean, adequate pumping facilities, to balance the pumping schedule with work demands, and to cope with coworkers who find the presence of a working maternal body disruptive or distasteful. For example, in an open letter to the American Board of Pediatrics, Niran S. Al-Agba describes her failed attempts to find suitable pumping facilities while sitting for her medical boards. She describes details of her struggle common to many pumping women: a lack of time, privacy, dedicated facilities (that are not bathrooms requiring one to "sit on the floor"), electrical outlets, and so on ("Humiliation"). Appropriately so, Al-Agba's letter is, as Stearns would say, full of complaints, especially since she assumes that the American Board of Pediatrics should do more to support the very same breastfeeding goals that they endorse. Despite facing unsupportive workplaces, women who nurse and work are by necessity women who pump, and the image of the pumping worker tends to dominate academic research on pumping.

In addition to helping women to continue breastfeeding after reentering the traditional workforce, breast pumps also enable a return to leisure activities. In her study of representations of breastfeeding on television, Kathryn Pallister has found that "numerous references to pumping clearly illustrate that nursing mothers can return to work or enjoy a night out, even drink alcohol, and still provide breast milk for their children" (231). Similarly, Stearns notes that nonworking mothers occasionally pump for leisure ("shopping, going to the hairstylist" ["Work" 73]). Likewise, Boyer notes that "pumping can serve as a means of returning to 'normal' (e.g. prebirth) activities ... or as a means of obviating ... the loss of corporeal control and spatial freedom" (272). Pumps enable women to put literal distance between themselves and their infants, and the benefits of pumping for leisure seem to make enduring its negative aspects worthwhile. In popular media, Pallister claims, "pumping, while ostensibly constructed as a bit of an annoyance, also shows the viewers that breastfeeding does not necessarily tie a mother to her infant 24/7. Rather, with the use of a breast pump, she can enjoy some of the pleasures of her previous child-free life" (231). In exchange for coping with a minor "annoyance," nursing women use the pump to regain control of both their bodies and their leisure time.

Whether used for work or for play, breast pumps become equated with maternal autonomy: whereas nursing binds mother to child, the breast pump loosens those ties, a fact that is especially important given the growing pressure on women to nurse. As Stearns explains, "breastfeeding is now essential to a woman's performance as a mother" ("Breast Pump" 14): in order to be considered a good mother, a woman must breastfeed. The good-mothering practice of breastfeeding has long been constructed as antithetical to maternal autonomy. According to Robyn Lee, "Breastfeeding continues to be viewed by some feminists as a challenge to women's freedom because it requires ongoing responsiveness to an infant and restricts mobility" (95). A woman chooses either breast or bottle, infant or self. Although the pump could be seen as a sought-after middle ground, a liberatory technology that melds body and machine so to meet the needs of both mother and infant, it is not. Instead, pumps are seen as following the letter but not the spirit of the law: they allow women to provide their children the superior nutritional benefits of breast milk, yet they use an intermediary piece of equipment that forgoes the additional benefits of breastfeeding—such as the near-constant physical contact between mother and child in the first weeks and months of the feeding relationship. Pumping, thus, becomes an undervalued form of both feeding and labour. Stearns's study, for example, finds that "pumping (whether an exclusive or partial food source) is not ideal mothering, and its performance is always secondary to hands-on (or breasts-on!) mothering" ("Breast Pump" 19). The ideal mother nurses her child directly, regardless of the sacrifice of self, work, or leisure this act requires. Pumping mothers, according to Stearns, pump in part so that they may lay some claim on the title of "good mother": "Pumping ... is a symbol and a practice used to construct the compensatory mother, who is culturally positioned as at least better than the mother who does not pump at all and far superior to the mother who provides formula" (19). In other words, nursing mothers are good; nursing-pumping mothers compensate for their lack of "the good" by providing expressed breastmilk; and formula-feeding mothers have no access to "the good" at all. EPers, meanwhile, are completely absent from this construction. For most women, pumping is only one part of the breastfeeding experience; existing pumping research always assumes an ideal breastfeeding relationship to which a woman returns when the workday ends or the fun is over. Associations between pump and autonomy—and the slippery slope of "bad mothering" on which women who pump occasionally perch—are remediated by the work of nursing. Exclusive pumpers, thus, devote themselves to an activity considered by most researchers to be second best to breastfeeding because it is understood as both supplemental and compensatory—an act that supports the difficult work of nursing, not an act that fully replaces it.

MANUFACTURING SHAME: EXCLUSIVE PUMPERS, INVISIBLY PUMPING

Although they rarely appear in academic research, EPers do share their personal narratives online, and their stories of pumping deviate significantly from any assumptions regarding their work. Tales of EPing follow a stunningly similar arc: during pregnancy, the EPer envisions an empowering and blissful breastfeeding relationship with her child. In a typical version of this vision, a woman named Chastity writes, "I wanted to feel the inseparable bond that breastfeeding mothers talked about. I wanted my heart to warm as my son gave me a milky smile" ("Pumping Journey"). Although their intention is to nurse, at or shortly after birth a medical event occurs: sometimes the mother's body fails, as when a very long labour, emergency C-section, or birth injury occurs. In other stories, it is the baby who somehow "fails": an illness requires a stay in the NICU, or an undiagnosed tongue-tie makes feeding ineffective. In some cases, everything goes wrong at once, as Swati Marquez details: "Three days after I gave birth—following fifty-four hours of labor, including eighteen hours of IV fluids that left me ... swollen with edema—my daughter was jaundiced, listless, losing weight, and not producing wet diapers [due to ineffective latch]." Marquez confesses that she was "a reluctant pumper" who "couldn't wait to breastfeed," claims that are quite typical among EPers.

Following some disruption of their expected narratives, women who had been so determined to breastfeed that they refuse even to buy pacifiers find themselves in an unexpected world: they must pump either to stimulate or maintain supply. At this point in their stories, EPers describe an almost immediate sense of relief: the milk is flowing, the baby is growing, and the pump enables the infant to successfully, though indirectly, breastfeed. Yet success does not mean ease. In "Breastfeeding without Nursing," Kristina Johnson writes, "EPers deal with the same time demands and worries over supply that a nursing mother would, with the added headaches of tons of washing, prepping, and packing." As many women report, pumping combines all of the effort of breastfeeding with all of the requirements of formula feeding: special diet, bodily devotion, pain, risk of infection, supplements to maintain supply, bottles, sterilization, ounce counting, and storage systems.

Tellingly, in addition to an emphasis on the desire to nurse and the difficulties pumping entails, most stories of EPing have another common thread: women who pump exclusively state that they had no idea EPing was an option until they discover references to it online. According to Johnson, "Exclusively pumping is not something I knew existed before I started doing it." Likewise, Chastity explains that after a lactation consultant tells her "formula isn't so bad," she "went online looking for answers, and I found a community of exclusive pumpers. These women pumped for three, six, nine, twelve months!" Perhaps for the very simple reason that exclusive pumping is not studied, let alone supported, by lactation professionals, women who pump exclusively lack the terminology they need to describe their work, not to mention the resources they need to perform it. Thus, each woman who exclusively pumps, despite sharing so much in common with other EPers, must discover EPing on her own. As Brittany Minor writes in "Exclusively Pumping Moms Exist Too," "Exclusively pumping mamas are hardly ever thought about because who in their crazy mind would choose to pump?" Yet she rightfully claims, "It's a hidden world, yes, but this world does exist."

How is it that an entire method of infant feeding remains a "hidden world"? The online stories and conversations of EPers reveal that they struggle to self-identify—to even admit that they exclusively pump—because they experience a great deal of shame associated with "failing" to breastfeed.[4] Of course, shame is in no short supply in the parenting world. Every parenting choice, from diet to diapers, the availability of screens to the schedule of vaccinations, can be divided into a number of sides, each of which declares that the others are terribly wrong. In the EP world, shame and invisibility have (at least) three sources: cultural understandings of the pump as a tool of autonomy, the association between pump and dis/ability, and the perception of the pump as overtechnologization of natural feeding. First, since we understand pumping as a means by which women regain autonomy after childbirth, EPers often choose not to admit they EP because they fear their doctors and families will assume they have chosen themselves over their infants. In a BabyCenter post titled "Midwife Shamed Me about EP," the women discuss times when they were subtly shamed or outright attacked for pumping. One woman writes, "I get this sort of response from women in my family, weird looks and pointed questions that imply I'm being lazy." EPers feel they are judged for putting their own needs before the needs of their children, casting off the bonds of direct breastfeeding in favour of the assumedly lighter bonds of the pump. In a terrible trap of logic, then, EPing labour is underrepresented and misunderstood because women prefer not to admit they EP, and this preference stems from the very fact that EPing is misunderstood and often maligned.

An overassociation with errant bodies stands as another explanation for the invisibility of exclusive pumpers. As evidenced in their personal narratives, women who turn to the pump most often do so after a medical trauma affecting mother and/or child. But even absent these more obvious events, women who pump often admit that they feel they have the wrong kind of body for breastfeeding. Although breastfeeding is most certainly possible for women with flat or inverted nipples, larger bodies, or surgically modified breasts, it is undoubtedly more difficult and requires some level of intervention (extensive lactation consultation, modified cushions and support devices, silicone shields, etc.). Indeed, it is often not major trauma but minor bodily difference that results in EPing: women experience initial latching difficulty leading to infant weight loss or jaundice, which results in the use of the pump to retrieve milk that the infant cannot access. If women are embarrassed to talk about their "flawed" breasts, they are even more reluctant to admit that pumping makes nursing significantly easier when the breastfeeding body does not perform as planned. In posts with titles like "Prefer Pumping over BFing?" and "Is pumping easier than breastfeeding?" women discuss their bodily differences (e.g., flat and/or inverted nipples, misshapen breasts, nonaverage body weight, vasospasm) and those of their children (e.g., cleft palate, tongue/lip tie, reflux, developmental oral motor deficiencies) that led them to the pump. In the "Prefer Pumping" discussion, a user named Yenafa writes, "If I had the beautiful storybook BFing relationship I envisioned, I would prefer BFing. But I didn't, I hated BFing. My LO [little one] arched his back, grunted and screamed whenever he went to the breast.... I vastly prefer pumping over what was going on back then [reflux]." The relative ease of pumping when compared to a difficult breastfeeding experience runs counter to the more popular narratives of EPing struggles that I detail in the next section. When an EPer admits she prefers the pump, she seemingly admits to choosing her comfort over her child's—the very assumption those outside the EP world make about women who pump exclusively. The acknowledgment of this so-called easier choice can be as shameful as the acknowledgment of the failure of one's body. Rather than explain the flaws that made nursing impossible and pumping (shamefully) easier, EPers choose silence and invisibility.

Finally, EPers sometimes feel embarrassed because pumping is associated not only with medicalization[5] but also with the technologization of a supposedly natural body process. Boyer calls pumping a "transgression of motherhood" because of the fact that infant feeding becomes a "wholly individuated socio-technical system of breast pumps, lactation rooms, refrigerators, and working mothers willing to discipline their bodies to the rigors of pumping at work" (284). Described in this way, working-pumping mothers become little but a cog in the feeding machine, tools rather than masters of the technology that supposedly enables their autonomy. To add a layer of complication (and guilt) to the subject, some studies implicitly hold women who pump at work responsible for the problem of inadequate maternity leave in the United States; that is, because they are too efficient at supplying their children with expressed breast milk, women who pump inadvertently prove extended leave and related policies to be unnecessary. For example, Maia Boswell-Penc and Kate Boyer state, "we are concerned that by providing a personalized, technical fix to the question of workplace lactation, breast pumps may lessen possibilities for receiving paid maternity leave, or remove any incentive for employers to come up with more—and perhaps better—alternatives for women trying to combine work and nursing" (563). Thus EPers carry a double load of shame: making milk via the pump alone, they depend solely on machines that, according to some, make life more difficult for all women. And unlike women who pump only for work or leisure, the EPer enjoys no redemption in the form of nursing and so seemingly cannot remedy all the bad she does in her quest to be a good mother.

EPERS AND OPDS, MOTNS AND PISAS: EXPLORING BABYCENTER'S "THE EXCLUSIVE PUMPERS!"

Women who pump exclusively find few readily available resources to support their version of the breastfeeding journey. Yet when EPers go online, they find the "hidden world" they were missing, especially when they stumble upon established communities like those on BabyCenter.com. A resource for expectant and new parents, BabyCenter hosts virtual meeting places related to pregnancy, parenting, and family life. Perhaps more importantly, individual-user-created boards unite families facing a variety of challenges—from VBACs, PCOS pregnancies, and fertility issues to NICU stays, developmental differences, and behavioural concerns. As Michelle Moravec has found in her studies of online parenting communities including BabyCenter, online communities meet a "need for support, shared reference points, and normalization of emotions" (17). Specialized online communities are especially critical for women who find themselves outside normalized mothering culture.

"The Exclusive Pumpers!", formed on 21 January 2009, is BabyCenter's largest and most active group for pumping women, with over 32,000 members, 76,000 posts, and 452,000 user responses to posts. New user posts appear every several hours.[6] To compare, a similarly active board formed in 2013, "Exclusive Pumping," hosts about 3,200 members and 1,300 posts. With such a large number of users, it would seem that exclusive pumping is not so exclusive at all, especially when one considers that a popular breastfeeding board, "Breastfeeding Support and Help," hosts 112,000 members and 168,000 posts. But further investigation shows that many members of "The Exclusive Pumpers!" are women who pump to supplement nursing. They join "The Exclusive Pumpers!" because they recognize that good pumping instruction is lacking, and women who must pump effectively to breastfeed at all have become, by necessity, their own best sources of instruction.

I surveyed a typical month of posts on "The Exclusive Pumpers!" at the end of July 2016. As usual, the board was quite active, with a total of 333 posts for the month. In addition to user-posted questions, the board moderators oversee monthly chats geared toward community building: a general interest chat, a MOTN chat for women performing their "middle of the night" pump, and a monthly weaning chat. In the user-generated posts, common questions and concerns include: pumping schedules and timing; the appropriate time to drop pumps; pump types and parts, including troubleshooting defective equipment; medical problems; increasing or decreasing supply; dietary advice; pumping in the workplace; managing newborn, infant, or child care while pumping; coping with unsupportive family; coping with emotions related to pumping, including embarrassment, guilt, and regret; and congratulatory posts reporting attained goals.

Surveying the July 2016 posts reveals important trends common to the community as a whole and critical to an understanding of the EP mindset. As with the writers of the EP stories discussed earlier, BabyCenter users carefully construct narratives of pumping difficulty—starting with their immense struggles to breastfeed and lingering in the "constant now" of pumping, where round-the-clock expression efforts combined with bottle-feeding and childcare duties add up to a form of maternal labour that is, according to EPers, far more intensive than nursing. According to Stearns's study, pumping mothers "typically viewed their mothering through pumping as second best ... a good effort, but never the best effort" ("Breast Pump" 19). Yet the women of "The Exclusive Pumpers" reject this notion entirely, claiming instead that their work exceeds the best efforts of nursing mothers. When a woman who does not yet EP comes to the board to discuss how one transitions from nursing to the pump, users strongly caution against the transition. In one typical post, a mother who successfully nurses asks if she should make the switch to pumping because it seems easier. In response, EPers write: "my only tip is don't do it unless you have to"; "EPing is generally more work and more of a chore"; "I'm sure most of us here would BF if we could"; "EP is not fun, not easy and there is really no advantage to it that I can see"; "EPing is incredibly difficult, time-consuming, and stressful"; "It is damn hard both ways but EPing is harder. It's double the work." This conversation among mothers who pump typifies self-representation on "The Exclusive Pumpers!": EPers define EPing as an act of double-labour, a combination of breastfeeding and bottle-feeding that requires more effort but receives less respect because it is supposedly not true breastfeeding. Unlike other forms of domestic technology—washing machines, dishwashers, vacuums—the breast pumps in these women's stories ultimately create more work for the women who use them, not less, and are undoubtedly depicted as such in order to counter the notion that women choose exclusive pumping because it is more convenient and requires less effort than breastfeeding.

Even as EPers emphasize the difficulty of the EPing process, they commend and congratulate themselves for enduring that process. That is, they consider the work as separate from the worker, disassociating women who pump from the negativity associated with pumping and repurposing that negativity as evidence of their extreme commitment to the work of breastfeeding. As evidenced by its very name, with the added exclamation point after "Pumpers!", women who join and become active members of the board may at first feel shame, guilt, and regret over their inability to nurse, but as a part of the community they find comfort in an acknowledgment of their efforts. In "To All of Us," a post written in January 2014 and commented on as recently as June 2017 (with a total of over 180 comments), one woman explains why she thinks EPers should take pride in their work. She begins by referring to every EPer's assumed intent to nurse: "From the time we were pregnant, we had an image in our mind of how life with a baby would be.... But then reality happened and LO couldn't nurse.... Maybe your LO was premature and couldn't come home. Maybe LO couldn't latch." As is typical of the EPing narrative, this woman claims for the community a commitment to breastfeeding disrupted by unexpected medical difficulties. She continues, "So here you are, a crusader for your LO. You never gave up hope that LO would have the best start to life, including BM [breast milk]. You do so much extra work, often with people not understanding how hard it is.... You continue through cracked nipples, clogged ducts, illness, and lack of sleep." In this paragraph, the writer denies the claim that expressed milk is "second best"; instead, she considers expressed milk to be the equivalent to nursed milk and then goes on to detail the difficulty of pumping itself. She concludes, "Even if nobody out there understands why you do it.... I understand. We all understand here.... We chose the hardest road to travel because we just could not give up. We want what is best for our child, even if it means great sacrifice for ourselves." Here, in a complete rebuttal of common misconceptions regarding pumping, she calls EPing an active choice of the "hardest" work of good mothering: EPers provide their children not second best but the best, sacrifice their own comfort and leisure to do so, and deserve to take pride in their labour.

GOOD SACRIFICES MAKE GOOD MOTHERS? THE INEVITABLE PROBLEMATICS OF EMBRACING DIFFICULTY

To this point, this chapter has endeavoured to identify and champion the exclusive pumpers, and to find a place for them in the field of breastfeeding studies. But we must openly confront the fact that EPers stake their claim to maternal legitimacy on the grounds of their own bodies: at a time when pumps should, and do, represent a claim to freedom (of time, employment, and/or leisure), EPers seemingly roll back the clock, using their attachment to the pump, extreme effort, lack of freedom, even lack of health and happiness as a claim on the territory of good mothering. If breastfeeding is good, they seem to say, then exclusive pumping is better because it is difficult, even because it is neglected, derided, and misunderstood. We therefore run the risk of equating good mothering with this elision of self and pump so that "the good" of pumping necessarily becomes equated with the negative effects of pumping on the EPer's life.

Where do we go from here? In part, we return to the EPers, who in one post might say "never quit on a bad day!" but in another post reassure each other than any breast milk is good breast milk, that a month of pumping is an achievement, that a fed baby is a happy baby, and that all food is good food. EPers strike a unique balance between pride in commitment to pumping and understanding of the need to wean. Despite the militancy with which EPers defend themselves to the outside world, among themselves this militancy disappears, replaced by kindness and acceptance of the hardships each woman endures. Although the length of time that one endures the physical and psychological demands of exclusive pumping becomes a point of pride for many women, EPers discuss the achievement of breastfeeding milestones in terms at once congratulatory and noncompetitive. In part because long-term pumpers carry so much knowledge that is not available from lactation consultants, mothers' groups, or midwives, one woman's ability to pump long term becomes the seed that allows other women to likewise continue pumping. By calling all infant feeding good infant feeding and actively working to build and promote a supportive, instructive community, EPers push back against inherently sexist constructions of competitive motherhood.

Furthermore, EPers endeavour to build egalitarian relationships with their partners. If exclusive breastfeeding is "solely maternal" with an "unequal division of labor" (Stearns, "Work" 70), then EPing is by necessity "inclusively paternal": the women often speak of how vital their (usually male) partners are to their success.[7] Although Stearns has found that even among pumping mothers, "opportunities for father involvement in bottle feeding are often not part of a daily routine" (74), the same is not true for EPers. Rather, EPers often advise women who are struggling to pump that they need to enlist more help from their husbands or partners. In a post titled "Convincing Husband I Need Help," one woman explains, "I always tell my DH [dear husband] he's my partner in this.... He does not 'help' me out as that implies a favor being done. He needs to pull his own weight." Just as pumping often requires more work than nursing, the co-parents of women who exclusively pump also must work harder, usually handling the majority of infant feeding and care during the first weeks and beyond so that the EPer can maintain her pumping schedule. Thus, although EPers do use their devotion to the pump as evidence of good mothering, by including their partners in their labour, EPers advocate for an image not of the good mother but of the good parent—a liberatory act that shares the work of breastfeeding not simply between partners but among the entire EPing community. Although the relationship between the pumping mother and the technologies she uses remains imperfect—she cannot, at this point in time, see or speak of the pump as a source of emancipation—the act of exclusive pumping, nonetheless, contributes to an equitable, communal experience of infant feeding.

ENDNOTES

[1]I examine online communities formed by mothers of full-term, healthy infants and so focus on bottle-feeding as opposed to feeding via nasal or gastronomy tubes. There is significant overlap among the exclusive pumping and tube-feeding communities, since the mothers of children who receive expressed milk via tube are, by necessity, exclusive pumpers. However, mothers who pump for medically fragile children tend to form their own communities online because their concerns and needs are often condition specific (e.g., pumped milk for a premature infant can only be refrigerated for forty-eight hours, versus three to eight days for a full-term infant).

[2]I use EP (exclusively pump), EPing (exclusive pumping), and EPer (exclusive pumper) interchangeably for brevity and variety. I have adopted these acronyms from the online communities in which they originate.

[3]Boyer notes: "In 2011 the right to express breast milk at work began to be protected by federal law in the US, under the 'Reasonable Break Time for Nursing Mothers' provision of the Patient Protection and Affordable Care Act, which mandated that workplaces of over fifty employees must provide lactation rooms and breaks during the workday to express milk" (270). NB: at this time (February 2018), it is unclear whether the Trump administration will support the federal protections for breastfeeding women that are tied to the Affordable Care Act.

[4]If exclusive pumping is difficult, then EPing by choice as opposed to circumstance is more burdensome. Even among EPers, it is assumed that one starts pumping only after breastfeeding has failed. Pregnant women who ask for advice on how to begin pumping at the hospital are strongly cautioned against choosing "the pumping life" and are advised instead to at least attempt breastfeeding because it is comparatively easier. Unfortunately, this preference for nursing neglects the needs of women who choose the pump either because of simple preference or because they wish to preserve their bodily autonomy for a complex reason, such as past history of emotional or sexual trauma. Because nursing is so strongly advised and the desire to pump is so quickly brushed aside, women who choose to pump without nursing first rarely self-identify, and those who do tend not to explain their reasons. Unfortunately, then, the exclusive-pumpers-by-choice remain the most invisible members of the breastfeeding community. Additionally, another group of women that I do not discuss here are those mothers who pump after a late-term pregnancy loss or infant loss. Although they occasionally visit online pumping communities for information on how to stop or continue pumping, they do not appear to frequent those communities.

[5]According to Glenda Walls, even nursing has become "medicalized," "something that women must be retaught through scientifically based professional intervention" (594-95). Without question, women must be taught how to pump effectively, but unlike nursing mothers, they enjoy no "professional intervention"—there are no EP consultants, though nurses do provide basic instructions on how pumps work.

[6]I also reviewed other online communities, including Reddit's r/

bbpumpers and r/BreastPumps. However, these communities are significantly less active than those on BabyCenter, despite Reddit's greater popularity overall. Bbpumpers sees, on average, four posts per month with a range from one to thirteen discussion comments per post. The interests and assertions evident in the BabyCenter community are also present in its Reddit counterparts, with women discussing their struggles, pumping tips, and reasons for pumping. Because the Reddit boards are so sparsely populated, users occasionally direct posters to "The Exclusive Pumpers!" for more advice.

[7]The women of "The Exclusive Pumpers!" almost always speak of male partners, and those partners are usually DHs ("dear husband"). My survey of the community found only one mother with a female partner. This finding is typical of BabyCenter communities as a whole, where users most often identify as heterosexual women. Similarly, single mothers infrequently appear in the community, though they frequently post on breastfeeding boards.

WORKS CITED

Al-Agba, Niran S. "The Humiliation a Nursing Physician Experienced During Her Board Exams." *KevinMD.com,* 2 July 2016, www.kevinmd.com/blog/2016/07/humiliation-nursing-physician-faced-board-exam.html. Accessed 24 Feb. 2018.

Boswell-Penc, Maia and Kate Boyer. "Expressing Anxiety? Breast Pump Usage in American Wage Workplaces." *Gender, Place and Culture*, vol. 14, no. 5, 2007, pp. 551-67.

Boyer, Kate. "'Neoliberal Motherhood': Workplace Lactation and Changing Conceptions of Working Motherhood in the Contemporary US." *Feminist Theory*, vol. 15, no. 3, 2014, pp. 269-88.

Chastity. "My Exclusive Pumping Journey (9 Months and Going Strong)." *The Badass Breastfeeder*, 13 Aug. 2013, www.thebadassbreastfeeder.com/my-exclusive-pumping-journey-9-months-and-going-strong-by-guest-blogger-chasity/. Accessed 24 Feb. 2018.

Firestone, Shulamith. *The Dialectic of Sex*. Bantam, 1972.

Happyhealthyloved. "Midwife Shamed Me about EP." *BabyCenter.com,* 28 Mar. 2013, Johnson and Johnson, community.babycenter.

com/post/a40982593. Accessed Feb. 24 2018.
Ischmidb. "Convincing Husband I Need Help." *BabyCenter.com,* 30 June 2016, Johnson and Johnson, community.babycenter.com/post/a63244957. Accessed Feb. 24 2018.
Johnson, Kristina. "Breastfeeding Without Nursing: What It's Like to Be an Exclusive Pumper." *Parent.co,* 3 Aug. 2016, www.parent.co/breastfeeding-without-nursing-what-its-like-to-be-an-exclusive-pumper/. Accessed 24 Feb. 2018.
KLa786. "Prefer Pumping Over BFing?" *BabyCenter.com,* 27 June 2016, Johnson and Johnson, community.babycenter.com/post/a63214021. Accessed 24 Feb. 2018.
Lee, Robyn. "Breastfeeding and Constraints on Mothers' Agency." *Journal of the Motherhood Initiative*, vol. 3, no. 2, 2012, pp. 93-102.
Marquez, Swati. "Op-Ed: When a Mother Chooses the Pump." *Feminist Wire,* 25 Aug. 2013, www.thefeministwire.com/2013/08/op-ed-when-a-mother-chooses-the-pump/. Accessed 24 Feb. 2018.
Minor, Brittany. "Exclusively Pumping Moms Exist Too." *Mom.me*, 12 Aug. 2014, mom.me/baby/14091-exclusively-pumping-moms-exist-too/. Accessed 24 Feb. 2018.
Momtocole&milo. "Is pumping easier than Breastfeeding? *BabyCenter.com*, 25 Aug. 2012, Johnson and Johnson, community.babycenter.com/post/a35959648. Accessed 24 Feb. 2018.
Monki929. "To All of Us." *BabyCenter.com,* 12 Jan. 2014, Johnson and Johnson, community.babycenter.com/post/a47025460. Accessed 1 Dec. 2016.
Moravec, Michelle. "Expectant Motherhood: How Online Communities Shape Pregnancy." *Motherhood Online*, edited by Michelle Moravec, Cambridge Scholars, 2011, pp. 2-22.
Pallister, Kathryn. "And Now, the Breast of the Story: Realistic Portrayals of Breastfeeding in Contemporary Television." *Mediating Moms: Mothers in Popular Culture*, edited by Elizabeth Podnieks, McGill-Queen's, 2012 pp. 221-35.
Rowland, Robyn. "Crumbling Motherhood: Reproductive Technology Creating Women's Procreative Alienation." *FINRRAGE,* 29 Oct. 1987, www.finrrage.org/wp-content/uploads/2016/03/Crumbling_Motherhoo_Rowland.pdf. Accessed 24 Feb. 2018.
Stearns, Cindy A. "The Breast Pump." *Giving Breastmilk: Body*

Ethics and Contemporary Breastfeeding Practice, edited by Alison Bartlett, Demeter, 2010, pp. 11-23.
Stearns, Cindy A. "The Work of Breastfeeding. *Women's Studies Quarterly*, vol. 37, no. 3-4, 2009, pp. 63-80.
Wall, Glenda. "Moral Constructions of Motherhood in Breastfeeding Discourse." *Gender and Society*, vol. 15, no. 4, pp. 592-610.

14. Surrogacy and Breastfeeding— A Puzzle to Solve

A Case Study on the Surrogacy Industry in India

ANINDITA SENGUPTA

Breastfeeding has always attracted the attention of feminist scholarship as it is an integral part of a woman's experience of motherhood, her maternal and personal choices, and her child's health. In recent years, with the medicalization of pregnancy and childbirth, it has also become an important public health issue all over the world. Breastmilk is now recommended by the medical fraternity, and childcare advocates as the ultimate source of nutrition for babies. Breastfeeding is also known as an excellent way of developing maternal bond with the newborn. As the new mother snuggles her baby close to her breast, she not only provides the child with the best nutrition possible but also develops an eternal nurturing relationship. Interestingly, therefore, although most mothers are encouraged and educated to breastfeed their babies, surrogate mothers in India are often denied the opportunity to do the same because of the apprehension that it may lead to an unnecessary emotional bond with the baby. Denial of breastfeeding is part of the process of controlling and disciplining the medicalized bodies and minds of these surrogates so that they do not claim the baby. Through a rigorous counselling process, clinics try to convert the surrogates into reproductive workers who produce healthy babies to whom they are emotionally unattached. Interestingly, even though the definition of an ideal mother is one who diligently breastfeeds her baby, a perfect surrogate, mother, and worker (Pande, "Commercial Surrogacy") is one who does not want to breastfeed and who gives the baby away without objection. In this chapter, using interviews with six surrogates, five medical practitioners, and three intending mothers in Kolkata and Delhi, India, I explore the dilemmas related to breastfeeding within the context of surrogacy. The interviews were conducted in Hindi, English, and Bengali. I observed most of my interviewees including surrogates in many occasions used English medical terms to describe their own experiences of pregnancy. The frequent use of medical parlance in their conversation demonstrates how medicalized these pregnancies are.

Assisted reproductive technologies, such as in-vitro fertilization (IVF), have led to the fragmentation of reproductive experiences. Their existence has opened up immense possibilities for reproduction, family, and kinship. In this collaborative birthing process, as many as three women can participate in producing one child, which complicates the question of motherhood (placing discussions of genetic motherhood alongside those of egg donorship, gestational surrogate motherhood, and social and/or legal motherhood). With these new options, assisted reproductive technologies (ARTs) have also led to new tensions in society between the local meanings of morality, family, and kinship, on the one hand, and discourses of modernity, the free-market economy, and bioethics on the other. This division of the reproductive process has also led to debates over who has the strongest claim over the baby. Since breastfeeding is a process through which the baby develops initial physical and emotional bonds, an important question to ask is who should be allowed to breastfeed and bond with a newborn? In India, there has not been any registered case of surrogates claiming any baby, yet an imagined environment of fear has been created, since these women carry these babies in their wombs for nine months.

Motherhood and women's reproductivity are always subjects of surveillance, as the creation of future citizens depends on them. Although the good mother is sometimes conceptually defined by her ability to breastfeed, mothers' choices and options to feed their babies are also limited by their social positions, as well as their privilege in terms of race, class, sex, caste, and other factors. Feminist literature (Apple; Baumslag and Michels; Blum, "Mothers"; Davis; Dettwyler; Maher; Palmer; Reissman; Van Esterik) surrounding breastfeeding demonstrates how varied women's positions and experiences are on this topic. Breastfeeding has been a tool for subordinating women as well as a means of resistance. The highly medicalized bodies of surrogates do not fit into the narratives of motherhood. Although good mothers are expected to breastfeed to bond with their babies and to provide necessary nutrition to the infants, there is an attempt to alienate the surrogate from the resultant baby by denying her to breastfeed. Feminists have claimed that breastfeeding should be considered as part of women's reproductive rights and her right to motherhood. The third annual Breastfeeding and Feminism Symposia in 2007 echoed the same sentiment (Labbok et al.). Surrogacy in India is not a relationship of equals, and the denial of the right to breastfeed demonstrates an extreme kind of scientific and medical colonization of reproduction and of women's bodies. Prohibited from breastfeeding, surrogates are denied the right to motherhood, whereas intending mothers claim a right over the baby by inducing lactation artificially.

Most clinics have formulated their own policies based on the essentialist understanding that breastfeeding establishes a so-called natural bond with the baby and that refusing the right to breastfeed will easily sever that connection. Severing the right of motherhood from Indian surrogates occurs not only with the help of technology but also with effective use of narratives. This chapter is divided into two parts. In the first part, I introduce the surrogacy industry in India and provide an overview of my research by asking these questions. Who are these surrogates? Are they considered mothers or reproductive workers in commercial surrogacy? How do cultural norms of compulsory parenthood in India create the narratives around assisted reproduction? In the second part of the chapter, I discuss the narratives around breastfeeding extant in the surrogacy industry using my interviews with surrogates, doctors, and intending mothers. The intent of the chapter is to show how breastfeeding is used in the surrogacy industry to colonize and commodify women's bodies by both the medical industry and market economy. The breastfeeding discourse in the surrogacy industry is efficiently deployed in an attempt to render surrogates as "other," not just from the women who hire them but from the fetuses they carry as well. However, some of the surrogates I interviewed claimed that the "maternal instinct" extends beyond the act of breastfeeding only. They develop the connection with the fetus from the first day of their pregnancy.

THE DEVELOPMENT OF THE SURROGACY INDUSTRY IN INDIA

Reproductive technologies, such as IVF, lead to the externalization of reproduction, and move beyond a conventional biological understanding of reproduction to create new possibilities of kinship and family. Ideas of kinship get even more muddled with respect to surrogacy and donor-inseminated births. Nowadays, through the use of gestational surrogacy and donor births, the process of having a baby has become more than a biological one dependent on heterosexual intercourse, and, instead, involves the creation of alternative families and the breaking of traditional norms. IVF offers the potential to split the genetic mother from the birth mother, and by the 1990s, this technology was already being used in gestational surrogacy arrangements, in which a surrogate is impregnated with another woman's eggs, which enables her to give birth to a genetically unrelated child. Within a few years, India had become the "surrogacy capital" of the world; fertility clinics mushroomed everywhere, in both small and large cities, and invited both local and foreign clients. The fertility industry in India grew organically without state intervention, and, therefore, commercial surrogacy developed in a space where surrogacy was neither legal nor illegal. Gradually, an established transnational network developed with medical tourism agencies, clinics, and surrogacy hostels, which made the fertility business an unregulated billion-dollar industry. Good medical facilities, the availability of women willing to work as surrogates due to poverty, and an unregulated market led to a thriving business environment for the fertility industry (DasGupta and Dasgupta; Pande, "Commercial Surrogacy," *Wombs in Labor*; Sama, *Birthing a Market*). Indian clinics started to offer surrogacy to all, and India became a popular destination for couples from the West opting for surrogacy.

Among all reproductive arrangements through ART, transnational surrogacy has received the most media attention. Indian surrogates are inexpensive—charging a fraction of what their Western counterparts charge—and they do not have any rights over the baby. Indeed, critics say that it is nothing but cheap surrogate wombs that led to the popularization of commercial surrogacy in India, but the medical fraternity claims that this is a win-win situation for both the intending parents and the surrogates; the commissioning couples get the child of their dreams, and the surrogate receives the money that she desperately needs. But is it an equal relationship of two equally informed parties? Alison Bailey argues that the rhetoric of "mutual help" silences the inequality embedded in the system. In the transnational commercial surrogacy industry, Indian surrogates' wombs are viewed as saleable commodities, which makes these women cheap reproductive labourers of the Global South. In this context, Sayantani DasGupta and Shamita Dasgupta argue, "While the general discourse of surrogacy frames it as a matter of mutually beneficial exchange between women who have money but are infertile, and women who are poor but can produce children, the barter effectively secretes the power differentials between the inhabitants of the First and Third Worlds to the detriment of Indian surrogates" (xiii). Surrogates and donors seldom have any bargaining power in the reproductive market, even with respect to decisions about the compensation they receive. During my fieldwork, I noticed that most surrogates are not aware of the medical procedures that they need to go through, nor do they understand the potential risks associated with those treatments when they sign the contract with the clinics.

THE RESEARCH LANDSCAPE

I conducted most of my interviews in two clinics in Kolkata and one clinic in Delhi. These clinics were attracting patients from all across India, including from small and large cities and from different countries. The clinics in Delhi that I visited were very different from those in Kolkata. Delhi clinics attract more Western clients and are, therefore, more equipped to provide services to an international clientele. Kolkata clinics get more local clients and patients from small towns. They also receive many clients from West Bengal's neighbouring states and countries such as Bangladesh and Nepal. Although I interviewed the major stakeholders (surrogates, doctors, and clients) involved in surrogacy arrangements, I also wanted to hear predominantly from women (infertile mothers and surrogates), since their bodies primarily become the medium of medical and scientific inquiry and experimentation during fertility treatments. I met these women mostly in doctor's clinics. The intending mothers shared their experiences of infertility, the familial pressure they faced to have a child, and their experiences receiving fertility treatments. Most of these women opted for surrogacy as a last resort to have a baby after long periods of fertility treatments. The surrogates also shared their stories about why they agreed to become surrogates, their experiences of pregnancy, and how they saw themselves in the reproductive arrangements—as mothers or as reproductive labourers renting their wombs. The women I interviewed (both clients and surrogates) were not members of two monolithic groups; they were from diverse sociocultural backgrounds, with diverse experiences. Most of the clients, however, were upper or middle class, whereas surrogates came from poor families. In India, the social stigma associated with infertility and assisted reproduction is significant, and, therefore, intending mothers did not want to disclose to their extended families and friends that they were opting for surrogacy. They wanted to hide the process of surrogacy as much as they could. Pregnancy out of marriage is also a huge social taboo, so surrogates did not want to reveal their identities publicly either. As a result, before the interviews, almost all the women (both surrogates and intending mothers) ascertained with me that I would use pseudonyms for them.

Most surrogates are driven to surrogacy because of desperate financial need. The majority of the surrogate women I interviewed came from the slums that have developed in the peripheries of the big cities, and many were day labourers from rural communities with few or no marketable skills. Surrogacy provides these women with an opportunity to earn a substantial amount of money in a relatively short period of time. Namita, a surrogate, said,

> We have severe financial problems at home. My husband got badly injured when he was working in a factory that made spare parts for cars. They had to amputate one of his legs. That was the worst time of my life. Everyone was tense at home. We didn't know how to pay our bills. It was literally a hand-to-mouth existence for us. When we learned about surrogacy, it was like a godsend.

For some women, surrogacy will provide their children a better life: "We want to send our children to an English-medium school," said Nisha. "Giving my children a good education is most important to us, and this is not possible with my husband's income [he sells *chaats*, a popular Indian snack, near Sarojini Market]. Otherwise, no woman bears a child and gives it away for no reason." Nila became a surrogate because her alcoholic husband left her for another woman. She was working as a maid, and her husband continued to come and take away her wages. Surrogacy, thus, provided an opportunity for her to earn and save some money. She explained her situation: "I am not concerned about anyone, only my children. Neither my husband nor our neighbours are going to give me anything to eat. I have to do this for my sake, for the sake of my children." Surrogate women have several reasons to take up the job of surrogacy, but all of those I interviewed sought a better life for themselves and their families.

SURROGACY: WHO IS THE REAL MOTHER?

As with surrogates, the intending mothers I interviewed were also under tremendous social pressure for not being able to produce a child after many years of marriage. In Indian society, motherhood is still considered an integral part of womanhood, and childbirth is perceived as a natural progression after marriage (Patel; Singh). Men and women experience pressure to marry and have a child in order to fulfill the social norms (Chadda and Deb; Gupta; Patel; Singh): A marriage without children is conspicuous and aberrant (Sama, *Birthing a Market*) and hence socially stigmatized. My research participants narrated similar experiences. To deal with infertility, desperate couples do whatever they can to have a child. The popularity of ART is therefore no surprise—the demand existed even before its inception. The advent of IVF, gamete donation, surrogacy, and other reproductive technologies provide new family-building options to these infertile couples and give them the opportunity to fulfill the cultural norms of family and kinship (Strathern, *After Nature*, "Future Kinship"; Franklin and Ragone; Thompson). My interviews revealed that once a child was born through surrogacy, parents did whatever they deemed necessary to erase the presence of the surrogate in the reproductive arrangements to establish a claim over the baby to the point of publicly pretending that there was no third-party involvement in the birthing arrangement.

Moreover, the clinics do everything they can to make sure the surrogates do not develop emotional connections with the babies. Sociologist Amrita Pande refers to these surrogates as "perfect mother-workers." According to her, "Surrogacy is remarkable as a form of labor in the way it requires the laborer to be both a mother and a worker. The disciplinary project exploits this duality in intriguing ways" (*Wombs in Labor*, 22). The surrogate is expected to be a disciplined contract worker who takes care of the fetus as a caring mother but also gives up the baby without any objection. These disciplinary techniques are implemented by counselling and controlling these women's bodies and minds. Almost all the clinics have their own counsellors, but some doctors take it more seriously and assume the role of the counsellor themselves. Dr. Banerjee from Delhi said, "I counsel all my patients and surrogates myself. Counsellors are not doctors; they do not know the medical conditions. We tell them [surrogates] clearly that they will get money just for gestating the child. It is not their child. The child is just a guest in her womb." The medical narratives, along with the use of technology, determine who deserves to claim the baby. The surrogates are made to believe that they are disposable reproductive machines necessary to create perfect babies without any emotional ramifications.

When discussing surrogates' rights to breastfeed it is important to remember that the options and experiences of breastfeeding are also embedded in questions of race, class, and caste, just like other reproductive rights. Linda Blum ("Mothers") points out how black women's breastfeeding rights in the United States, just like their reproductive rights, have historically been limited and controlled from the time of slavery. Black women's bodies fed white babies, sometimes even at the expense of their own children. In the Indian context, such issues as surrogacy and surrogates' reproductive rights need to be evaluated with a perspective on caste and class, which often intersect in this part of the world. Surrogate women in India often come from poor economic backgrounds—and hence also from lower-caste communities—and are, therefore, encouraged to give birth for rich clients and, if necessary, to pump their milk for the health of the infant, but they must give up basic rights of motherhood. In India, upper-caste and upper-class Hindu women's reproductivity has always been celebrated (Ahluwalia; Puri). In contrast, poor and lower-caste women's reproduction has been viewed with suspicion, especially within the mainstream birth control discourse, as it is believed that such women pose a challenge to the nation's development and economic modernization. Hence, it is economically and socially made acceptable by the surrogacy industry to use the bodies of these poor women to create babies for rich and international clients. Surrogates' wombs gestate the babies, and if the intending parents want, surrogates pump their breastmilk as well. The bodies of the surrogates are commodified and dismembered to provide services according to the customers' wishes.

THE ACT OF BREASTFEEDING AND THE CLAIM OVER THE BABY

In India, even while opting for surrogacy, couples, along with the help of the clinic, try to replicate the heterosexual biological parenthood model after the child is born; they, therefore, want to erase the presence of the surrogates from the birthing process as quickly as possible. All the doctors I interviewed expressed reservations and skepticism about allowing surrogates to breastfeed the newborn. Some even expressed doubts about letting the surrogate meet the baby after its birth. Dr. Srikanth from Kolkata said the following:

> Most of the time parents do not want to keep in touch with the surrogate once the child is born. Couples here go through a lot before they go for surrogacy; mothers feel the pain of being deprived of the pleasures of pregnancy. Therefore, once the baby is born, they don't want to share him/her with anyone. Now, we can induce breast milk in intending mothers with hormonal treatments. They could not enjoy the pregnancy; why should we deprive them from the joy of feeding the baby? On the other hand, if the surrogate has milk, she will want to see the baby all

> the more. Therefore, we give injections to the surrogates to dry up their milk.

The intent of the doctors in these fertility clinics is not only to provide medical treatments to infertile couples and give them technological solutions to create babies, but also to produce a narrative around these surrogate babies that mirrors the traditional heterosexual biological norms of family and kinship.

In an attempt to reproduce the existing socially acceptable traditional heterosexual biological family narrative, doctors go through different dilemmas and challenges. They are aware of the nutritional value of breastmilk, but at the same time, they are equally skeptical about the possibility of the surrogates breastfeeding the babies. Moreover, doctors also need to satisfy their clients. Dr. Banerjee from Delhi did not encourage the surrogates to breastfeed the newborn but acknowledged the importance of the health benefits of their breastmilk. In surrogacy arrangements, "the baby is the most prized possession," he remarked. "Couples here do everything just to be a parent. They sometimes spend all their savings to have a baby." For him, taking care of the health of the baby was important, but at the same time, it was equally important to see that the surrogate did not claim the baby. Therefore, an easy solution was to "pump the initial milk for the child": although the baby got the essential nutrients, the surrogate did not get the chance to bond with the child. Dr. Dipika from Kolkata said the following:

> I do think colostrum is super important, but all my surrogates happily pump and provide the initial milk to intending couples anyway. I want the babies to bond with their parents. Nursing is a very intimate bonding experience. If the surrogate pumps and gives the milk to the couple, it's also healthier for the surrogate's postpartum recovery. Once they start breastfeeding, giving away the baby is very difficult. I don't want my surrogates to go through the pain.

Another doctor in the same clinic, Dr. Paul, reiterated these views and insisted, "We ask the surrogate to pump the initial milk, and in cases where the intending mother is keen to breastfeed, lactation can be induced. We follow up on the surrogate baby's health status long term, and if required, we introduce formula. I think this is a better option than allowing surrogates to breastfeed the baby." In surrogacy arrangements, after the child is born, by denying surrogates the right to breastfeed and inducing lactation in intending mothers, doctors try to establish the initial kinship ties. The breastfeeding right given to the intending mother facilitates her claim over the baby, whereas the surrogates get the message that their responsibilities are over and they do not have any future relationship with the baby.

Some doctors argued that they were quite flexible about the idea of surrogates breastfeeding after birth. These doctors claimed that surrogacy arrangements basically take place between adults (commissioning couples and the surrogates) without interference from the clinic. Dr. Mukherjee from Kolkata was herself a mother of two, and she thought that the experience of breastfeeding was not that pleasurable for all women and that Indian society over romanticizes it. She explained by sharing her own experience: "I actually had a rough time breastfeeding my own girls, so I don't see it as a bonding activity. I don't think surrogates should complain about it. I really think it's a personal decision, and there is no right or wrong here; to each their own. We give options to the intending parents." She further added that even though they gave that option to their clients, most parents were not comfortable with the idea of surrogates breastfeeding their babies, and those who agreed also did not keep in touch with the surrogates after the first few months. The doctors claimed that the surrogacy arrangement is a contract between adults, but Dr. Mukherjee's words indicated that surrogates and intending couples were not equal participants in surrogacy arrangements. In commercial surrogacy, the customer's (here the intending mother's) word is the last word, and the surrogates rarely have any power to negotiate the contract. The other doctor I interviewed in Kolkata, Dr. Giri, echoed a similar point of view. According to Dr. Giri, it was not uncommon for surrogates to breastfeed the child, especially in cases where the clients were gay couples. In fact, in those cases, surrogates are paid extra for breastfeeding. In Kolkata, there is also the practice of surrogates living in the same house with the commissioning couples. They cosleep with the mother and the baby and feed the baby when she or he is hungry. In few cases when surrogates breastfeed the babies, it is also then viewed as if they are selling their breast milk just like their uteruses. By assigning a market exchange value to breast milk, the attempt is to undermine the possibility of emotional bonding. Dr. Giri left it to the commissioning couples to decide what they wanted. The surrogates are not equal participants in the surrogacy arrangements and therefore must agree to do whatever the clinic says without question.

The intending mothers I interviewed also had mixed feelings about surrogates breastfeeding their babies. They expressed fear that the surrogate could claim the baby and that the baby might develop a bond with the surrogate, but at the same time they could not overlook the health benefits. Some women regretted that they could not experience the pregnancy, but since the technology was available, they didn't want to let go of the pleasures of breastfeeding. Intending mother Smrita tried to get pregnant for five years, going through several rounds of intrauterine inseminations (IUIs) and IVFs, only to realise that she would need to resort to surrogacy to have a child. She didn't want to lose the opportunity to breastfeed and bond with the baby, and therefore the doctor induced her breast milk. As she put it at the time,

> It will break my heart to watch my baby being nursed by someone else. When people talk about their concerns about surrogacy, they always talk about the fear of surrogates getting emotionally attached to the baby. What if my baby starts bonding with her as well? I dread that thought. Not carrying your own child means missing special moments in life. Like that first kick, or the flutter of the baby in the womb. It is a mind-blowing experience. I always wanted to experience pregnancy.

But since she could not enjoy that, she felt that breastfeeding was the only process available to her to bond with the child: "It establishes the necessary exchange of sensory information. The doctor is inducing lactation in me. Therefore I can breastfeed my baby. The surrogate will pump her milk for the first few weeks. But that's it." Gender socialization and cultural expectations of motherhood are so strong for these women that failing to give birth is considered as a matter of personal loss and shame. Infertility is a matter of social stigma. The new reproductive technologies give them the joy of parenthood while the related social narratives enable the couple to claim the baby as their "own." Sometimes they do not reveal to their extended families that the baby is a result of a surrogacy arrangement and, therefore. they want to erase the presence of the surrogate as early as possible.

The fear of sharing the baby with the surrogate after it is born is daunting for most intending mothers. Since they could not enjoy pregnancy, some of my participants wanted to compensate by breastfeeding the baby. Nivedita had gotten her uterus removed because of fibroids at an early age. She knew surrogacy to be the only option for her. She had accepted that a long time back, but like Smrita, she still regretted that she could not enjoy pregnancy. She was appreciative of the fact that she could now be a mother because of her surrogate and the egg donor, but she was of two minds about breastfeeding: "Now good formula milk is available in the market. Many working women are not able to breastfeed, and their children get their nutrition from the formula milk. The doctor said the surrogate can pump the milk for us as well for the initial few weeks. I am skeptical about the surrogate breastfeeding the child." She feared that because her surrogate carried the baby for nine months, she would already have bonded with the child and that the baby may bond with the surrogate in a maternal way outside of the womb, as well, particularly because the child would not be genetically linked to her. She could not carry the baby in her womb, but once the baby was born, she did not want to share the baby with anybody.

Moreover, some women fear that the child will not recognize them as a mother if the surrogate stays in their lives. Rekha, for instance, tried to get pregnant several times. She had one abortion and several IUIs and IVFs before deciding on surrogacy. There was huge family pressure on her to conceive; this was, therefore, a coveted child for her, as she thought that this baby would reinstate her status in the family. Most of her extended family members did not know about surrogacy, and so she wanted to cut off her ties with the surrogate as soon as she could. She said,

> Not being able to carry your child is hard. You don't get to know that experience. I feel like a total loser. I would not dream of making it any harder by having someone else breastfeeding my child. I can't be pregnant with a child, but I have breasts, so I can nurse my baby. I know breastfeeding will be an extremely rewarding experience. I don't care about colostrum. We have formula milk for that.

For many women like Rekha, the social pressure of motherhood is so intense that they do not want to waste any time sharing the child with the surrogate. In their haste to hold their babies in their arms, many commissioning parents tend to overlook the infant's need for mother's milk, even though it has been scientifically established that mother's milk is a critical source of nutrition for the infant.

In commercial surrogacy arrangements, doctors work under pressure to satisfy their clients. Clients go to any extent to have a baby. Sometimes more than three women (egg donor, surrogate, and interned parent) take part in creating a baby, which leads to the fragmentation of reproduction and motherhood. In such arrangements, therefore, determining who is going to claim and bond with the baby is so convoluted that it complicates many other conventional motherhood narratives, such as association of breastfeeding with so-called good and bad motherhood. In surrogacy arrangements, in my research, I witnessed that breastfeeding is considered more of a bonding exercise than a means of providing nourishment or nutrition to the baby. The surrogacy process is so medically orchestrated and monitored that mother's breastmilk can be easily substituted by market-manufactured formula milk in order to disconnect the link between the surrogate and the baby. Commercial surrogacy arrangements operate within the market economic system where the consumer is always right, and, therefore, the intending mothers are not vilified if they choose formula milk over breastmilk.

Although surrogates do not have much of a voice in surrogacy arrangements, they did express their own opinions on breastfeeding when I interviewed them. Most of the surrogates, during the time of the interview, were either receiving fertility treatments to conceive or were pregnant with their surrogate babies. But most of them appeared to me to be uninformed about the entire surrogacy process. They generally tended to accept the doctors' words as final, since they did not have the education or information to challenge them. Many were doing surrogacy for the first time, and they only knew that this process was very different from their own experiences of pregnancy and childbirth. As was the case with the surrogacy procedures, they were not properly informed about breastfeeding. According to surrogate Nisha, "Doctor *didi* told me that the parents do not want me to breastfeed. I will be given some sort of injection to dry my milk. I am not sure about this. When I had my own babies, I breastfed them for years. I have no clue how the baby will survive without my milk. That is the most 'natural' thing, right?" She shared her own experience of pregnancy and breastfeeding:

> I knew that as a mother, it was my utmost responsibility to breastfeed the baby. When my son was born, he was a weak child, and the doctor in the hospital had told me that he will get all his strength from my breast milk. He actually grew bigger and stronger within a few months. That's the magic of my breast milk … but doctors here say they don't want me to breastfeed. I don't understand. I know it is not my baby, but she is going to stay in my womb for nine months. Do I have no responsibility towards her? What about my own health and recovery? I have no clue. Well we have to do whatever the doctor says.

Breastfeeding is seen as the natural part of birthing, an integral part of the mother-child relationship, and it is often considered a mother's responsibility toward the baby. But in the surrogacy arrangement, doctors try to sever that natural relationship and opt for an extreme scientific and medical colonization of reproduction so that surrogates do not start developing emotional ties with the baby.

Some of the surrogates thought that whether the intending parents agreed or not, they still had a connection with the baby. They argued that the experience of gestating a child in the womb established a strong bond that was difficult to disconnect. Namita said

> I was not thrilled to get up and feed my own girls every night. But I did it since this is a part of my experience of pregnancy and having a child. I didn't mind it, but I was not too ecstatic about it either. I thought it is my duty as a mother to do it, so I did it. Here the doctors tell me that I don't have to breastfeed the baby since that might develop emotional connection. Well, but I am already attached to the baby. The baby will grow up in my womb, she will get food from my blood. We already have a connection. Whether I breastfeed or not doesn't really matter for me. I know the baby is not mine, but no one can deny the fact that she is also a part of me.

Sometimes even surrogates who do not want to breastfeed still believe that the baby is a part of them. These women challenge the entire notion that breastfeeding is a natural maternal instinct present in every woman. Regardless the clinic's attempt to prevent them from breastfeeding, they still developed an emotional bond with the baby. The surrogate Nila, who was also pregnant during the interviews, echoed a similar point of view: "I certainly didn't view it as a bonding experience. It was so different from my own kids. With my own kids, I would just look at their faces lovingly and admire how adorable they were. With my surrogate babies, my mind knows that they are not my own. But the baby is already getting his food from my body. So the connection is still there."

Although all the surrogates I interviewed went through an intensive counselling process, many of them agreed that it was difficult to forget the experience and deny the emotional bond with the baby (whether they breastfed the baby or not). Mala in Delhi was the only surrogate I interviewed who was undergoing treatment for her second surrogacy. The first time, she surrogated for a gay couple from Germany. Mala not only gave birth but also breastfed the twins for a month. She said, "I still remember them. The day I last breastfed them, I gave them a lot of kisses and hugs as I knew I was never going to see them again. But those sirs [the gay couple] are really nice. They send me gifts and pictures of the babies once in a while." As she was narrating, she took a pause, her voice choked, and her eyes became moist. Counselling and the medical narrative try to create an efficient reproductive labourer who will produce healthy babies without any emotional claim. Surrogates are told that they are nothing but a womb or an incubator where the baby stays as a guest, but for many surrogates, the bond with the child is more powerful than the mere act of breastfeeding. As Mala explained, "How can I forget? They were my blood. They stayed here [pointing at her stomach] for nine months." Similarly, Bina, another surrogate, said, "Even though I know they are not my babies, I am still curious to know how the babies would look. I am not going to breastfeed the babies, but I feel their kicks, all their movements, but their real mother will never be able to experience that." Interestingly, even though the clinics try to render the surrogates as dismembered reproductive organs, Bina's words show that the surrogates understand their contribution in the reproductive arrangement; they do not claim themselves as the "real mothers," but they are not emotionless reproductive organs or incubators either. Denying the surrogates the right to breastfeed has failed to be successful as a means of disconnecting the emotional link with the baby.

CONCLUSION

Although the popularity of surrogacy is growing and providing new reproductive options to many, advocates of surrogacy still have not solved many puzzles that come with surrogacy; one of them is whether surrogates should be allowed to breastfeed or not. On the one hand, doctors fear the emotional bond that the surrogate may develop because of breastfeeding, while, on the other, they do not want to deny the baby the nutritional value of breastmilk. Interestingly, India's own breastfeeding campaign for reducing child mortality encourages all mothers to breastfeed their infants at least in the initial months ("Health Minister"). Even though the government of India is planning to place a lot of emphasis on promoting the utility of breastmilk as important for a child's early nutrition and health, surrogates are denied the opportunity to breastfeed, while surrogacy as a practice continues to increase.

Although feminist literature on the subject of breastfeeding explores how varied women's positions and experiences are, the emergence of commercial surrogacy adds new complexities to feminist scholarship on breastfeeding. Commercial surrogacy compels us to think differently about the association of breastfeeding and such ideas as "good motherhood" (Blum; Davis). The cultural and medical script for a "good mother" is often associated with her ability to breastfeed efficiently. Breastmilk provides the necessary nutrition, develops the infant's immune system, and establishes the mother-child bond, and hence a good mother must try to breastfeed her child. However, in contrast, a good surrogate should never want to breastfeed; her duty is limited to giving birth to a healthy baby. In cases of commercial surrogacy, surrogates' reproductive rights or the newborn's right to receive breastmilk are secondary; the primary concern is who gets to claim the baby. The essentialist discourse that breastfeeding establishes a natural mother-child bond has also been appropriated by the surrogacy industry with a deeper meaning. The act of breastfeeding is looked at from the perspective of family and kinship arrangements, and it determines who is the real mother and who will get the opportunity to bond with the newborn. Hence, surrogates are refused the right to breastfeed, whereas some of the intending mothers look at their right to breastfeed by hormonal therapy as a claim to motherhood. Breastfeeding policies in reproductive clinics also demonstrate that when childbirth, motherhood, and reproductivity become part of a market system and market logic prevails, consumer choice prevails over social justice and reproductive rights.

WORKS CITED

Ahluwalia, Sanjam. *Reproductive Restraints: Birth Control in India, 1877-1947*. University of Illinois, 2008.

Apple, Rima. *Mothers and Medicine: A Social History of Infant Feeding 1890-1950*. University of Wisconsin Press, 1987.

Bailey, Alison. "Reconceiving Surrogacy: Toward a Reproductive Justice Account of Indian Surrogacy." *Hypatia*, vol. 26, no. 4,

2011, pp.715-41.

Banerjee, Anindita. "The Rhetoric of the Womb: The Representation of Surrogacy in India's Popular Mass Media." *Globalization and Transnational Surrogacy in India: Outsourcing Life,* edited by Sayantani DasGupta and Shamita Das Dasgupta, Lexington Books, 2014, pp. 107-125.

Baumslag, Naomi, and Dia L. Michels. *Milk, Money and Madness: The Culture and Politics and Breastfeeding.* Bergin & Garvev, 1995.

Bharadwaj, Aditya, and Peter E. Glasner. *Local Cells, Global Science: The Rise of Embryonic Stem Cell Research in India.* Routledge, 2009.

Blum, Linda. *At the Breast: Ideologies of Breastfeeding and Motherhood in the Contemporary United States.* Beacon, 1999.

Blum, Linda. "Mothers, Babies, and Breastfeeding in Late Capitalist America: the Shifting Contexts of Feminist Theory." *Feminist Studies,* vol.1, no.9, 1993, pp. 291-311.

Chadda, Rakesh K., and Koushik Sinha Deb. "Indian Family Systems, Collectivistic Society and Psychotherapy." *Indian Journal of Psychiatry Indian J Psychiatry,* vol. 55, no.6, 2013, pp. 299-309.

DasGupta, Sayantani, and Shamita Das Dasgupta. *Globalization and Transnational Surrogacy in India: Outsourcing Life.* Lexington Books, 2014.

Davis, Joanna R. "Bad Breast-Feeders/Good Mothers: Constructing the Maternal Body in Public." *Berkeley Journal of Sociology,* vol. 48, 2004, pp. 50-73.

Dettwyler, Katherine A. "Beauty & the Breast: The Cultural Context of Breastfeeding in the United States." *Breastfeeding: Biocultural Perspectives,* edited by Dettwyler and Patricia Stuart-Macadam, Aldine de Gruyter,1995, pp. 167-216.

Franklin, Sarah, and Helena Ragone. *Reproducing Reproduction: Kinship, Power, and Technological Innovation.* University of Pennsylvania Press, 1998.

Gupta, Jyotsna Agnihotri. "Reproductive Biocrossings: Indian Egg Donors and Surrogates in the Globalized Fertility Market." *International Journal of Feminist Approaches to Bioethics,* vol.5, no.1, 2012, pp. 25-51.

"Health Minister Launches MAA Programme to Promote Breastfeeding." *UnicefIndia*, 5 August 2016, unicef.in/PressReleases/416/Health-Minister-launches-MAA-programme-to-promote-breastfeeding. Accessed 24 Feb. 2018.

Maher, Vanessa. *The Anthropology of Breast-Feeding: Natural Law or Social Construct*. Berg Press, 1992.

Labbok, Miriam H., Smith, Paige Hall, and Taylor, Emily C. "Breastfeeding and feminism: A focus on reproductive health, rights and justice." *International Breastfeeding Journal*, vol. 3, no. 8, 2008, pp. 1-6.

Palmer, Gabrielle. *The Politics of Breast-Feeding*. Pandora, 1988.

Pande, Amrita. "Commercial Surrogacy in India: Manufacturing a Perfect Mother? Worker." *Signs: Journal of Women in Culture and Society* , vol.35, no.4, 2010, pp. 969-992.

Pande, Amrita. *Wombs in Labor: Transnational Commercial Surrogacy in India*. Columbia University Press, 2014.

Patel, Tulsi. *Fertility Behaviour: Population and Society in a Rajasthan Village*. Oxford University Press, 1994.

Puri, Jyoti. *Woman, Body, Desire in Post-Colonial India: Narratives of Gender and Sexuality*. Routledge, 1999.

Reissman, Catherine Kohler. "Women and Medicalization: A New Perspective." *The Politics of Women's Bodies: Sexuality, Appearance, and Behavior*, edited by Rose Weitz, Oxford University Press, 1998, pp. 3-18.

Sama—Resource Group for Women and Health. *Birthing A Market: A Study on Commercial Surrogacy*. Sama, 2012.

Sama—*Constructing Conceptions: The Mapping of Assisted Reproductive Technologies in India*. Sama, 2010.

Singh, Holly Donahue. "Fertility Control: Reproductive Desires, Kin Work, and Women's Status in Contemporary India." *Medical Anthropology Quarterly*, vol. 30, no.3, 2016.

Strathern, Marilyn. *After Nature: English Kinship in the Late Twentieth Century*. Cambridge University Press, 1992.

Strathern, Marilyn."Future Kinship and the Study of Culture." *Futures* vol. 27, no.4, 1995, pp.44-64.

Thompson, Charis. *Making Parents: The Ontological Choreography of Reproductive Technologies*. MIT, 2005.

Van Esterik, Penny. *Beyond the Breast-Bottle Controversy*. Rutgers University Press, 1989.

15.
Framing Breastfeeding as "Natural"

Implications for Mothers' Identities

LAURA FITZWATER GONZALES

To use "natural" to describe breastfeeding highlights the elasticity of the term, as it can be stretched to fit many different definitions (Faircloth). In interviews with first-time parents, I found that they defined "natural" to mean biological, social, historical, instinctual, animalistic, and—as one participant indicated—a term used for marketing goods. Individuals feel strongly about breastfeeding being natural, yet because of the elasticity and ambiguity of the term, they often struggle to give a clear definition of what it means. For example, one participant, Jill, said, "Feeding your baby however you can is natural. I know lots of people who can't breastfeed and so it's not natural for everyone to be able to breastfeed. It's had different connotations. Historically, upper class people didn't breastfeed and then other people did, so it's just, the term natural just doesn't mean anything to me anymore." In my interviews, participants often talked about breastfeeding as natural, many of them relying on the notion that breastfeeding was inherent to women's abilities and bodies. In this chapter, I discuss how participants constructed breastfeeding as "natural." I then apply this framework to breastfeeding, and argue that when breastfeeding is framed as natural, it can negatively affect the identities of mothers who struggle to breastfeed and discourage women from seeking breastfeeding support.

THEORETICAL FRAMEWORK

Although the medicalization of childbirth and breastfeeding

through hospitalization and formula use peaked in the mid-1900s (Apple; LaRossa), Glenda Wall documents in her article, "Science, Nature, and 'The Nature of Things,'" how the end of the twentieth century saw not only a shift to a return to nature and the natural, but also a reverence for nature and natural experiences. Wall finds that breastmilk is characterized as nature's "perfect food" and understood to be "pure and good" ("Moral Constructions of Motherhood" 596-97). Current breastfeeding and parenting discourses link women, motherhood, and breastfeeding with being natural (Blum). The implication of a breastfeeding discourse framing breastfeeding as natural is that it implies that all women have the inherent capacity to breastfeed successfully, and, thus, breastfeeding and mothering require little support. When breastfeeding is presented as natural, convenient, simple, and enjoyable, it creates a picture of a relatively easy process that any mother should be able to succeed at and find rewarding (Braimoh and Davies), yet this discourse does not often match women's experiences (Schmied and Lupton). Many women do not find breastfeeding to be easy or enjoyable, and some women feel like failures if they cannot breastfeed (Avishai; Blum; Braimoh and Davies; Knaak; Lupton; Simonardottir; Taylor and Wallace). Breastfeeding has, thus, become a marker of a mother's identity: breastfeeding reaffirms the "good mother" identity for those who do it, and stigmatizes mothers who do not or who do it inappropriately (Faircloth; Hausman; Tomori et al.). When mothers practise breastfeeding, they accomplish identity work (Schwalbe and Mason-Schrock), which helps to affirm their identities as good mothers.

As I discuss in my findings, when participants framed breastfeeding as natural, their definitions revolved around considering breastfeeding to be an embodied practice with embodied knowledge. Cindy Stearns explains the embodied perspective on breastfeeding as "[centring] the analysis on the doing of breastfeeding: how mothers go about and think about breastfeeding within the immediate social context and structural constraints of their lives" (361). I focus on the idea of how mothers (and in my analysis, fathers) think about breastfeeding. Chris Bobel uses the term "embodied knowledge" to describe how the mothers in her study discussed their own parenting choices. Embodied knowledge occurs when "mothers regard their bodies as sources of knowledge" (103). She interviewed "natural mothers," women who merged the lifestyles of voluntary simplicity and attachment parenting, and were also inspired by cultural feminism. When Bobel questioned her participants on their parenting choices, mothers often relied on "just knowing":

> This notion of ideas coming from the heart, of "just knowing" something to be true but lacking the ability to express it, pervaded natural mothering discourse. Over and over again, women described the sensation of "knowing deep inside" or understanding something that defied description but was nonetheless strongly felt... It was clear that "just knowing" defied further description. (89)

The mothers in Bobel's study implied that their decisions, which were beyond explanation or reason, were intuitive and, more importantly, that they felt right. The mothers' reasoning did not rest on thinking; instead, they discussed feeling the "power of nature" (98) as they cared for their children. Similarly, the participants in my study rely on their embodied knowledge when discussing why breastfeeding is "natural."

Charlotte Faircloth also documents how the mothers in her study used the concept of "natural" to account for their parenting decisions, and because of the power of nature, their actions went unquestioned. Her participants, as with Bobel's, discussed knowing through "gut feelings" (120) or feeling that something was right. Faircloth argues that the concept of natural is elastic, which means, it could be stretched to accommodate a number of different ideas. I find, too, that the ways people described natural and the meanings they ascribed to natural highlight the term's elasticity. To rely on embodied knowledge to understand breastfeeding as natural the idea to go unchallenged.

This is the framework I use to analyze my findings below. The participants in my study also used the word "natural" to describe breastfeeding, and, as with the mothers in both Bobel and Faircloth's studies, the perceived naturalness relied on feelings and defied further definition. It simply was natural. My participants additionally framed the naturalness of breastfeeding as a part of the design of women's bodies, and contrasted it with things they considered unnatural. I argue that when this framework of breastfeeding as natural is used as a reason to breastfeed, it can negatively affect the identities of mothers who struggle to breastfeed and discourage struggling mothers from seeking breastfeeding support.

RESEARCH METHODS

The data presented here come from a larger project examining first-time parents' expectations and experiences with breastfeeding. As I have noted, in this chapter, I focus on how participants use the term "natural" in connection with breastfeeding. Beginning in 2013, I recruited and interviewed twelve couples who were planning to breastfeed their first child, and followed them from before the birth of their child until the child was about six months old. I used grounded theory methods to guide my data collection and analysis (Charmaz).

Because I focused on participants' expectations and experiences over time, my method of data collection was longitudinal qualitative interviews (Hermanowicz) with multiple family members (Reczek). Data were gathered through three waves of in-depth interviews with both parents at three distinct time-points (*n*=60). In-depth interviews offer a way to capture a full range of meanings, beliefs, and ideas people hold about a certain topic. In the first wave, couples were interviewed individually and sequentially (when possible) before the birth of the baby, typically in the third trimester of pregnancy. In the second wave, I again interviewed couples individually and sequentially after the birth of the baby, when the baby was between two to seven weeks old. In the third wave, I interviewed couples jointly. The babies were between six and seven months old at the time of the final interview. Dyadic or group interviews with multiple family members are another way to see how families co-create and co-construct their reality in a collaborative way (Reczek).

The participants were relatively affluent and educated, white, married, and identified as heterosexual. Only one participant did not hold at least a bachelor's degree, and fifty-eight percent had a master's degree or PhD. All participants were working full- or part-time jobs or attending school fulltime for advanced degrees at the onset of the study. Additionally, I assigned pseudonyms to all the participants in order to maintain confidentiality. Due to the narrow demographic scope of my sample, as well as the qualitative research design, my findings are not generalizable, nor can I draw conclusions about all breastfeeding mothers and their partners. However, qualitative analysis provides insight into the meanings that people give to their experiences (Corbin and Strauss). The interviews were transcribed verbatim, and I read all transcripts, wrote memos, and coded the data to develop the following analysis.

FINDINGS

In the first wave of interviews, before the birth of the baby, the term "natural" emerged as an important concept when participants described why they were choosing to breastfeed their baby, or what breastfeeding meant to them. One-third of participants said that one of the reasons they were choosing to breastfeed was because breastfeeding was natural, and one-fourth of participants used the word "natural" to describe breastfeeding. In total, just over half of the participants talked about breastfeeding as natural in some way. As this became a pattern in interviews, I began asking about it in subsequent interviews, following theoretical sampling (Charmaz). By focusing specifically on what "natural" meant to different people, I developed further analysis on its meaning in the context of breastfeeding.

In this chapter, I argue that when breastfeeding is perceived as natural, it negatively affects the identities of mothers who struggle to breastfeed, and it also discourages mothers who struggle from seeking out breastfeeding support. Three prominent definitions emerged from the interviews as participants attempted to describe what it meant that breastfeeding was "natural": something that just exists, an inherent design of women's bodies, and a contrast to something unnatural. First, I describe each of these definitions in detail. Next, I consider how they contribute to the moral meanings of breastfeeding and good mothering. I argue that each of these ways of constructing breastfeeding as natural contributes to the idea that women should be able to accomplish breastfeeding without help or support—sometimes without effort—and that needing any form of breastfeeding support may signal to them that they are a failure: if breastfeeding is "natural," support should not be necessary.

NATURAL JUST EXISTS: AN AMBIGUOUS DESCRIPTION

The first definition that emerged when I analyzed the interview data was how new and expectant parents described what "natural" meant. They said that breastfeeding was just natural, came naturally, or would become natural. These ambiguous descriptions continued from before the birth of their child throughout their breastfeeding experiences. For example, Emily said in describing what she thought breastfeeding would be like, "I kind of have this mindset ... this is something natural that you're supposed to do, and that ... hopefully you and your child will just click and you'll be able to figure it out." Catherine said she was worried that breastfeeding would feel uncomfortable but hoped it would become "a natural little scene" between her and her baby. On deciding to breastfeed, Ashley said, "I just didn't really consider the other option, it just seems kind of more natural ... It just seemed like this is what you do when you have children." Her husband Pat agreed: "it's kind of a natural way [to feed]."

Some participants said breastfeeding seemed natural because when they were growing up, they saw others breastfeeding. Andrea said, "everybody I knew that had babies breastfed, so I've always seen it as the normal and natural thing to do." Robert, in addition to describing breastfeeding as "a natural process," said the decision to breastfeed their baby was "just a natural [decision], based on how we were raised, and what seems to be the norm of what's healthy for your child ... Something that was really less of a decision than just something that was, you know; it's logical." Like Robert, few participants could describe a process of discussing and deciding how they would feed their new baby. Instead, the decision to breastfeed just seemed to occur without considering other infant feeding options, and at least part of the reason for this decision was because breastfeeding was natural.

After the birth of their baby, couples continued to characterize breastfeeding in this ambiguous way. It "seemed to be just kind of natural" Josh said of his wife Andrea and their baby, immediately after the birth. Nick also described breastfeeding as something that "seems pretty natural." Likewise, Molly said that breastfeeding came "so naturally to [the baby] ... he knew what he was looking for." Catherine, who had at first been worried about it being uncomfortable, said at her third interview said, "It's nothing weird; it's completely natural now."

When I asked participants to explain what they meant by "natural," many of them struggled to do so. I argue that these ambiguous definitions are significant because of the lack of a clear meaning. As Wall shows in her study, "Moral Constructions of Motherhood," the culturally constructed concept of nature is infused with moral authority that goes unquestioned. In her analysis of breastfeeding literature, Wall has found the implication that it "is mothers' moral obligation to breastfeed, an obligation that is lent authority through its connection with cultural constructions of nature and motherhood" (605). Similarly, the participants in my study did not question or challenge their ideas of why they thought breastfeeding was natural. Rather, when breastfeeding was constructed as "natural," there did not need to be any further description. As with the natural mothers in Bobel's study who described "just knowing" what was right for themselves and their children, my participants seemed to just believe or feel that breastfeeding was natural. This embodied knowledge made breastfeeding the best option for their families, and this was reason enough for them to breastfeed.

When some of the women in my study were faced with breastfeeding difficulties that challenged this notion of natural, it rendered them confused and feeling as they had done something wrong. Before I discuss this point further, I first turn to the second definition that emerged from the interviews—the idea that breastfeeding is inherent to women's bodies.

"NATURAL" AS BIOLOGICAL: THAT'S WHAT WOMEN'S BODIES DO

The second most prominent definition of the meaning of breastfeeding as natural was the way that participants connected it to women's bodies' ability to produce milk and breastfeed. Participants used such terms as "instinctual," "animalistic," "design," and "biology" to further describe this connotation. Overall, many participants expressed that they perceived women as mammals with bodies designed to produce life and produce sustenance for that life. The meaning of "natural" was embedded in the design of women's bodies. Several participants relied on their academic background in the sciences for their reasoning. For example, when I asked Holly what it meant to say that breastfeeding was natural she said, "I think that we're mammals, and they're mammary glands, and that's what they're there for." When I asked her if she meant it was biological, she continued: "Yeah, but maybe that's because I'm in science that I think that way. But yeah, that's kind of what I think, that's their purpose, and I almost feel like, gosh, they were so useless before, but now they're doing what they're supposed to do." Through breastfeeding, Holly felt that she found the purpose of her breasts and focused on the function of her breasts: producers of breastmilk.

Others continued along this line of thinking. Rachel described breastfeeding as "one of the most animalistic things that you do as a human." Both Michelle and Catherine, after having breastfed their babies, described breastfeeding as an instinct. Catherine said, "It really was instinct, it was like, I need to do this, this is what feels right ... it was really surprising to me that it felt that natural." Andrea and her husband Josh discussed breastmilk supply and demand in their third interview: how Andrea's body responded to the baby's need for milk, and that when the baby nursed more often, Andrea's body would produce more milk. Josh pointed to "the connection [with the baby]" that made breastfeeding natural, whereas Andrea also included a religious element: "Your body—we are Christians—we believe that God designed us, and we were designed to have milk for our babies ... And all mammals, they feed their babies with their milk." Both of Andrea's reasons reflect

Wall's findings in, "Science, Nature, and 'The Nature of Things:'" "natural" suggests both a connection to nature (through her example of being mammals) as well as a connection to her religious faith.

One husband, Chris, provided a lengthy description of breastfeeding as natural, which encompassed much of how others connected breastfeeding to bodies and/or biology. He notes the following:

> It's kind of a natural thing to do. It's how our bodies were designed and there's very few opportunities in our life these days; there's just so much technology and so many things we rely on but, to have something like [breastfeeding], it really kind of takes you back to the roots of, this is what we're kind of designed to do. Not me specifically, but that Desiree as the mother is capable of doing that ... I think it does increase the attachment to the child and vice versa because you really are responsible for its nourishment and its wellbeing in a very direct sense ... knowing that you're capable of doing that I think is one thing ... as a parent, I think it helps us kind of attach ourselves to the child better.

Chris's narrative reveals not only multiple ideas about how breastfeeding is connected to women's bodies, but also the tensions that several male participants felt when talking about breastfeeding. First, Chris uses breastfeeding as an answer to reliance on technology. Other research discusses how a "return to nature" can be a response to growing technical advances, such as the return to natural childbirth movement as a response to obstetric interventions in childbirth and the medicalization of pregnancy (Moscucci). Chris's narrative seems to echo this sentiment, as he indicates that breastfeeding takes people "back to the roots" of being human. Second, Chris stresses that the design of women's bodies makes them capable of breastfeeding and that by breastfeeding, women are better attached to their children. Breastfeeding provides a direct link between mother and baby—literally connecting them and thus holding the mother responsible for the infant's wellbeing. Third, Chris acknowledges the tension between male and female bodies: he begins by using first-person pronouns—we, ours, us—to describe bodies and breastfeeding, but then he admits that his body cannot do the same as Desiree's. Yet at the end of his narrative, he returns to the idea that breastfeeding will help both parents be attached to the child. Here, and throughout his interviews, Chris reveals himself to be a very active parent, but by "design," he remains excluded from the act of breastfeeding.

These last two points signal another conflict expressed by several participants. Many of the fathers wanted to be involved in parenting activities and decisions; however, if breastfeeding was something only the mother was capable of doing, then the men could not make the breastfeeding "choice."[1] Several male participants acknowledged this tension: they advocated breastfeeding, and they wanted to support their wife's breastfeeding, but they also knew they could not do it themselves. This made them feel as though they had no right to make the final decision regarding feeding. Men often said they would leave the decision about breastfeeding up to their wives. As Chris said in his first interview, "Ultimately [Desiree] has a decision-making power in what she wants to do."

In one sense, the men seem to be able to abdicate responsibility when it comes to infant-feeding choices. Examining couples' negotiations over moving for a career, recent research finds that when men defer to women's desires, it became the woman's duty to accomplish the necessary emotional and practical work to coordinate the couples' current life decisions (Wong). I argue this occurs in decisions regarding infant feeding as well. Although the women in my study generally found their partner's encouragement or support to be positive, women were often the ones ultimately responsible for devising infant-feeding strategies, which resulted in women's mental labour (Walzer) that was unequally shared with their spouse. When men frame supporting their wives' breastfeeding choices using "her body, her choice" rhetoric, they are, in a sense, able to distance themselves from the responsibility of that choice. Men appear to walk a fine line between offering support and respecting their partner's decisions because, as they frame it, it's about her body and not his. Rather than using the idea of women's "natural" caring abilities to justify their unequal parenting arrangements (Deutsch), the men and women in my study remain committed to breastfeeding as natural; thus, parents experience tension in wanting men to be involved in making decisions and taking responsibility for their children while acknowledging that women are in control of their own bodies.

As the above quotes illustrate, framing breastfeeding as natural is connected to ideas about the capabilities and purposes of women's bodies, and the relationship with and attachment to their baby. But women's bodies do not always function in the ways that women want them to. Indeed, many of the participants faced physical breastfeeding challenges, including low milk supply, flat nipples that made latching difficult, or babies who struggled to breastfeed. Thus, in the context of this understanding of "natural," the women who faced breastfeeding challenges often felt like they were failing to achieve something essential to their identities as women and as mothers. I will expand on this idea further after I discuss the final definition that emerged in the interviews: contrasting natural breastfeeding with other unnatural feeding options.

NATURAL IS NOT UNNATURAL: FORMULA, PUMPING, AND PAIN

The third most prominent definition in participants' narratives about breastfeeding being natural emerged as participants identified different feeding options that they described as unnatural: using infant formula, pumping breast milk, and challenging or painful breastfeeding experiences.

Several participants contrasted breastfeeding and breastmilk with infant formula, a product most participants hoped to avoid. Michelle said breastmilk was "a natural product. Formula is obviously synthetic, even if it's made from natural things … if you have a choice between something that is physiologically designed to do what it's supposed to do and something that has been synthetically made … it's maybe preferable to use the biologically relevant thing." Chris said that he and his wife Desiree felt they would be "short changing" their baby if they decided to feed him formula over breastmilk and that they had "a pretty strong reticence to having dependency on something that wasn't entirely natural." Additionally, Michael said he would be concerned if all the baby was eating was formula: "I feel good about [breastmilk] coming from [the mother] … that's been tried and tested over thousands of years, versus formula I kind of wonder, ok what's the difference between this brand and that brand?" Michael acknowledged that "pretty much everything we eat is manufactured, but we have it spread out across all these different things that we eat, but [the baby's] just eating this one thing, so … if he's going to get all his food from one source, I'd rather know exactly what the source is." These narratives serve to underscore both the hesitancy to be reliant on something considered unnatural, but also the desire to control what goes into their child's body.

Another way that breastfeeding was framed as natural was by comparing it with the unnaturalness of pumping breastmilk. Although participants generally favoured breastmilk over formula, doing so through a pump and a bottle was not considered natural, whereas breastfeeding clearly was. Allie described her frustration with pumping like this:

> And then you got … the equipment, and it's loud and it's uncomfortable and … it's unnatural, and it's just like, god, all you can do is think how much it sucks, figuratively and literally … it's just awful … If you breastfeed and you're able to take care of your child better because you're not strapped down by the equipment and you're just more free to be a mom and not just a milk machine.

Allie was adamant that pumping was not natural and that pumping turned her into an object—"a milk machine" rather than a human mother. When she was hooked up to the pump she said, "Yeah, you're not a mom. You're trying to produce. You're trying to force it, and that's not what it's about. It's just supposed to happen naturally." As I discussed earlier, when breastfeeding was framed as natural, it was often described as inherent to the design of women's bodies. Allie relied on her body to produce milk, but including the breast pump in that production reduced her humanity. Thus, for Allie, her ability to breastfeed was linked to her identity as a mother. When Allie was unable to breastfeed, she did not feel like a mother, and instead felt like a machine.

Finally, breastfeeding was framed as natural when it was contrasted with painful, challenging breastfeeding. Natalie faced challenges with breastfeeding that she described as "more of a burden" than a problem, and during the first few months of her baby's life, she did not look forward to breastfeeding. She experienced pain in her breasts, and her baby was fussy, would cry, and would yank away from her breasts. When the pain subsided after several months, she described breastfeeding as starting to "become more natural" and that "now it just flows, it just seems natural, it just kind of happens, so it's been easy." Natalie used her challenging breastfeeding experiences to define her easy breastfeeding experiences as natural. This shift to understanding easy breastfeeding as natural contributes to the difficulties women face with their identities as mothers when they struggle to breastfeed. In light of this, I turn now to my argument of how women's identities as mothers are challenged when they perceive breastfeeding as natural but struggle to breastfeed.

FAILING BODY, FAILING MOTHER

The connection of natural to women's bodies, biology, and identity is important for exploring this term. If women's bodies are naturally able to breastfeed, then what does it mean when they cannot breastfeed or, as in Natalie's situation above, when breastfeeding is challenging? To explore this issue, I draw heavily from two participants who struggled with breastfeeding: Allie and Natalie. Both of their stories demonstrate that if breastfeeding is framed as natural, women's identities as good mothers are challenged when breastfeeding does not easily occur.

Out of all the participants, Allie was one of the most committed to breastfeeding. She spoke passionately about breastfeeding: "It's the right thing to do, it's the best thing for your child, it's what your body is meant to do, it's just one of those things that ... shouldn't be that difficult ... I'm a mammal; it's what we do." Although she acknowledged that breastfeeding would require effort to figure out, she was confident that she would be able to do what she needed to do to make it work.

However, for Allie, breastfeeding was a challenge. She discovered that she had flat nipples, and her newborn baby was unable to latch. She spent time wrestling with nipple shields to help him nurse, and then she began pumping and feeding him with a bottle. She said that bottle-feeding made her "feel guilty" because she worried he was not "getting that connection that he needs" with her and that pumping made her feel like "not a mom" but rather "trying to produce." Although she said in her first interview that breastfeeding would not necessarily be easy, in reflecting on her experience in her second interview she said, "I was not prepared for how difficult and all the trials that I was going to face. I just thought I was just going to be naturally equipped for it and, 'cause everybody told me ... it's just so natural and wonderful and easy and like, no it's not. It's not. It's hard. It's really hard. And it's not natural." Allie felt blindsided by people who described breastfeeding as wonderful and magical: "I just was under the illusion that it was just going to go great and be easy," but she blamed her naiveté on not taking a breastfeeding class before the birth of her baby. When the baby was about three months old, breastfeeding caused Allie so much pain that she almost quit. Each day that she continued became an accomplishment, and when the baby was about six months old she said:

> For me it has not been a natural, easy thing. It's been a work in progress. It's been hard. It's been really, really, hard and so it's kind of, I don't want to give it up just for the sheer fact that I've had to work so hard to do it and make it this long ... If you can, you should try to make it to the six-month mark. But if you can't, I now understand. There are no solids in this baby world ... it's just do what you can.

For Allie, breastfeeding was hard work, and it was not a natural, magical, or easy process as she said she was led to believe. She struggled mentally and physically, yet remained committed to breastfeeding despite these trials. Her identity as a mother was negatively affected by her challenges with breastfeeding, coupled with the belief that breastfeeding was supposed to be natural. Rather than breastfeeding being an effortless experience, Allie said she had to work hard to breastfeed her son. Although her "good mother" identity was compromised through her breastfeeding challenges, the work she put into breastfeeding helped rebuild her identity as a mother. A few other women in my study also faced breastfeeding challenges that required them to engage in emotional identity work (Fields et al.; Wolkomir) to recreate their identities as good mothers—changing both what they thought it meant to be a good mother as well as changing how they felt about being a good mother. Although the things they did and the choices they made were not the same in each situation, the purpose was the same: to recraft a "good mother" identity when the first option, breastfeeding, failed.

Natalie was another mother deeply committed to breastfeeding her child, but she struggled from the beginning. Her baby was diagnosed with tongue-tie—a condition where the tissue connecting the tongue is tightly connected to the floor of the lower jaw, affecting the baby's latch on the mother's breast. An improper latch then affects the woman's breast in a variety of ways, such as causing blistering or interfering with emptying ducts, which can become blocked or infected. These can be very painful for the mother and very frustrating for the baby.

In their third interview, Natalie and her husband Dave talked about how breastfeeding became more natural when the baby was around three to four months old. For Natalie, it was not natural when she dreaded breastfeeding her baby, nor was it natural that she had to pump through mastitis and pain. During these times, Dave told Natalie that they should use formula because he thought it was "crazy" that she kept breastfeeding. It upset Natalie when Dave encouraged formula use, and she said it felt as if Dave were telling her, "You're failing, let me just go get the next option … formula." One time, when the baby spit up blood, Natalie rushed her to the pediatrician but found out that it was blood from her own nipples, and she said, "It crushed me that that's what she was taking in from me." She described the first few months of breastfeeding as "one of the hardest things I've ever had to do, but I didn't want to give up."

Natalie was hesitant to share some of the details of her breastfeeding experiences with her friends because she did not like hearing negative stories when she was pregnant. When she was struggling to breastfeed she said, "Sometimes I felt I had to say, 'Breastfeeding's going great,' and you're just gritting through it because you hear of all the successes, and you're struggling." When I asked Natalie how she felt others perceived her when she shared her challenges, she said the following:

> As I shared it, I felt like I was failing. I told [Dave] that one day, that I was failing as a mom. I can't do this, why is [breastfeeding] not happening, why does this keep happening to me, why do I keep bleeding, why do I keep getting mastitis, why am I still so engorged? I thought that my body was failing me, and I was failing [the baby] ... I don't think anybody likes sharing a failure of any kind, and especially one that is being so pushed for. Breastfeed, breastfeed, breastfeed, but you're failing. Just knowing how long everybody else had done it, falling short of that on the timeline, that was always in the back of my head.... You are falling short of what they accomplished, it's a failure. It's less, it's less than they did and maybe in their eyes it would be a failure. I don't think they'd ever say that, but I think I would just feel it right here [points to heart]. Just kind of ugh, I just shared that, boom, they think I failed.

For Natalie, the challenges that she experienced before being able to describe her breastfeeding as natural were experiences that indicated her failure. Her body failed to do the natural thing: breastfeed. And by failing to breastfeed, she was failing her baby. Natalie also compared herself to other women whom she knew had breastfed longer than she anticipated being able to. This made her hesitant to share her struggles for fear of being judged as a failure. The only way for Natalie to be a good, successful mother, was to have a breastfeeding experience she felt was natural. The implications here point to a vicious cycle for women who struggle to breastfeed: women may feel shame when they cannot breastfeed in the way they thought they could, and this shame prevents them from seeking out breastfeeding support. As Natalie indicated, she had a breastfeeding timeline that she had planned to follow, but her experience caused this to be an unattainable standard. She felt shame that she did not live up to this standard. Until breastfeeding was no longer a challenge, Natalie felt like a failure.

CONCLUSION

As the narratives of the participants in my study indicate, breastfeeding is framed as natural— meaning that it is inherent to the biological design of women's bodies, and it is distinct from unnatural types of feeding, such as formula or pumping breastmilk. I argue here that when breastfeeding is framed in this way, it can be internalized by women as something easy or as something that just occurs. Men, too, may internalize these messages. One father, Shawn, said before the birth of his son: "As far as I know you just put a baby [at the breast] and it just kind of takes care of itself." Yet Allie and Natalie's stories reveal the amount of work it can take to do something natural. If framing breastfeeding as natural means it should be instinctive, easy, and essential to women's physical bodies, then women may feel they should be able to accomplish it without help or support. Needing breastfeeding support may signal a failure to them because if something is supposed to be natural and easy, support should not be necessary.

In line with feminist breastfeeding advocacy that reframes breastfeeding as a reproductive right rather than a choice (Labbok et al.), these narratives can provide insight on how breastfeeding promotion should occur. In describing the goals that developed out of the 2007 Breastfeeding and Feminism Symposium, Miriam Labbok and her colleagues listed several suggestions for women's reproductive health goals and different levels of strategic action. For example, they suggested reinforcing breastfeeding as the normative approach to infant feeding within the healthcare system, engaging communities in broad-based breastfeeding education, providing access for all women to unbiased information regarding their reproductive goals, and supporting family practices in the healthcare fields to increase attention to the reality of the mother-child dyad. I argue that within this framework of feminist breastfeeding advocacy, breastfeeding should be framed as a learned experience between mother and baby, rather than a natural experience. I also argue that breastfeeding education should focus on how the breastfeeding journey does not occur in isolation and that mothers and babies can benefit from the support of others.

ENDNOTE

[1]Framing breastfeeding as a choice falsely assumes that everyone has equal access to that choice. This is an important issue for feminist breastfeeding advocacy; however, it is beyond the scope of this chapter to discuss this point further. For additional references on breastfeeding and the rhetoric of choice, see Hausman's articles about "Women's Liberation and the Rhetoric of Choice" and "Breastfeeding Rhetoric and the Politics of Feminism."

WORKS CITED

Apple, Rima D. *Perfect Motherhood: Science and Childrearing in America*. Rutgers University Press, 2006.

Avishai, Orit. "Managing the Lactating Body: The Breast-Feeding Project and Privileged Motherhood." *Qualitative Sociology*, vol. 30, no. 2, 2007, pp. 135-52.

Blum, Linda. *At the Breast: Ideologies of Breastfeeding and Motherhood in the Contemporary United States*. Beacon Press, 1999.

Bobel, Chris. *The Paradox of Natural Mothering*. Temple University Press, 2002.

Braimoh, Jessica, and Lorraine Davies. "When 'Breast' is No Longer 'Best': Post-Partum Constructions of Infant-Feeding in the Hospital." *Social Science & Medicine*, vol. 123, 2014, pp. 82-89.

Charmaz, Kathy. *Constructing Grounded Theory: A Practical Guide through Qualitative Analysis*. Sage, 2006.

Corbin, Juliet, and Anselm Strauss. *Basics of Qualitative Research*. 3rd ed. Sage, 2008.

Deutsch, Francine M. *Halving It All: How Equally Shared Parenting Works*. Harvard University Press, 1999.

Faircloth, Charlotte. *Militant Lactivism? Attachment Parenting and Intensive Motherhood in the UK and France*. Berghahn Books, 2013.

Fields, Jessica, et al. "Symbolic Interactionism, Inequality, and Emotions." *Handbook of the Sociology of Emotions*, edited by Jan E. Stets and Jonathan H. Turner, Springer, 2006, pp. 155-78.

Hausman, Bernice L. "Breastfeeding, Rhetoric, and the Politics of Feminism." *Journal of Women, Politics & Policy*, vol. 34, no.

4, 2013, pp. 330-44.

Hausman, Bernice L. "Things (Not) to Do with Breasts in Public: Maternal Embodiment and the Biocultural Politics of Infant Feeding." *New Literary History*, vol. 38, no. 3, 2007, pp. 479-504.

Hausman, Bernice L. "Women's Liberation and the Rhetoric of 'Choice' in Infant Feeding Debates." *International Breastfeeding Journal*, vol. 3, no. 10, 2008, doi: 10.1186/1746-4358-3-10. Accessed 1 Jan. 2017.

Hays, Sharon. *The Cultural Contradictions of Motherhood*. Yale University Press, 1996.

Hermanowicz, Joseph C. "The Longitudinal Qualitative Interview." *Qualitative Sociology*, vol. 36, no. 2, 2013, pp. 189-208.

Knaak, Stephanie J. "The Problem with Breastfeeding Discourse." *Canadian Journal of Public Health*, vol. 97, no. 5, 2006, pp. 412-14.

Labbok, Miriam H., et al. "Breastfeeding and Feminism: A Focus on Reproductive Health, Rights and Justice." *International Breastfeeding Journal*, vol. 3, no. 8, 2008, doi: 10.1186-1746-4358-3-8. Accessed 1 Jan. 2017.

LaRossa, Ralph. *Becoming a Parent*. Sage, 1986.

Lupton, Deborah. "'A Love/Hate Relationship': The Ideals and Experiences of First-Time Mothers." *Journal of Sociology*, vol. 36, no. 1, 2000, pp. 50-63.

Moscucci, Ornella. "Holistic Obstetrics: The Origins of 'Natural Childbirth' in Britain." *Postgraduate Medical Journal*, vol. 79, no. 929, 2003, pp. 168-73.

Reczek, Corinne. "Conducting a Multi Family Member Interview Study." *Family Process*, vol. 53, no. 2, 2014, pp. 318-35.

Schmied, Virginia, and Deborah Lupton. "Blurring the Boundaries: Breastfeeding and Maternal Subjectivity." *Sociology of Health and Illness*, vol. 23, no. 2, 2001, pp. 234-50.

Schwalbe, Michael, and Douglas Mason-Schrock. "Identity Work as Group Process." *Advances in Group Processes*, edited by Barry Markovsky et al., Emerald Group Publishing Limited, 1996, pp. 115-49.

Simonardottir, Sunna. "Getting the Green Light: Experiences of Icelandic Mothers Struggling with Breastfeeding." *Sociological Research Online*, vol. 21, no. 4, 2016, doi: 10.5153/sro.4149.

Accessed 9 Mar. 2017.
Stearns, Cindy A. "The Embodied Practices of Breastfeeding: Implications for Research and Policy." *Journal of Women, Politics, and Policy*, vol. 34, no. 4, 2013, pp. 359-70.
Taylor, Erin N., and Lora Ebert Wallace. "For Shame: Feminism, Breastfeeding Advocacy, and Maternal Guilt." *Hypatia*, vol. 27, no. 1, 2012, pp. 76-98.
Tomori, Cecilia, Aunchalee E.L. Palmquist, and Sally Dowling. "Contested Moral Landscapes: Negotiating Breastfeeding Sigma in Breastmilk Sharing, Nighttime Breastfeeding, and Long-Term Breastfeeding in the U.S. and the U.K." *Social Sciences & Medicine*, vol. 168, 2016, pp. 178-85.
Wall, Glenda. "Science, Nature, and 'The Nature of Things': An Instance of Canadian Environmental Discourse, 1960-1994." *Canadian Journal of Sociology*, vol. 24, no. 1, 1999, pp. 53-85.
Wall, Glenda. "Moral Constructions of Motherhood in Breastfeeding Discourse." *Gender and Society*, vol. 15, no. 4, 2001, pp. 592-610.
Walzer, Susan. *Thinking about the Baby: Gender and Transitions into Parenthood.* Temple University Press, 1998.
Wolkomir, Michelle. "Emotion Work, Commitment, and the Authentication of the Self: The Case of Gay and Ex-Gay Christian Support Groups." *Journal of Contemporary Ethnography*, vol. 30, no. 3, 2001, pp. 305-34.
Wong, Jaclyn S. "Competing Desires: How Young Adult Couples Negotiate Moving for Career Opportunities." *Gender & Society*, vol. 31, no. 2, 2017, pp. 171-96.

About the Contributors

Katherine Foss is an associate professor of media studies at Middle Tennessee State University. She is the author of *Breastfeeding and Media: Exploring Conflicting Discourses That Threaten Public Health* (2017), *Television and Health Responsibility in an Age of Individualism* (2014), and articles in *Journalism & Mass Communication Quarterly*, *Critical Studies in Media Communication*, and other journals.

Lee Ann Glowzenski is an editor of *WLN: A Journal of Writing Center Scholarship*. She received her Ph.D. in English literature from Duquesne University in 2014. Her current research focuses on community building among formula-feeding mothers.

Laura Fitzwater Gonzales is a visiting assistant professor of sociology at Pacific Lutheran University in Tacoma, WA. She received her PhD in sociology from North Carolina State University in 2017. Her current research examines breastfeeding experiences of new parents.

Dionne Irving's work has appeared in *The Missouri Review, Boulevard Magazine, The Normal School, The Crab Orchard Review*, and other places. She is an assistant professor of English at Saint Mary's College, a women's college in Notre Dame, Indiana. Currently, Irving is working on a novel set in Jamaica.

Elizabeth Johnston has a PhD in eighteen-century British literature and is an associate professor at Monroe Community College in Rochester, NY. Her scholarship and poetry tend to focus on representations of women in literature, myth, and popular culture. You can read more about her publications and the writing group she co-founded at http://strawmatwriters.weebly.com/.

Dana Lloyd is a PhD candidate in the Department of Religion at Syracuse University and holds degrees in law and philosophy from Tel Aviv University. Her publications include "Politicizing Kierkegaardian Repetition," in *Kierkegaard and Political Theology*, edited by Roberto Sirvent and Silas Morgan (forthcoming, Pickwick Publishing), and "Paradoxes of Dignity in Israel/Palestine" (forthcoming, *Law, Culture and the Humanities*).

Elaine McDevitt recently graduated with a master's degree in design history and material culture from the National College of Art & Design, Dublin. In 2016, she co-edited issue twelve of the Irish Institute of Creative Advertising & Design's journal, Campaign, which had last been published in 1963. Her central research interest is the cultural manifestation of twentieth century and contemporary objects, with a particular focus on infant feeding, gender issues, and Irish identity.

Abigail L. Palko is the director of the Maxine Platzer Lynn Women's Center at the University of Virginia. Her scholarship focuses on cultural and literary representations of mothering practices. Her book, *Imagining Motherhood in Contemporary Irish and Caribbean Literature*, is available from Palgrave Macmillan. She co-edited *Mothers, Mothering and Globalization* with Dorsía Silva Smith and Laila Malik for Demeter Press. Her work has appeared in a number of journals and Demeter Press publications.

Tatiana Prorokova holds a PhD in American Studies from the University of Marburg, Germany, and is an academic editor at Pod Academy, United Kingdom. Her research interests include war studies, ecocriticism, gender studies, and race studies. She is a co-editor of *Cultures of War in Graphic Novels: Violence, Trauma, and Memory* (forthcoming in 2018 with Rutgers University Press).

Sucharita Sarkar is an associate professor at D.T.S.S College of Commerce, Mumbai, India. She is currently pursuing her doctoral degree from Mumbai University on contemporary mothering narratives in India. She has written on the intersections of motherhood, media, diaspora, memoir, and food and culture studies.

Anindita Sengupta received her PhD from the Department of Women, Gender, and Sexuality Studies at the Ohio State University in May 2017. She completed her undergraduate studies in Political Science and her master's degree in international relations at Jadavpur University Kolkata, India. Her areas of research interests are postcolonial and critical race theory, feminist reproductive politics, global and transnational feminisms, neoliberalism, science and feminism, women and conflict, and modern South Asia. She is currently a visiting assistant professor of Women's, Gender, and Sexuality Studies at the University of Connecticut.

Ann Marie A. Short is an associate professor of English at Saint Mary's College in Notre Dame, Indiana, where she also teaches gender and women's studies and intercultural studies. Her previous publications have appeared in *Literature Compass*, *MELUS: The Society for the Study of Multi-Ethnic Literature of the United States* and *Anthurium: A Caribbean Studies Journal*. In addition to motherhood studies, her scholarship focuses on Anglophone postcolonial and immigrant women writers.

Patty Sotirin is professor of communication at Michigan Technological University. She co-authored with Laura L. Ellingson, *Aunting: Cultural Practices that Sustain Family and Community Life* and *Where the Aunts Are: Family, Feminism, and Kinship in Popular Culture* and co-edited the collection *Feminist Rhetorical Resilience* with Elizabeth Flynn and Ann Brady.

Jutta Sperling teaches early modern European history at Hampshire College, MA. Her research interests include lactation imagery, female property rights in Portugal, Italy, and the wider Mediterranean, and convent studies. Among her recent publications are *Roman Charity: Queer Lactations in Early Modern Visual Cul-*

ture (transcript Verlag and Columbia University Press, 2016) and "Address, Desire, Lactation: On a Few Gender-Bending Images of the *Virgin and Child* by Jan Gossaert," *Wallraf-Richartz Jahrbuch* 76 (2015): 49-77.

Eileen Sperry is a visiting assistant professor of English at the College of Saint Rose in Albany, NY. She received her PhD from Stony Brook University in 2016. Her current research explores corporeality and mortality in early modern English literature.